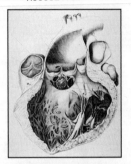

Timothy Wm. Smith, DPhil, MD, FACC, FHRS

Associate Professor of Medicine
Director, Cardiac Electrophysiology Laboratory
Washington University School of Medicine
Saint Louis, Missouri

Duane S. Pinto, MD, MPH, FACC, FSCAI

Associate Professor of Medicine, Harvard Medical School
Associate Director, Interventional Cardiology Section
Director, Cardiology Fellowship Training Program
Beth Israel Deaconess Medical Center
Boston, Massachusetts

JONES & BARTLETT
LEARNING

World Headquarters
Jones & Bartlett Learning
5 Wall Street
Burlington, MA 01803
978-443-5000
info@jblearning.com
www.jblearning.com

Jones & Bartlett Learning books and products are available through most bookstores and online booksellers. To contact Jones & Bartlett Learning directly, call 800-832-0034, fax 978-443-8000, or visit our website, www.jblearning.com.

Substantial discounts on bulk quantities of Jones & Bartlett Learning publications are available to corporations, professional associations, and other qualified organizations. For details and specific discount information, contact the special sales department at Jones & Bartlett Learning via the above contact information or send an email to specialsales@jblearning.com.

The authors, editor, and publisher have made every effort to provide accurate information. However, they are not responsible for errors, omissions, or for any outcomes related to the use of the contents of this book and take no responsibility for the use of the products and procedures described. Treatments and side effects described in this book may not be applicable to all people; likewise, some people may require a dose or experience a side effect that is not described herein. Drugs and medical devices are discussed that may have limited availability controlled by the Food and Drug Administration (FDA) for use only in a research study or clinical trial. Research, clinical practice, and government regulations often change the accepted standard in this field. When consideration is being given to use of any drug in the clinical setting, the health care provider or reader is responsible for determining FDA status of the drug, reading the package insert, and reviewing prescribing information for the most up-to-date recommendations on dose, precautions, and contraindications, and determining the appropriate usage for the product. This is especially important in the case of drugs that are new or seldom used.

Production Credits
Executive Publisher: Christopher Davis
Senior Acquisitions Editor: Nancy Anastasi Duffy
Associate Editor: Laura Burns
Production Assistant: Sarah Burke
Marketing Manager: Rebecca Rockel
Manufacturing and Inventory Control Supervisor: Amy Bacus
Composition: Cenveo
Cover Design: Kate Ternullo/Kristin Parker
Cover Image: © Courtesy of National Library of Medicine
Printing and Binding: Cenveo
Cover Printing: Cenveo

ISBN: 978-1-4496-1516-1

6048
Printed in the United States of America
16 15 14 13 12   10 9 8 7 6 5 4 3 2

Tarascon Pocket Cardiologica

Contents

Contents

Contents

■ CONTRIBUTORS

Suzanne V. Arnold, MD, MHA
Fellow in Cardiovascular Medicine
Department of Medicine,
    Cardiovascular Division
Washington University School
    of Medicine
St. Louis, Missouri

Nathalie Bello, MD
Clinical Fellow in Medicine
Department of Medicine,
    Division of Cardiology
Beth Israel Deaconess
    Medical Center
Boston, Massachusetts

Anjan Chakrabarti, MD
Clinical Fellow in Medicine
Department of Medicine,
    Division of Cardiology
Beth Israel Deaconess
    Medical Center
Boston, Massachusetts

Daniel H. Cooper, MD
Assistant Professor of Medicine
Department of Medicine,
    Cardiovascular Division
Washington University School
    of Medicine
Staff Cardiac Electrophysiologist
Barnes-Jewish Hospital
St. Louis, Missouri

Andre Dejam, MD, PhD
Clinical Fellow in Medicine
Department of Medicine, Division
    of Cardiology
Beth Israel Deaconess
    Medical Center
Boston, Massachusetts

Jennifer Giuseffi, MD
Cardiology Fellow
Department of Medicine, Division
    of Cardiology
Vanderbilt University
Nashville, TN

Faizul Haque, MD
Staff Cardiologist
John Muir Hospital
Walnut Creek, CA

Susan Joseph, MD
Assistant Professor of Medicine
Department of Medicine,
    Cardiovascular Division
Washington University School
    of Medicine
Staff Cardiologist
Barnes-Jewish Hospital
St. Louis, Missouri

Andrew J. Krainik, MD
Staff Cardiologist
Missouri Baptist Medical Center
St. Louis, Missouri

Thomas K. Kurian, MD
Fellow in Cardiac Electrophysiology
Department of Medicine,
    Cardiovascular Division
Washington University School
    of Medicine
Barnes-Jewish Hospital
St. Louis, Missouri

Jefferson H. Lee, MD
Fellow in Cardiac Electrophysiology
Department of Medicine,
    Cardiovascular Division
Washington University School
    of Medicine
Barnes-Jewish Hospital
St. Louis, Missouri

Michael Levy, MD
Interventional Cardiology Fellow
Department of Medicine, Division
    of Cardiology
Beth Israel Deaconess
    Medical Center
Boston, MA

Jose Madrazo, MD
Assistant Professor of Medicine
Department of Medicine,
    Cardiovascular Division
Washington University School
    of Medicine
Staff Cardiologist
Barnes-Jewish Hospital
St. Louis, Missouri

Christopher Umberto Meduri, MD
Clinical Fellow in Medicine
Department of Medicine, Division
    of Cardiology
Beth Israel Deaconess
    Medical Center
Boston, Massachusetts

Yonathan Felix Melman, MD
Clinical Fellow in Medicine
Department of Medicine, Division
    of Cardiology
Beth Israel Deaconess
    Medical Center
Boston, Massachusetts

Hassan Pervaiz, MD
Interventional Cardiology Fellow
Department of Medicine, Division
    of Cardiology
Beth Israel Deaconess
    Medical Center
Boston, MA

Tarascon Pocket Cardiologica

SECTION I

DIAGNOSTICS AND EVALUATION

1 ■ INTRODUCTION: SIGNS AND SYMPTOMS OF CARDIOVASCULAR DISEASE

INTRODUCTION

Some texts have an introductory chapter concerning "The Approach to the Patient with Cardiac Disease." The title implies an assumption that heart disease is known to be present. Yet a large portion of the cardiologist's and internist's efforts is expended on establishing (or excluding) the presence of heart disease. (What good is an entire book about management of coronary disease if the patient has none and his/her chest pain is caused by pulmonary disease, anxiety, musculoskeletal injury, or supraventricular tachycardia?) Refinement of the diagnosis and then consideration and management of therapy follow. Therefore, the clinician must assimilate the patient's presentation and chief complaint(s) with initial diagnostic testing (preferably noninvasive and inexpensive) to assess:

- The probability that the patient has heart disease
- What further testing is indicated
- What treatment is indicated

At each step, decisions must be tempered by considerations of risk (including the risk of further testing or treatment prompted by a false positive test). Therefore, much of cardiology is risk analysis and balancing risk–benefit ratios. The cardiologist must constantly ask: "What is the risk of pursuing a diagnosis or treatment compared to the risk of an alternative strategy (or no further action)?"

GOALS OF EVALUATION AND TREATMENT

As in all of medicine, the goal of evaluation and treatment in cardiology is one or both of the following:

- Make the patient feel better
- Prevent a bad outcome (e.g., death, stroke, progression of heart failure)

These goals have strong implications for choosing therapy. If there is no predicted mortality benefit to a treatment, and the patient does not feel ill, risky steps are inadvisable. It is therefore essential to educate the patient as well as possible about the goal of therapy. Examples include:

- Defibrillator implantation is *not* designed to make the patient feel better or to make the heart stronger. Defibrillators are not even intended to prevent arrhythmias or palpitations. The defibrillator's job is prevent sudden death by terminating a life-threatening arrhythmia when (if) it happens. Defibrillator implantation should be recommended when judgment says the risk (and inconvenience) of defibrillator therapy is outweighed by the likelihood of preventing sudden death.

- On the other hand, occasional, well tolerated reentrant supraventricular tachycardias are not associated with increased mortality. Treatment, whether pharmacological or procedural, has some risks, and these must be weighed against the potential benefit. In this case, improvement of mortality is not one of the potential benefits. Talking with the patient about severity of the syndrome is critical.
- Heart transplants are intended to prevent deterioration in heart failure patients and death and to make the patient feel better. But it is (obviously) a very intense therapy (utilizing limited resources) that is not desirable to a patient who feels well.

To reiterate: The goals of therapy must be clear in the physician's mind, and the patient must also be educated on expected outcomes and risks.

In all, there may be surprisingly few presentations of cardiac disease. In almost all cases, symptoms alone are not diagnostic and require corroboration from other evaluation.

SYMPTOMS

Symptoms are sensations experienced by the patient. They are not observed by the physician, though they may be named and/or interpreted by the physician.

- **Chest Pain** is the classical presentation of cardiac ischemia, but all chest pain is not *angina pectoris*. Qualitative assessments (PQRST: position of the pain; precipitating factors—like exertion, palliative factors; quality of the pain; radiation; severity; timing) can assist but are not specific in themselves. Other investigations such as ECG, enzyme analysis, echocardiography, or even cardiac catheterization may be required.
  - Classic descriptions of angina seem to be based on men's presentations. So it has been said that women are more likely to have so-called "atypical" angina, especially dyspnea on exertion.
  - Many patients appear to have their own personal "anginal equivalents". Some are expected, but some seem highly atypical. Examples are: right-sided pain, isolated jaw pain, arm pain, palpitations, atrial fibrillation (or other arrhythmias), lightheadedness, syncope, isolated dyspnea.
    - **Nausea** may be an anginal equivalent specifically associated with inferior ischemia.
- **Palpitations.** For practical purposes, palpitations are any sensation of the heart beat. They may fast or slow, strong or weak, regular or irregular. They may be severe or not bothersome. They may occur due to arrhythmias or they may occur in normal sinus rhythm. Evaluation almost always starts with recording the ECG during symptoms.

- **Dyspnea** is a hallmark of congestive heart failure. It may represent pulmonary congestion or (particularly with exertion) hypoperfusion. It may also proceed from other inefficiencies of cardiac output, including arrhythmias (fast and slow), and valve disease. Dyspnea may also represent pulmonary disease, anxiety.
  - **Cough** may be a sign of pulmonary congestion due to heart failure, but may result from a number pulmonary processes.
- **Lightheadedness** may be a result of hypoperfusion of the brain due to poor cardiac output, but many other factors may lead to lightheadedness.
- **Fatigue and malaise** and highly nonspecific, but may result from arrhythmias, ischemia, or heart failure.

SIGNS AND SYNDROMES

Signs and Syndromes. Signs can be observed by someone other than the patient. A syndrome is a collection of signs, symptoms, and other features, sometimes with an established pathogenesis (a disease), sometimes more ill defined.

- **Vital signs** typically include heart rate, blood pressure, and respiratory rate. Some include oxygen saturation, since it is now easily and noninvasively measured. The vital signs are so-called because they reflect vital status. Abnormalities of vital signs may be part of virtually any cardiac disease process.
- **Shock** is generalized hypoperfusion of the end organs, resulting in dysfunction and injury, which may become irreversible. There are cardiac and noncardiac causes of shock.
- **ECG abnormalities** are part of many cardiac disease processes. The ECG is an essential part of initial cardologic evaluation (like auscultation).
  - Some abnormalities even without direct symptoms demand further evaluation, treatment, or at least follow-up.
    - Examples include ventricular pre-excitation, hypertrophic changes, some arrhythmias, prolonged QT interval, and conduction disease.
  - Conversely, some syndromes can occur without ECG changes.
    - SVT may occur in patients whose baseline ECG is entirely normal
    - Classically, a left circumflex acute myocardial infarction may fail to produce ST segment elevations on a standard 12-lead ECG.
- **Syncope** is a transient loss of consciousness with loss of postural tone. Syncope may have cardiologic/arrhythmic cause and implications. But there are a large number of noncardiac syncopal syndromes. Syncope is a difficult clinical problem and is addressed in its own chapter.

- **Sudden cardiac arrest (sudden cardiac death)** is not syncope. It includes collapse and loss of consciousness However, recovery is not spontaneous, and resuscitation is required. Sudden cardiac arrest is most commonly caused by ventricular fibrillation or polymorphic ventricular tachycardia. Other rhythms, such as monomorphic VT and bradycardia/asystole are also possible causes. There are also nonarrhythmic causes of pulseless electrical activity, such as pericardial tamponade and massive pulmonary embolism.

ORGANIZATION OF THIS BOOK

Cardiology is a highly diagnostic specialty. There are many diagnostic modalities, both invasive and noninvasive. Similarly, there are multiple different types of therapies. This book is arranged into three major sections for clarity and ease of reference:

- *Diagnostics and Evaluation* is the first section; it includes noninvasive techniques and invasive procedures.
- *Cardiovascular Syndromes* is a separate discussion of several common cardiologic disease processes.
- The final section discusses an array of modalities of *Cardiovascular Therapeutics*.

2 ■ THE PHYSICAL EXAMINATION OF THE HEART

INTRODUCTION

The cardiovascular examination begins with assessment of general condition, vital signs, pulse, clubbing, edema, signs of malperfusion such as cool extremities, and signs of associated disorders.

ARTERIAL PULSE EXAMINATION

The carotid, radial, femoral, and pedal pulses should be examined for symmetry and contour. The presence or absence of carotid, supraclavicular, aortic, and femoral bruits should be noted. Depending upon the clinical situation, asymmetry may indicate obstruction of the upstream vessel such as with atherosclerosis, dissection, or coarctation.

There are several abnormalities in the contour and timing of the arterial pulse:

- *Pulsus parvus:* Weak upstroke due to decreased stroke volume (hypovolemia, LV failure, aortic or mitral stenosis).
- *Pulsus tardus:* Delayed upstroke (aortic stenosis).
- Bounding (hyperkinetic) pulse: Hyperkinetic circulation, aortic regurgitation (Corrigan's pulse), patent ductus arteriosus, marked vasodilatation.
- *Pulsus bisferiens:* Double systolic pulsation in aortic regurgitation, hypertrophic cardiomyopathy.
- *Pulsus alternans:* Regular alteration in pulse pressure amplitude (severe LV dysfunction).
- *Pulsus paradoxus:* Exaggerated inspiratory fall (>10 mmHg) in systolic BP (pericardial tamponade, severe obstructive lung disease).

JUGULAR VENOUS PULSATION (JVP)

Jugular venous distention (JVD) develops in right-sided heart failure, constrictive pericarditis, pericardial tamponade, and obstruction of superior vena cava. JVP normally falls with inspiration but may rise (Kussmaul's sign) in constrictive pericarditis.

Abnormalities in examination of the JVP include:

- Large or "a" wave: Tricuspid stenosis (TS), pulmonic stenosis, AV dissociation (right atrium contracts against closed tricuspid valve ("cannon 'a' wave").
- Large "v" wave: Tricuspid regurgitation, atrial septal defect.

7

- Steep "y" descent: Constrictive pericarditis.
- Slow "y" descent: Tricuspid stenosis.

Inspection. Note chest wall deformities or abnormalities in chest wall excursion.

Palpation. The point of maximal impulse is the apical impulse and is normally localized in the fifth intercostal space at the midclavicular line.

Abnormalities include:

- Sustained "lift" at lower left sternal border: Right ventricular hypertrophy.
- Forceful apical thrust: Left ventricular hypertrophy.
- Prominent presystolic impulse: Hypertension, aortic stenosis, hypertrophic cardiomyopathy.
- Double systolic apical impulse: Hypertrophic cardiomyopathy.
- Lateral and downward displacement of apex impulse: Left ventricular dilatation.
- Dyskinetic (outward bulge) impulse: Ventricular aneurysm, large dyskinetic area post MI, cardiomyopathy.

HEART SOUNDS

S1 is formed by closure of the mitral and tricuspid valves.

   S1 Loud: Mitral stenosis, short PR interval, hyperkinetic heart, thin chest wall.

   S1 Soft: Long PR interval, heart failure, mitral regurgitation, thick chest wall, pulmonary emphysema.

   S2 is formed by closure of the aortic (A2) and pulmonic (P2) valves. Normally, A2 precedes P2 and splitting increases with inspiration; abnormalities include:

- Increased split S2: Right bundle branch block, pulmonic stenosis, mitral regurgitation.
- Fixed split S2 (no respiratory change in splitting): Atrial septal defect.
- Decreased split S2: Pulmonary hypertension.
- Paradoxically split S2 (splitting decreases with inspiration): Aortic stenosis, left bundle branch block, CHF.
- Loud A2: Systemic hypertension.
- Soft A2: Aortic stenosis.
- Loud P2: Pulmonary hypertension.
- Soft P2: Pulmonic stenosis.

   S3 Low-pitched: heard best with bell of stethoscope at apex, following S2; after age 30–35 years, likely indicates LV failure or volume overload.

   S4 Low-pitched: heard best with bell at apex, preceding S1; reflects atrial contraction into a noncompliant ventricle; found in AS, hypertension, hypertrophic cardiomyopathy, and CAD.

   Opening snap (OS): High-pitched; follows S2 (by 0.06–0.12 s), heard at lower left sternal border and apex in mitral stenosis (MS); the more severe the MS, the shorter the S2-OS interval.

Ejection clicks: High-pitched sounds following S1; observed in dilatation of aortic root or pulmonary artery, congenital AS (loudest at apex) or PS (upper left sternal border); the latter decreases with inspiration.

Midsystolic clicks: At lower left sternal border and apex, often followed by late systolic murmur in mitral valve prolapse.

HEART MURMURS

Systolic murmurs:
- May be "crescendo–decrescendo" ejection type, pansystolic, or late systolic; right-sided murmurs (e.g., tricuspid regurgitation) typically increase with inspiration.

Diastolic murmurs:
- Early diastolic murmurs: Begin immediately after S2, are high pitched, and are usually caused by aortic or pulmonary regurgitation.
- Mid-to-late diastolic murmurs: Low pitched, heard best with bell of stethoscope; observed in MS or TS; less commonly due to atrial myxoma.
- Continuous murmurs: Present in systole and diastole. This type of murmur is found with patent ductus arteriosus. Continuous murmurs can also be seen with coarctation, ruptured sinus of Valsalva aneurysm, and other less common disorders.

TABLE 2-1. Clinical Response of Auscultatory Events to Physiologic Interventions

Auscultatory events	Intervention and response
Systolic murmurs	
Valvular aortic stenosis	Louder following a pause after a premature beat
Hypertrophic obstructive cardiomyopathy	Louder on standing, during Valsalva maneuver; fainter with prompt squatting
Mitral regurgitation	Louder on sudden squatting or with isometric handgrip
Mitral valve prolapse	Midsystolic click moves toward S_1 and late systolic murmur Starts earlier on standing; click may occur earlier on Inspiration; murmur starts later and click moves toward S_2 during squatting
Tricuspid regurgitation	Louder during inspiration
Ventricular septal defect (without pulmonary hypertension)	Louder with isometric handgrip

(continues)

TABLE 2-1. (Continued)

Auscultatory events	Intervention and response
Diastolic murmurs	
Aortic regurgitation	Louder with sitting upright and leaning forward, sudden squatting, and isometric handgrip.
Mitral stenosis	Louder with exercise, left lateral decubitus position, coughing
	Inspiration produces sequence of A_2-P_2-OS ("trill")
Continuous murmurs	
Patent ductus arteriosus	Diastolic phase louder with isometric handgrip
Cervical venous hum	Disappears with direct compression of the jugular vein
Extra heart sounds	
S_3 and S_4 gallops	Left-sided gallop sounds: accentuated by lying in left lateral decubitus position; decreased by standing or during Valsalva. Right-sided gallop sounds usually louder during inspiration, left-sided during expiration
Ejection sounds	Ejection sound in pulmonary stenosis fainter and occurs closer to the first sound during inspiration
Pericardial friction rub	Louder with sitting upright and leaning forward, and with Inspiration

Reprinted from *Curr Probl Cardiol*, Vol. 33, Issue 7, Chizner MA, Cardiac auscultation: rediscovering the lost art, pages 326-408, Copyright 2008, with permission from Elsevier.

3 ■ ELECTROCARDIOGRAPHY

INTRODUCTION

Introduced by Willem Einthoven in 1903, the electrocardiogram (ECG, EKG) remains the central instrument of cardiac diagnosis. It is noninvasive, quick, easy, and inexpensive. It provides reliable information about the heart rhythm and rate. It also yields remarkable insight into anatomy (including enlargement and hypertrophy) and physiology (including ischemia and metabolism), even at the cellular and molecular levels.

WHAT IS THE ECG? WHAT ARE THOSE WAVES?

The electrocardiogram is a graphical representation of changes in electrical potential recorded from the body surface (**Figure 3-1**). When skeletal muscle is at rest, changes in surface potential reflect propagation of the cardiac depolarization, then repolarization. The *y*-axis is the potential—the amplitude of the waves. The *x*-axis is time. What is recorded is the propagation of the wave of action potentials through the heart (not the action potential itself, which is a transmembrane phenomenon).

- Atrial depolarization: the *P-wave* (or a variant) represents atrial activity. Its axis and conformation can be revealing about the source of the impulse.
  - Atrial repolarization is not seen, nor is activation of the AV node or His bundle.

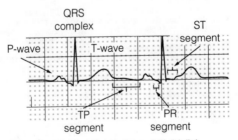

FIGURE 3-1. Single ECG lead. Waves and segments are labelled.

- Ventricular depolarization is registered as a *QRS complex*, almost always of higher amplitude than the P-wave.
  - The QRS is comprised of more than one wave, which varies with lead examined, the axis, the rhythm, the presence of infarctions, and other things.
    - A *Q-wave* is any initial negative deflection.
    - An *R-wave* is any positive deflection, and there may be more than one.
      - A second positive deflection is typically labeled R' ("R-prime").
    - An *S-wave* is any negative deflection that occurs after an initial Q-wave or R-wave.
      - A QRS may be composed of a single negative deflection and is often called a *QS* to emphasize the lack of positive R-wave.
  - The QRS complex may then be labeled by the waves seen (sometimes with upper or lower case letters to suggest their amplitude). A *qR* is an initial negative followed by a positive. An *rSR'* is two positive deflections with a valley in between. An *rS* is a small positive deflection followed by a deep negative one. All of these are still QRS complexes representing ventricular depolarization.
- The period between completion of depolarization and the beginning of repolarization is represented by the *ST segment*. The ST segment is normally flat at the baseline, representing a period of stable potential (in the depolarized state—the ventricular myocytes are all in the plateau [phase 2] of the action potential).
- Ventricular repolarization is represented by the *T-wave*, usually of lower amplitude and frequency (it is "flatter") than the normal QRS complex.

RECORDING THE ECG

There are two electrode configurations used in standard ECG recording:
- **Bipolar surface electrograms** measured with one positive and one negative electrode placed on the body surface. Einthoven's original leads utilized electrodes placed on the right arm , the left arm, and the left leg. The bipolar leads are:
  - Lead I: negative electrode on the right arm, positive electrode on the left arm.
  - Lead II: negative electrode on the right arm, positive electrode on the left leg.
  - Lead III: negative electrode on the left arm, positive electrode on the left leg.
- **Unipolar surface electrograms** utilize a combination of right arm, left arm, and left leg electrodes attached to the negative pole of the recording device. This common electrode represents a zero po*tential point in the center* of the chest, *Wilson's central terminal*. The positive electrode then reports the surface electrogram relative to the zero at Wilson's central terminal. Unipolar leads are labeled with a "V."

- Unipolar limb leads use the same electrodes as I, II, and III, with one as the positive electrode and a combination of the other two as the zero point (a modification of Wilson's central terminal). These leads require augmentation, signified by an "a."
  - aVR, aVL, aVF
- Unipolar chest leads utilize Wilson's central terminal and electrodes at standard sites on the precordium. (Recall that the Angle of Louis [sternal angle] marks the level of the second ribs. The 2nd intercostal spaces, therefore are just caudal to the Angle of Louis):
  - V_1: right of the sternum in the 4th (not the 2nd) intercostal space
  - V_2: left of the sternum in the 4th (not the 2nd) intercostal space
  - V_3: in the 4th intercostal space, midway between V_2 and V_4
  - V_4: in the 5th intercostal space at the midclavicular line
  - V_5: midway between V_4 and V_6
  - V_6: in the 5th intercostal space at the mid axillary line
  - In addition to these standard locations, additional chest leads may rarely be used:
    - V_7, V_8, and so on
  - Right-side leads are placed in the mirror image location of their standard counterparts
    - Primarily used to detected RV abnormalities (such as ischemia/infarct)
    - Also used for *situs inversus* or dextrocardia
    - V_{1R} is the same lead as V_2
    - V_{2R} is the same lead as V_1
    - V_{3R} is opposite V_3, and so on
- Some special leads
  - The **Lewis lead** is used to emphasize atrial activity (particularly flutter) in the recording that may be low amplitude and/or obscured by ventricular activity.
    - The negative electrode is placed in the 2nd intercostal space, just to the right of the sternum; the positive electrode is placed in the 4th intercostal space, also just to the right of the sternum.
    - In practice, this is simply achieved by moving the right arm electrode to the to the 2nd intercostal space, and moving the left arm electrode to the 4th intracostal space, right of the sternum. In this configuration, the ECG labeled *Lead I* is the Lewis lead.
  - **MCL leads** are typically used in 3-electrode recording systems, as in hospital telemetry. They approximate the precordial leads.
    - The negative (indifferent electrode) is placed just caudal to the clavicle in midclavicular line.
    - The positive electrode corresponds to the desired precordial lead.
      - MCL1 is recorded when the positive electrode is placed in the 4th intercostal space, right of the sternum.
      - MCL2 is recorded when the positive electrode is placed in the 4th intercostal space, left of the sternum.
      - Recording continues as above.

○ Unfortunately, recordings labeled MCL are unreliable because of inconsistency of locating the electrodes at most hospitals.

- **Directionality of the leads.** The reason there is an array of leads is that each provides a different "perspective" on myocardial activation. A wave of depolarization proceeding along the axis of the lead (toward the positive pole) will produce a maximal positive deflection in that lead, and a less positive deflection in neighboring leads. A wave of depolarization propagating directly opposite the axis of the lead will produced a maximal negative deflection. With 12 standard leads, the progress of activation can be reconstructed in space.

  • **The frontal plane** is represented by the limb leads. It is traditionally described by a 360° compass (**Figure 3-2**).
    ○ 0° is directly to the patient's left.
    ○ 90° is directly caudal.
    ○ −90° is directly cranial.
    ○ 180° (and −180°) is directly to the patient's right.

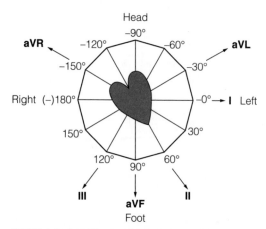

FIGURE 3-2. The Frontal Plane is divided into two 180° halves, with 0 degrees at the patient's left. Each of the frontal (limb) leads is shown superimposed on its own axis.

- Each limb (frontal) lead has its own orientation/axis corresponding to the placement of the electrodes:
  ○ Lead aVL is −30°.
  ○ Lead I is 0°.
  ○ Lead II is 60°.
  ○ Lead aVF is 90°.
  ○ Lead III is 120°.
  ○ Lead aVR is −150° (not surprisingly, this lead is frequently an outlier and an exception to rules, since it is so far away from all the other leads).
- Each of the **precordial leads** presents its own "perspective," from its chest surface location looking toward the center of the heart (Wilson's central terminal).
  ○ V_1 typically overlies the right atrium and ventricle.
  ○ V_2 typically overlies the left atrium and ventricle.
  ○ V_6 is more apical or lateral, but this depends on the heart position in the chest.

THE ECG OUTPUT

The ECG is rendered as a graph on paper or a computer screen with a grid of fine horizontal and vertical lines making boxes (**Figure 3-3**). The lines are typically said to demarcate "millimeters" (even if they are being projected on a large auditorium screen and each "millimeter" is really a few centimeters). Every 5th line is heavier to aid in measurement of 5-mm intervals.

- The *x*-axis represents time.
  - The most standard recording speed is 25 mm/second.
    ○ 1 mm (1 small box) = 40 ms
    ○ 5 mm (1 big box) = 200 ms
    ○ 25 mm (5 big boxes) = 1 second
  - Faster or slower speeds are occasionally used for specialized purposes.
    ○ In the electrophysiology (EP) laboratory, it is common to use sweep speeds of 100 mm/second or 200 mm/second.
- The *y*-axis represents potential ("voltage").
  - The most standard recording scale is 10 mm/mV
    ○ Interestingly, wave amplitudes are almost always discussed in "millimeters" rather than in units of potential. (As above, the term *millimeters* is often used, even if the ECG is enlarged and each millimeter is really several centimeters).
    ○ Like the *x*-axis, the scale can be adjusted. A halved or doubled scale can cause errors in interpretation if not considered.
- **Formats.** ECGs may be presented in multiple formats, with different patterns of leads and different scales. The savvy ECG reader always examines the format carefully to avoid pitfalls of misunderstanding.
  - Telemetry and ambulatory monitoring leads usually show one or more leads on a standard scale of 25 mm/sec and 10 mm/mV.

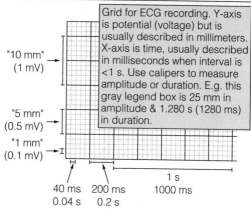

"10 mm"
(1 mV)

"5 mm"
(0.5 mV)

"1 mm"
(0.1 mV)

Grid for ECG recording. Y-axis is potential (voltage) but is usually described in millimeters. X-axis is time, usually described in milliseconds when interval is <1 s. Use calipers to measure amplitude or duration. E.g. this gray legend box is 25 mm in amplitude & 1.280 s (1280 ms) in duration.

40 ms   200 ms   1 s
0.04 s   0.2 s   1000 ms

FIGURE 3-3. Standard ECG recording graph, enlarged.

- ○ Standard lead positioning, however, is rarely used, limiting interpretation of waveforms and other things requiring standard leads, such as:
  - ■ Ischemia
  - ■ Axis
  - ■ Origin of ventricular tachycardia (VT)
- ○ Telemetry and ambulatory monitoring tracings are therefore best used for evaluating the rate and rhythm
- • **The standard 12-lead ECG** is the common rendering of the ECG. An example of a normal adult 12-lead ECG is shown in **Figure 3-4**.
  - ○ One standard page with 3 continuous tracings, but with switches in the leads at intervals across the page.
    - ■ This makes for three row of leads in four columns, typically arranged:

I	aVR	V_1	V_4
II	aVL	V_2	V_5
III	aVF	V_3	V_6

    - ■ There are often 1–3 additional leads across the bottom of the page to allow more full analysis, particularly of the rhythm, typically called "rhythm strips." Occasionally, all 12 leads are in "rhythm strip format," all the way across the page.

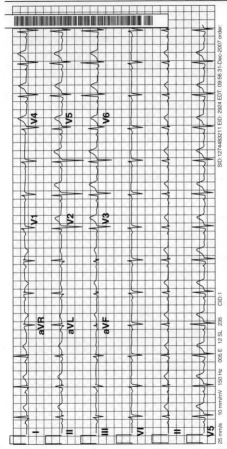

FIGURE 3-4. A normal 12-lead ECG in standard format, including 3 "rhythm strips."

- Leads II and V_1 are particularly useful for analyzing atrial activity.

READING THE ELECTROCARDIOGRAM: bRRAICE YOURSELF

Skilled reading of the ECG requires an algorithm to avoid omissions and errors. The algorithm should be followed faithfully, and soon becomes quick and second nature, allowing the reader to concentrate on expanding his or her fund of knowledge.

- The algorithm presented here is designed to be a flexible approach to reading the ECG for beginners and more experienced readers.
  - It cannot be followed without thought. The findings in one step may lead to skipping a step or even backtracking to a previous step.
  - Some steps (e.g., "extras") ultimately contain a vast array of findings to seek, but just a few examples are offered. The learner will add many with experience.
  - Practice is experience, and experience is vital to expert ECG interpretation.
- The **bRRAICE** algorithm consists of:

  basics

  Rate

  Rhythm

  Axis

  Intervals

  Conformations of the waves

  Extras/everything else

The bRRAICE algorithm is presented here step by step with relevant pointers, diagnoses, and findings.

- **basics**
  - Correct patient identification and date
  - Check the format
    - 12 leads? Rhythm strips?
    - Standard time and voltage scales? Or something different?
      - The scale should be labeled and often there is a standardizing pulse (usually of 1 mv for 200 ms—but not always!).
    - Is the recording quality high, or is there artifact that limits interpretation?
- **Rate** usually refers to ventricular rate, but the atrial rate may be different. So both should be considered.
  - Rate (units: s^{-1} or minutes^{-1}) is the inverse of *cycle length* (units: seconds or minutes), which can be measured on the x-axis. Thus, measure the cycle length and then convert to frequency.
    - Measuring the cycle length is easy, knowing that a small box is 40 ms and a large box is 200 ms.
      - There are 60,000 ms in a minute. This means that:

60,000 ms/minute ÷ cycle length (in ms) = rate (minute⁻¹)

- Two additional (and easier) ways to determine the rate are:
  - Memorize the rates associated with the big boxes:
    - **300 (bpm), 150, 100, 75, 60, 50, 42.9 (really!)**
      - If the cycle length is 1 big box, the rate is 300 bpm.
      - If the cycle length is 4 big boxes, the rate is 75 bpm.
      - Cycle length: 5 big boxes (1 second); rate: 60 bpm.
      - If the cycle length is somewhere between big boxes, esti-
        mate the interpolation.
  - Utilize the fact that the standard 1-page 12-lead page repre-
    sents *10 seconds.*
    - **Count the events (QRSs, P-waves, etc.) across the page
      and multiply by 6 to get cycle per minute.**
      - Very useful for slow rates and irregular rates
- Normal and abnormal
  - Normal: 50 bpm (some say 60) to 100 bpm
  - Bradycardia: less than 50 bpm
  - Tachycardia: greater than 100 bpm

- **Rhythm** is an entire subject unto itself, but some basics must be estab-
  lished early on.
  - Is it normal sinus rhythm with 1:1 AV conduction, a P-wave preceding
    every QRS?
    - Is the P-wave upright in lead II and biphasic in V₁, suggesting a
      sinus origin?
  - If it is not obviously sinus with 1:1 conduction (normal sinus rhythm,
    sinus tachycardia, or sinus bradycardia), what is the relationship of
    the QRSs to the P-waves?
    - First, find the P-waves (or flutter waves, or the chaotic baseline of
      atrial fibrillation). Look at their conformation (particularly in leads
      II and V₁ to assess the origin.
      - What is their rate?
      - Are they faster or slower than the QRSs?
      - Are they "driving" the QRSs or vice versa, or are the Ps and
        QRSs *dissociated*?
        - If the P-waves are faster than the QRSs but there is still
          some conduction, there is some sort of AV block (see
          Bradycardia chapter).
        - If the atrial activity is driving the rhythm and it is tachy-
          cardic, there is some type of rhythm originating from the
          atrium (see Tachycardia chapter), including atrial fibrilla-
          tion, atrial flutter, and atrial tachycardia.
        - If the QRSs are driving the rhythm, its origin is junctional
          (narrow QRS) or ventricular (wide QRS). If the QRSs are
          faster than the Ps, there is said to be "VA dissociation" and
          the diagnosis is nearly always ventricular tachycardia.

- If there is a tachycardia with AV association, but it is difficult to distinguish whether the Ps or the QRSs are driving the rhythm, it may be a reentrant supraventricular tachycardia (SVT). (See Tachycardia chapter.)
- If the diagnosis is unclear, report what you see and consider the differential diagnosis. For example:
  - "A narrow complex tachycardia. P-waves are difficult to discern."
    - Likely one of the reentrants SVTs
  - "A wide, complex tachycardia."
    - VT or possibly a supraventricular rhythm with aberrant conduction
  - "A rapid irregular rhythm with variable atrial activity"
    - Atrial fibrillation, flutter, or an atrial tachycardia
- Watch out for *paced* rhythms, discussed in more detail in Extras, pp.23.
- **Axis** typically refers to the frontal plane axis of the QRS, though the P-wave and any other waves have an axis, too. The axis is estimated by looking at the net amplitude of each lead.
  - Use the limb leads (the left half of the 12 lead). Look for the most positive deflections. A lead that has a primarily positive deflection must be in the same half of the compass as the axis.
    - If lead I (0°) is positive, the axis must be between −90° and 90°.
    - If lead II (60°) is positive, the axis must also be between −30° and 150°.
  - Also look for a lead that is roughly *isoelectric*; that is, one with net amplitude roughly 0°.
    - The axis is roughly perpendicular to a roughly isoelectric lead.
  - **Normal and abnormal.**
    - The normal QRS axis is between −30° and 90°.
      - *Left axis deviation*: axis < −30°.
      - *Right axis deviation*: axis > 90°.
      - Many call an axis between −90° and −180° *extreme axis deviation*, since it is hard to tell whether it is deviated in the extreme right or left direction.
    - Tip for quick analysis.
      - *If the QRS is net positive in Lead I and in Lead II the axis is normal.*
        - If the net QRS is positive in Lead I but negative in Lead II, there is usually left axis deviation.
        - If the net QRS is negative in Lead I but positive in Lead II, there is usually right axis deviation.
- **Intervals** (other than the RR interval, which yields the heart rate, see above) describe the rate and/or pattern of conduction through the heart. (See Figure 3-1.)
  - **PR interval**, measured from the beginning of the P-wave to the beginning of the QRS, represents conduction through the atria, the AV node, and the His bundle.

- ○ **Normal: 120 ms to 200 ms.**
  - ▪ >200 ms suggests slow conduction, common in the AV node with a long *PR segment* (the isoelectric portion of the PR interval between the P-wave and the QRS)
  - ▪ <120 ms is uncommon and suggests one (or more) of:
    - ▫ Very rapid conduction through the AV node
    - ▫ Origin of the impulse near or in the AV node
    - ▫ *Pre-excitation*: The slow conduction properties of the AV node are bypassed by via an *accessory AV pathway*, as in the Wolff-Parkinson-White Syndrome.
- • **QRS duration** is measured from the beginning of the QRS to the beginning of the ST segment (the J-point). The normal QRS is narrow because the His-Purkinje system spreads activation rapidly throughout the ventricles.
  - ○ **Normal: < 100 ms**
  - ○ Prolonged QRS implies slow conduction through the ventricle due to failure or circumvention of the His-Purkinje system. Conduction through ventricular myocardium is relatively slow.
    - ▪ A wide (long) QRS should prompt further analysis: See Conformations, pp. 30.
- • **QT interval** is measured from beginning of the QRS to the end of the T wave (which may be hard to pinpoint).
  - ○ Traditionally, lead II is recommended.
  - ○ If there is beat-to-beat variability, an average is desirable.
  - ○ The normal QT interval varies with the heart rate. Therefore, a corrected QT (QTc) is typically calculated.
    - ▪ Bazett's formula is:

$$QTc = \frac{QT(\text{in seconds})}{\sqrt{(RR \text{ interval [in seconds]})}}$$

  Note that QTc = QT when the heart rate is 60 bpm.

  - ○ Prolonged QTc: Men: > 450; Women > 470
  - ○ **Quick analysis:** If the QT is less than half of the RR interval, it is likely normal.
- • **Conformations.** The morphology of the P-waves, QRS complexes, ST segments, and T-waves should be examined.
  - ▪ **The P-wave.**
    - ○ The best leads for examining the P-wave are II and V_1.
    - ○ In sinus rhythm P-waves are usually upright in lead II (and in I, III, and aVF) and biphasic in lead V_1.
    - ○ Left atrial enlargement:
      - ▪ Lead II: Bifid P-wave with an early (right atrial) phase and a delayed (left atrial phase).

- Lead V_1: Total area of the negative portion of the P-wave is greater than 1 small box.
  - Right atrial enlargement: P wave amplitude in lead II > 2.5 mm.
  - Biatrial enlargement: Criteria for both right and left atrial enlargement are met.
- **The QRS complex** normally is narrow (< 100 ms).
  - Except in aVR, significant Q-waves are not normal.
    - Significant Qs (suggesting completed *transmural* infarction):
      - ≥ 1mm wide
      - Depth ≥ 25% of the R wave
      - Not aVR
      - Should usually be in at least two leads reflecting the same territory. For example:
        - Inferior: II, III, aVF
        - Lateral I, aVL, and possibly V_4–V_6.
        - Anteroseptal: V_1–V_3.
        - Anteroapical: V_1–V_6.
  - **R-wave progression.** The frontal plane axis was discussed earlier (see **axis** section); there is also a normal QRS orientation in the precordial leads (see the normal 12-lead ECG). As you look from V1 to V6, there is an R-wave *progression*:
    - V1 has a small R-wave and a relatively deep S-wave
    - The R wave grows and the S-wave shrinks; the R-wave is usually larger than the S-wave by the time you reach lead V4.
    - In V6, the R-wave is relatively tall with a small S-wave.
    - Delayed R-wave progression is a nonspecific finding, but may occur:
      - With an anterior infarct, even if Q waves are not present.
      - With a shift of orientation of the heart.
  - **Widened QRS** occurs when conduction of the depolarization impulse through the ventricles is not mediated by a healthy His-Purkinje system, since myocardial conduction is slower than conduction through Purkinje fibers. There are three ways in which this may occur:
    (1) **Aberrancy**—part of the His-Purkinje system fails
    (2) **Ventricular origin**—the ventricles are activated from a ventricular source and the *His-Purkinje system is not used.*
    (3) **Pre-excitation**—An accessory pathway activates some of the ventricular myocardium prior to His-Purkinje conduction.
- These three mechanisms are discussed in more detail as follows:
  - **Aberrancy** refers to patterns of slowed conduction through the ventricular myocardium due to failure of part of the His-Purkinje system. There are some specific patterns of aberrancy:
    - Bundle branch blocks. The Purkinje fiber system branches distal to the bundle of His in the left and right bundle branches. The left bundle branch is further split into anterior and posterior *fascicles*. Bundle branch blocks are diagnosed when the QRS

duration (conducted from sinus or other supraventricular origin) is > 120 ms.

- Left bundle branch block (LBBB):
  - V_1: a small narrow R-wave (if any), and a deep wide S-wave.
  - V_6: a wide monophasic R-wave or RsR'
- Right bundle branch block (RBBB)
  - V1: Primarily positive deflection, classically rSR', "rabbit ears"
- Fascicular blocks typically prolong the QRS slightly, < 120 ms. and change the QRS axis (the axis has already been determined; see above).
  - Left anterior fascicular block:
    - Left axis deviation
    - Typically aVR will have a "late" R-wave (occurring after the R-wave in aVL)
  - Left posterior fascicular block:
    - Right axis deviation
    - Relatively rare, since the posterior fascicle is highly branched, and loss of all the branches is uncommon.
  - Nonspecific intraventricular conduction delay: Widening of the QRS that does not conform to a specific pattern
- **Ventricular origin.** If the depolarization impulse originates in the ventricular myocardium, the His-Purkinje system is not fully engaged and slows spread of activation through the ventricles, making for a wide QRS.
  - Ventricular tachycardia (VT): whether focal in origin or resulting from reentry within the ventricles. VT usually overdrives the sinus rate.
  - Accelerated idioventricular rhythm (AIVR): typically rhythm of focal origin (though slow reentry is possible) that is abnormally fast and overdrives the sinus node rate, but is not fast enough to be called VT.
    - Most commonly seen after acute infarcts and/or reperfusion.
  - Ventricular escape: In the event of complete heart block or profound sinus node dysfunction (with failure of the other subsidiary pacers—the AV node, the His bundle, and the distal conduction system).
    - Ventricular escape rhythms are usually between 20 and 40 bpm and are notoriously unreliable.
  - Ventricular pacing.
- **Pre-excitation.** Ventricular pre-excitation is mediated by an accessory atrioventricular pathway. Accessory pathways (usually) do not have the decremental (slow conduction) properties that the AV node does. Therefore, the portion of the ventricular myocardium at the insertion of the accessory pathway is activated early, relative to normal myocardial activation. Ventricular pre-excitation plus tachypalpitations is the Wolff-Parkinson-White (WPW) syndrome.
  - The PR interval is shortened since a portion of the ventricles is activated early.
  - The first portion of the pre-excited QRS is termed a *delta wave*.

- The deflection of the delta is gradual (some say "slurred"), less steep than a normal QRS.
  - This is because the spread of pre-excited activation is slow (since it does not utilize the rapid His-Purkinje system). The result is a widened QRS.
- The QRS becomes a *fusion* complex. Fusion occurs between the pre-excited portion of the myocardium followed by the normally activated remainder of the ventricle.
  - The 12-lead pattern of pre-excitation and the axis of the delta wave can aid in locating the accessory pathway.
  - At electrophysiology study, the accessory can be mapped and ablated, curing the pre-excitation and WPW syndrome.
- **The ST Segment** normally is flat at the baseline and joins the end of the QRS (the J-point) and the beginning of the T-wave. The ST segments' main utility is revealing ischemia and myocardial injury/acute infarction. Abnormal depolarization (aberrancy, VT, pacing) begets abnormal repolarization, so diagnosis from the ST segment is difficult in the setting or aberrancy or pacing.
  - **ST segment elevation** occurring in leads representing an identifiable coronary distribution (e.g., inferior, anterior), suggest acute/ongoing myocardial injury, as seen in acute coronary occlusion and myocardial infarction.
    - ST segments may become elevated in the chronic phase suggesting aneurysm formation.
  - **ST segment depression** is a nonspecific finding. It may suggest nontransmural (subendocardial) ischemia/injury.
    - The location of ST segment depression is less specific than ST elevation.
    - ST depressions may occur as **reciprocal changes** in leads "opposite" ST elevation injury.
      - For example, high lateral (I, aVL, V4-V6) ST elevations may be reciprocated by inferior (especially III, aVF) ST depressions.
    - ST segment depression in leads V_1–V_3 may be a reciprocal change to a posterior MI, which would be seen in leads V_7–V_9 (if recorded).
    - Downsloping ST segments may associated with left ventricular hypertrophy
- **The T-wave** represents the wave of ventricular repolarization. Most normal T-waves have a positive QRS (except aVR, where the normal T wave is negative) or the T wave is congruent with the QRS. Many findings are nonspecific. Abnormal depolarization (aberrancy, VT, pacing) begets abnormal repolarization, so diagnosis from the T-wave (like the ST segment) is difficult in the setting of aberrancy or pacing.
  - T-wave inversions may represent ischemia, but may also occur in the setting of left ventricular hypertrophy.

- - - After a long period of ventricular pacing, there is frequently a period of time that the T-wave stays inverted—post pacing T-wave inversions.
      - A similar phenomenon may occur after prolonged tachycardia. The mechanism is poorly understood.
      - Deep T-wave inversion (with some QT prolongation can be seen with elevated intracranial pressure, "cerebral T-waves." However, the specificity of the finding is low.
    - T-wave amplitude may change with serum potassium concentration.
      - Tall, peaked T-waves suggest hyperkalemia.
      - Flattened T-waves suggest hypokalemia.
  - o **U-waves** may occur after the T-wave. They may appear on the normal ECG, especially in V_2 and V_3.
    - U-waves may appear or grow in amplitude as the T-wave loses amplitude with hypokalemia.
- **Extras** should really be labeled **everything else**. It is ultimately a long list of patterns for which to be alert. They cannot all be discussed here. In most cases, features noted by following the rest of the analysis algorithm must be synthesized to detect the pattern.
  - o **Left Ventricular Hypertrophy (LVH)** usually occurs with left ventricular pressure overload. Hypertrophic cardiomyopathy may cause different ECG patterns from afterload-induced hypertrophy. There are numerous criteria for diagnosing LVH; they are more reliable in patients over 40 year of age. Some useful ones are:
    - The sum of the S-wave n V_1 or V_2 and the R-wave in V_5 or V_6 > 35 mm (3.5 mV)
    - R-wave in V_5 or V_6 > 26 mm (2.6 mV)
    - R-wave in aVL > 13 mm (1.3 mV)

    LVH may be accompanied by T-wave inversions and (usually) downsloping ST segments.
  - o **Right Ventricular Hypertrophy (RVH)** occurs with right ventricular pressure overload (due to pulmonary disease and/or congenital heart disease) and typically shifts the QRS axis to the right and causes increased R-wave amplitude in the right precordial leads.
    - Look for right axis deviation and R-wave > S-wave in V_1.
  - o **Atrial and Ventricular Ectopy.** When the rhythm is sinus with superimposed complexes (*extrasystoles*), ectopy is often the cause. There are multiple patterns of ectopy, for example:
    - Atrial ectopy (premature atrial complexes, PACs) occur when an action potential from atrial myocardium outside the sinus node initiates atrial depolarization.
      - The P-wave comes earlier than expected from the sinus rate.
      - The P-wave (if it is not obscured by the T-wave) usually will have a different axis/morphology than the sinus P-wave, reflecting its origin.
      - The PAC may be:

- Blocked (in the AV node) particularly if it is very premature
  - ▲ The most common "cause of a pause" in the ventricular rate. Pauses should induce a careful search for blocked PACs.
- Conducted normally (with a narrow QRS)
- Conducted with aberrancy, with a QRS of RBBB, LBBB, LAFB, FPFB, or a nonspecific conduction defect. The widened QRS may make the conducted PAC confused with a ventricular premature complex (VPC).

- Ventricular ectopy (ventricular premature complexes, VPCs; premature ventricular complexes [or contractions], PVSs; ventricular premature depolarizations, VPDs) occurs when an action potential from ventricular myocardium occurs before normal activation depolarizes the ventricles.
  - Since they are of ventricular origin, the QRS complex is wide.
  - There may be a retrograde P-wave.

- Junctional extrasystoles are presumed to occur when a narrow QRS complex (or a QRS that reflects conduction aberrancy) is seen with or without a preceding P-wave. There may be a retrograde P-wave.

- Patterns of ectopy:
  - Any of these ectopic beats may occur:
    - In bigeminy (every other complex is an extrasystole)
    - In trigeminy (every 3rd complex)
    - In quadriginimy (every 4th complex)
  - The term *couplet* means 2 consecutive ectopics, and triplet refers to 3 consecutive extrasystoles. Anything further is usually called:
    - A run of atrial tachycardia,
    - Accelerated junctional rhythm, or
    - Accelerated idioventricular rhythm (AIVR)
      - ▲ Usually seen in the setting of ischemia and/or reperfusion
      - ▲ Sometimes called "slow VT", though this is technically incorrect

- Electrolyte abnormalities
  - Potassium
    - Hyperkalemia is suggested by tall, peaked T-waves
      - Progressive hyperkalemia is marked by:
        - ▲ Loss of visible P-waves, though the rhythm is still thought to be sinus (sinoventricular conduction)
        - ▲ Loss of the ST segment, with the initiation of the T-wave occurring immediately after the QRS
        - ▲ Widening of the QRS, sometimes to an extraordinary extent
      - Severe hyperkalemia is associated with poor mechanical activity, shock, and death.

- The hyperkalemia pattern should not be confused with VT (since its rarely tachycardic) or AIVR.
  - Hypokalemia is suggested by decreased amplitude, broadened T-waves. U-waves may appear and increase in amplitude with progressive hypokalemia
- Magnesium and calcium
  - Hypomagnesemia and hypocalcemia tend to prolong the QT interval, specifically by lengthening the ST segment, usually with a normally appearing T-wave.
    - Prolonged QT can lead to *torsades de pointes*, magnesium infusion may help normalize the QT and prevent torsades de pointes (especially if serum magnesium is low)
  - Conversely, hypermagnesemia (rare) and hypercalcemia shorten the ST segment.
- Digoxin effect. Digoxin therapy causes a fairly specific "scooping" of the ST segments, usually with slight ST-segment depression, and usually in leads V_5 and V_6.
  - Digoxin effect is *not* indicative of digoxin toxicity, merely of the presence of digoxin.
  - *Digoxin toxicity* may result in:
    - Sinus node dysfunction
    - Conduction blocks and aberrancy
    - Automatic rhythms, such as:
      - Atrial tachycardia (classically atrial tachycardia with AV block suggests digoxin toxicity)
      - Accelerated junctional rhythms
      - Ventricular ectopy and VT, including:
        - Bidirectional VT, VT with alternating QRS complexes and axes
        - Due to alternating automatic foci at two different ventricular sites
- Combined aberrancy. The patterns of aberrancy discussed earlier consider the unifascicular blocks (each of the right bundle, the left anterior fascicle, and the left anterior fascicle are considered single fascicles).
  - *Bifascicular blocks* are loss of function in two fascicles:
    - Right bundle branch block and left anterior fascicular block
    - Right bundle branch block and left posterior fascicular block (much less common)
    - Left bundle branch block can theoretically occur with loss of the anterior and posterior fascicles, but is usually assumed to be due to more proximal left bundle branch block.
  - *Trifascicular block* is a term that is meant to describe a bifascicular block plus PR prolongation (1st-degree AV block) and to suggest risk of progression to high-degree AV block. It is a poor term (since PR prolongation is not a third fascicular block) and should be avoided.

- Pacemaker. Be alert for the presence of a pacemaker. Pacemaker stimulus artifacts may be very small. Most pacemaker programming results in inhibition of the pacemaker when the intrinsic rate is higher than lower pacing rate.
  - Since P-waves are of low amplitude, paced P-waves may have very little discernible difference from sinus P-wave. Look for a pacing artifact at the beginning of the P-wave.
  - Paced QRS complexes are wide and reflect the site of pacing. The most common ventricular pacing site is the RV apex, yielding a wide QRS with deep S-waves in the all the precordial leads. The axis is usually left superior.
  - Cardiac resynchronization pacing creates a fusion pattern between the left ventricular paced site and the RV pacing site (typically the RV apex). Usually there is a tall R-wave in V1, distinctly different from pacing at the RV apex alone.
  - Stimulus artifacts from bipolar pacing (most common in modern pacemakers) are frequently of low amplitude and may be difficult to detect.
    - Some ECG devices have a feature to enhance the pacing spike. They add an artificially high-amplitude spike to the recording.
      - Unfortunately, these enhanced pacing spikes are poorly reliable. They should always be viewed skeptically.
    - Other instruments place a marker above or below the actual ECG.
      - These are equally unreliable, but preferred since they do not change the ECG tracing itself.
- Pericarditis. The epicardial inflammation of pericarditis creates an injury pattern like an ST elevation MI. Some hints might help to distinguish between them:
  - Global ST elevation (ST depression in aVR) is not consistent with an acute MI due to occlusion of a single coronary.
  - Similarly, ST-segment elevation in a pattern of leads not consistent with a coronary distribution may be pericarditis, rather than an acute MI.
  - Pericarditic alterations in the PR segment may also occur.
    - PR depressions in any lead or all leads.
    - aVR (as always) is an exception. Look for PR elevation in aVR.
  - Pericardial effusion (which may appear with or without pericarditis).
    - Criteria for low voltage may be met.
    - **Electrical alternans** is the term for alternating QRS amplitudes (high and low) due to beat-to-beat changes in the position of the heart in the fluid-filled pericardium.
- Acute right ventricular pressure overload, from large **pulmonary embolism**:
  - RV hypertrophy pattern.
  - Right bundle branch block may occur.

- The classic ECG shows an "S1-Q3-T3" (S-wave in V_1, Q = wave in lead III and inverted T-wave in lead III).
  - This finding is poorly sensitive.
- The **most common** ECG abnormality in PE is sinus tachycardia.
- **Lead placement errors** are all too common, and the interpreter must be vigilant.
  - One common lead switch (and popular with examination writers) is left arm/right arm:
    - The frontal leads are affected, but not the precordial leads (because Wilson's central terminal is unchanged)
    - Negative P-wave and predominantly negative QRS are rare and left/right arm electrode switch is a common cause.
      - However, *situs inversus* (heart is in a mirror image of normal) is also a cause of an "upside down" lead I.
        - ▲ The key is to examine the precordial leads. If they are normal, lead switch is the likely culprit.
        - ▲ If the precordial leads are abnormal, with progressively decreasing amplitudes, *situs inversus* is likely.
  - There is an extraordinary number of patterns that could be included in "extras." The physician should constantly add to his mental library of ECG features. Where possible, time should be taken to discuss unusual patterns both with more and less experienced interpreters of ECGs, so that constant learning can occur.

4 ■ AMBULATORY ECG MONITORING

INTRODUCTION

The standard ECG captures only 10 seconds of cardiac electrical activity. Extended recording is required to capture transient events, particularly dysrhythmias. Extended monitoring has been used to monitor for the ST changes of ischemia, but provocative testing with a 12-lead ECG (stress testing) is more commonly used than monitoring for spontaneous ischemia. Ambulatory monitors usually require only a few electrodes and can monitor one or several leads, but usually not a full set of precordial leads. There are several available types of monitor.

HOLTER MONITORING

Holter monitoring is the oldest and most well known type of ambulatory monitoring.

- Continuous recording of the ECG, usually for 24 hours, though 48-hour and longer monitors are now available.
- The tracings are computer- and technician-analyzed for final reading by a cardiologist.
- Items analyzed include:
  - Dominant rhythm and episodic arrhythmias
  - Minimum, maximum, and average heart rates
  - Number/frequency of atrial and ventricular premature complexes, couplets triplets and runs of nonsustained arrhythmias
  - Episodes and type of AV block
  - Sinus pauses
  - Pacing
  - ST segment deviation
  - Correlation of ECG with symptoms kept in a diary by the patient

EVENT/LOOP MONITORING

Holter monitoring is limited by its still-brief duration. Patients' symptoms notoriously resolve while wearing a 24- or 48-hour monitor, only to "magically" reappear after taking it off and returning it! The event monitor is intended for longer use, but only records intermittently.

- Typically it is used for 30 days.
- While activated, it constantly records and over-records.
- The patient presses a button to indicate the presence of a symptom and the monitor commits a portion of the recording to a memory.

- When the memory is filled, the patient can upload the data from the episodes via telephone to a central recording location.
- Most monitors record in a "looping" fashion, so that when triggered, the data from several (e.g., 30) seconds before the trigger are recorded.
- Some monitors can detect tachycardia and bradycardia and self-trigger.
  - Subject to artifact and false positive recordings.
- Advantages:
  - Useful for monitoring symptomatic episodes that occur less than daily but more frequently than monthly.
- Disadvantages:
  - Some patients have trouble operating.
  - Patient noncompliance.

CONTINUOUS EXTENDED MONITORING

Continuous extended monitoring utilizes wireless technology to transmit a continuous ECG to a central recording/analysis site. The patient may also report specific episodes of symptoms. In addition to the advantages of an event monitor, continuous recording allows Holter-like analysis of rhythms and events. For example the patient's overall "burden" of atrial fibrillation can be established.

IMPLANTABLE LOOP RECORDER

Advancing technology and miniaturization has allowed packaging a loop monitor in a device small enough to be subcutaneously implanted. The casing of the device has two recording electrodes, and the device contains battery memory and circuitry much like a pacemaker generator.

- Battery usually lasts more than a year.
- The device can be triggered by a hand-held device held over the site of the implanted device, and the device auto-records tachycardia or profound bradycardia.
- Data can be retrieved from the device with a programmer, much like pacemaker interrogation.
- The device and implantation/explantation procedure are simple compared to use of a pacemaker.
  - No intravascular or intracardiac parts.
  - Infection is still a risk but should be limited to the subcutaneous pocket.
    - Immediate explant, along with antibiotics is the appropriate treatment.

5 ■ ECG EXERCISE STRESS TESTING

INTRODUCTION

Exercise stress testing is one of the fundamental tests in cardiology for the assessment of ischemia, and it also yields prognostic value and can aid in assessment of the patient's functional status. It may also be used to attempt to induce exertion-associated arrhythmias. Guidelines for exercise testing were updated in 2002 by the AHA and ACC.[1]

ECG is the basic modality for assessing ischemia. More advanced imaging with exercise (stress echo and nuclear perfusion) increase the sensitivity and specificity of the exercise test, but at additional expense.

INDICATIONS FOR ECG STRESS TESTING

- Assessing for hemodynamically significant (e.g., severe enough to cause myocardial ischemia) coronary stenosis.
  - Patients with new symptoms or a change in symptoms and suspected/ known CAD
  - Low- and intermediate-risk patients after presenting with anginal type symptoms after MI are excluded
  - For follow up after an MI to evaluate medical therapy and prognosis
- Factors limiting the utility of ECG exercise testing. Consideration should be given to additional imaging to allow evaluation for ischemia.
  - > 1 mm ST segment depression at baseline
  - Complete LBBB
  - Ventricular paced rhythm
  - Ventricular pre-excitation
- In some cases, treadmill testing is used to develop an exercise pre-scription prior to cardiac rehabilitation or to assess functional status in patients with valvular heart disease or to assess certain conditions (pre-excitation).

CONTRAINDICATIONS

- Absolute:
  - Acute MI within 2 days
  - High-risk unstable angina
  - Uncontrolled symptomatic arrhythmias
  - Symptomatic severe aortic stenosis
  - Uncontrolled symptomatic heart failure
  - Acute pulmonary embolus or pulmonary infarction

- Acute myocarditis or pericarditis
- Acute aortic dissection
- Relative:
  - Left main coronary stenosis
  - Moderate stenotic valvular heart disease
  - Electrolyte abnormalities
  - Severe hypertension
  - Tachyarrhythmias or bradyarrhythmias
  - Hypertrophic obstructive cariomyopathy (HOCM) or other outflow tract obstruction
  - Mental or physical limitation preventing exercise
  - High degree AV block

PREPARATION

- It is important to perform a history and physical examination, primarily to rule the contraindicating conditions described in the previous section.
- The patient should not eat or drink 2 hours before the test.
- Appropriate shoes should be worn.
- If possible, beta-blocking agents should be held in order to avoid interfering with achieving target heart rate unless the indication for stress testing is to assess for ischemia in the medically managed patient with known disease.

EXERCISE

Exercise is the best form of stress testing. It is the more physiological form of stress, and using a standardized protocol gives information about the patient's functional capacity. During the stress, the ECG is continuously recorded and the heart rate and blood pressure are tracked.

- A Bruce protocol is most commonly used. A treadmill is programmed to increase speed and incline in 3-minute stages.
- Protocols are also available for a bicycle ergometer, arm ergometer, and other exercises. Arm or bicycle ergometry can be combined with invasive catheterization to assess the severity of mitral stenosis.
- For maximum sensitivity it is desirable to reach 85% of the maximum predicted heart rate (maximum = 220 – age)
- Indications for ending the test:
  - Absolute:
    - Decrease in SBP by > 10 mmHg with increase in workload, if accompanied by other evidence of ischemia
    - Moderate to severe angina
    - Nervous system symptoms (ataxia, dizziness, near syncope)

- ○ Cyanosis or pallor
- ○ Patient desire to stop
- ○ Sustained VT
- ○ ST elevation > 1.0 mm in leads without diagnostic Q waves (not V_1 or aVR)
- Relative
  - ○ Decrease in SBP by > 10 mmHg with increase in workload, in the absence of other evidence of ischemia
  - ○ Marked ST depression (>2 mm horizontal or downsloping ST depression
  - ○ Marked QRS axis shift
  - ○ Arrhythmias, such as nonsustained VT, SVT, heart block, bradyarrhythmias
  - ○ Fatigue, dyspnea, wheezing, claudication, leg cramps
  - ○ Wide QRS complex difficult to distinguish from VT
  - ○ Increasing chest pain
  - ○ SBP > 250 mmHg and/or DBP > 115 mmHg

ECG INTERPRETATION

- Horizontal or downsloping ST segment depression ≥ 1 mm during exercise or recovery is indicative of ischemia.
  - No information is given concerning the location of the ischemia or vessel involved.
- Exertion-induced ST segment elevation suggests transmural ischemia. Unlike ST depression, ST elevation:
  - Suggests high risk for ventricular arrhythmias
  - Is localizing to the stenosed of infarct-related vessel
- Exercise-induced VT and ventricular ectopy (PVCs) are independent predictors of mortality.
  - However, idiopathic VT may be provoked by exercise or other adrenergic stimulation; it is not predictive of mortality.
- Nondiagnostic tests/features:
  - Upsloping ST segment depression.
  - Failure to achieve 85% of maximum heart rate without ST segment changes is not a negative test, but a nondiagnostic one.

EVALUATION OF FUNCTIONAL STATUS AND PROGNOSIS

- Number of metabolic equivalents (METs) is an estimate of intensity of exertion/stress.
  - 1 MET is approximately 3.5 mL $O_2kg^{-1}min^{-1}$ or 1 kcal kg^{-1} h^{-1} and is equivalent to the resting metabolic rate, sitting quietly.
  - Walking 2 mph is about 3 METs; 4 mph is about 4 METs; jogging is about 7 METs; jumproping is about 10 METS.

- Prognosis:
  - < 5 METs achieved carries a poor prognosis.
  - 13 METs achieved carries a good prognosis independent of other responses to exercise.
- The Duke Treadmill score is also used prognostically
  - = (exercise time (min)) − (5 × ST segment deviation (mm)) − (4 × angina index)
    - Angina index:
      - No angina = 0
      - Angina present = 1
      - Test stopped due to angina = 2
- Risk
  - Duke score ≥ +5: low risk (0.25% annual mortality)
  - −10 ≤ Duke score ≤ 5: intermediate risk (1.25% annual mortality
  - Duke score < 10: high risk (5% annual mortality

PHARMACOLOGIC STRESS TESTING

Pharmacologic stress is used as an alternative to exercise stress when exercise is not feasible. Pharmacologic stress testing usually incorporates imaging to improve sensitivity and specificity.

- Coronary vasodilators employ the principle that the coronaries distal to a significant stenosis are already maximally vasodilated. Dilation of the remaining coronaries will create a relative decrease in perfusion to myocardium served by a stenosed vessel.
  - Useful in left bundle branch block, paced rhythms, beta-blocker therapy, ventricular ectopy, poorly controlled HTN.
  - Nuclear perfusion imaging is usually used.
  - Adenosine is a direct vasodilator.
  - Dipyridamole inhibits adenosine reuptake:
    - Longer half-life than intravenous adenosine.
    - Side effects include flushing, headache nausea, chest pain.
    - Reversible with aminophylline.
  - Patient must not receive caffeine or theophylline 48 hours prior to the test.
  - Reactive airways disease is a contraindication.
- Inotropes. Dobutamine causes stress and increases myocardial oxygen consumption by increasing heart rate and inotropy.
  - Useful in COPD
  - Risk of arrhythmia
  - Less useful with pacemaker, ventricular ectopy, atrial ectopy/ arrhythmias, hypertension
  - Typically uses echo wall motion imaging to assess for ischemia

IMAGING

- Nuclear perfusion imaging can be used with exercise testing or with vasodilator infusion.
  - Thallium-201 is a congener for potassium, entering myocytes via the Na+/K+ pump in amount proportional to blood flow.
    - Over time, redistributes slowly to ischemic but viable myocardium, but not to nonviable myocardium, allowing viability assessment.
  - Technitium-99 (sestamibi) enters myocardial cells by passive diffusion. Uptake is directly related to perfusion.
    - No significant redistribution.
    - Images can be gated to cardiac cycle (using the ECG). Reconstruction of wall motion can be done, and the ejection fraction can be estimated.
- Echo examines wall motion at rest and then in response to stress. It can be used with exercise, and it is typically used with dobutamine infusion.
  - Response to exercise can help characterize the perfusion state of any wall.
    - Normal at rest and normal "recruitment" (increase in contractile function) is normal.
    - Normal at rest with initial recruitment then relative hypokinesis suggests an ischemic segment.
    - Hypokinetic at rest but increasing contractility with stress suggests damaged (e.g., infarcted) myocardium but with viability.
    - Hypokinetic at rest without recruitment suggests lack of viability.

6 ■ CARDIAC IMAGING

INTRODUCTION

Imaging technologies in the form of echocardiography (transthoracic [TTE] and transesophageal [TEE]), radionuclide imaging (RNI), computerized tomography (CT), and magnetic resonance imaging (MRI) have become key components in the diagnosis and management of heart disease. Given the additional risks and costs, it is important to understand the indications for and limitations of these technologies so that they can be applied appropriately to patients and help inform our clinical decisions and, ultimately, improve patient outcomes.

TRANSTHORACIC ECHOCARDIOGRAPHY (TTE)[2]

TTE is ultrasound imaging of the heart through the chest wall. It is excellent for both structural and functional assessment of the heart and has minimal risk involved. Resolution is highly dependent on the patient size and cooperation, lung pathology, and the sonographer's skill. See **Figure 6-1** for a diagram of some standard views.

- Utility of TTE.
  - Left ventricular (LV) size and function, including regional wall motion abnormalities.
    - Important for evaluation of symptoms of heart failure, syncope, and tachyarrhythmias.
    - Useful in the evaluation of active chest pain as a wall motion abnormality may impact the decision for an early invasive strategy.
    - Evaluation of LV function after an MI: aids in determining indication for:
      - ACE inhibitors (for any LV dysfunction).
      - Warfarin (for anterior wall/apical akinesis).
      - Implantable defibrillator (ICD) (see chapter 30).
    - LV wall thickness is prognostically important in various conditions, such as hypertension, aortic stenosis, amyloidosis, and others.
    - Can be used to monitor tolerance of cardiotoxic medications such as anthracyclines.
    - Often used in conjunction with exercise or dobutamine to evaluate for physiologically significant obstructive CAD, as these stressors will induce a new wall motion abnormality that can be visualized with TTE.
  - RV size and function
    - Evaluation and management of patients with pulmonary hypertension.

- ○ Determination of eligibility for thrombolytics for pulmonary emboli and monitoring recovery post-thrombolytics by assessment of right heart strain and pulmonary pressure.
  - ○ Evaluation of patients with primarily right-sided heart failure symptoms (e.g., peripheral edema and elevated jugular venous pulse without pulmonary edema).
- Atrial size
  - ○ Atrial fibrillation: assessment of atrial size can assist in choosing and planning treatment strategy.
  - ○ Assessment of the chronicity of valvular pathology as the atria will stretch over time.
    - For example severe mitral regurgitation with a normal left atrial size suggests the regurgitation is acute.
  - ○ Assessment of diastolic dysfunction. Left atrial enlargement suggests more advanced dysfunction with increase in left atrial pressure.
    - Large atria with very thick walls are characteristic of a restrictive cardiomyopathy.
  - ○ Enlarged atria may also be seen in septal defects.
- Valvular morphology and function
  - ○ Aids in the initial diagnosis of valvular pathology as the cause of a murmur, syncope, fever, heart failure, hemodynamic instability, and others.
  - ○ Serial TTEs are indicated in asymptomatic patients with severe valvular stenosis or regurgitation to help guide the timing of surgical intervention.
  - ○ Patients with nonsevere valvular pathology do not need routine-surveillance TTEs, which should be reserved for when there is a change in clinical status.
  - ○ A TTE in the immediate post-valve replacement or repair is indicated to establish a baseline with which future TTEs can be compared.
  - ○ TTE can be used to screen for infective endocarditis (particularly in the cases of bacteremia with a virulent organism, persistent bacteremia/fever, fever or bacteremia with a new murmur, fever or bacteremia with hemodynamic instability), and to monitor for clearance of the valve lesion when the endocarditis is high risk (e.g., virulent organism, aortic involvement).
- Fluid volume status
  - ○ In patients with hemodynamic instability, TTE can help determine fluid status and thereby guide diagnosis and management. For example, in a patient with hypotension, which could be from intravascular depletion or from heart failure, evaluating the caliber of the IVC, the LV chamber size, and other measures could help determine the fluid status of the patient and guide management of IV fluids.
- Pericardium
  - ○ TTE can reliably detect pericardial effusions and evaluate their physiologic significance of the effusion (e.g., tamponade physiology).

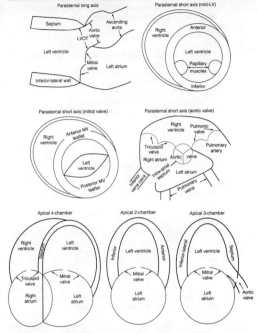

FIGURE 6-1. Standard TTE views.

- Loculated effusions, which most commonly occur post-cardiac surgery, may not be seen.
  - Presence of cardiac masses, such as tumors, thrombus, (most reliably LV thrombus), and others.
- Aortic root
  - Important in connective tissues diseases, such as Marfan's, and with a bicuspid aortic valve as both of these can cause root dilation.

- ○ Ascending aortic dissection can be seen in TTE, although this is not the test of choice for this diagnosis.
- **Limitations of TTE.**
  - ○ Patient factors
    - ○ Body habitus
      - Imaging in large patients may be limited by distance from transducer to heart.
      - Imaging in very small patients may be limited by poor transducer contact between the ribs.
    - ○ Severe obstructive lung disease:
      - Imaging through air-filled lung is limited.
      - Chronic obstructive pulmonary disease (COPD) may change heart's position, limiting normal views.
        - However, the subcostal window may be excellent in the vertically positioned heart.
    - ○ If a patient cannot lie down or turn on his side (e.g., illness, dyspnea, pain, confusion), images may be of limited quality.
    - ○ Contrast can improve image quality when determining LV size, LV function, wall motion abnormalities, and presence of LV masses.
  - ○ Posterior structures
    - ○ Loculated pericardial effusion along the posterior border of the heart will be unlikely to be seen with TTE.
    - ○ The left atrial appendage is rarely seen in adult TTEs.
    - ○ Coronary arteries
      - If the images are excellent, then the proximal portions of the coronary arteries and associated anomalies can be seen, but this degree of resolution is rarely achieved in adults.
    - ○ Right ventricular function, pulmonic valve regurgitation, and Qp:Qs ratios
    - ○ Quantification of RV stroke volume, RV ejection fraction, and pulmonic valve flow is difficult to do with TTE and is fraught with errors. However, both semi-quantitative and qualitative assessments of RV function can be done easily with TTE.
    - ○ Aorta
      - In some patients, portions of the root, proximal, arch, and abdominal aorta can be evaluated and abnormalities may be seen. However, TTE is not sufficient for ruling out aortic pathology such as dissection, atheroma, or aneurysm.

TRANSESOPHAGEAL ECHOCARDIOGRAPHY (TEE)[2]

TEE is ultrasound imaging of the heart with a flexible probe in the esophagus. Due to the short distance from the heart, TEE has excellent resolution, particularly for posterior structures. It is an invasive procedure, requiring sedation or anesthesia, and thus has an associated risk.

- **Utility of TEE.**
  - Aortic valve structure and function
    - Structure—in terms of number of cusps, leaflet excursion, calcification, vegetations—is easily seen with TEE.
    - Aortic regurgitation can be accurately quantified by the width of the regurgitation jet as compared with the width of the LV outflow tract.
    - Evaluation of aortic stenosis is more difficult. Aortic valve area can be planimetered, but valve gradients are more difficult to obtain (can be done from deep transgastric view but these are often underestimated).
  - Mitral valve structure and function
    - Morphology, prolapse, vegetations, and coaptation are all easily seen on TEE.
    - Mitral regurgitation—severity, eccentricity, and mechanism—are typically easily demonstrated.
    - Mitral valve gradients are easily obtained but planimetry of the valve area is often difficult. Thickening/calcification of the leaflets and subvalvular structures to determine candidacy for valvuloplasty can be done with TEE.
  - Tricuspid and pulmonic valves
    - Structure of the valve and valvular vegetations can typically be seen with TEE, although image quality of these valves, given their anterior position and resultant distance from the probe, are often not as good as the mitral and aortic valves.
    - Amount of regurgitation and gradients across the valves are often underestimated as compared with TTE.
  - Atrial structures
    - TEE is the test of choice for identifying clots in the atria or atrial appendages, which is often necessary prior to cardioversion or ablation of atrial arrhythmias.
    - The intra-atrial septum can be interrogated for defects (PFO, ASD), although due to patient sedation, the sensitivity for identifying tiny PFOs is lower than with a saline bubble study on TTE. In addition, the size and location of the defects can be determined, and TEE can guide the placement of percutaneous closure devices.
  - Aorta
    - Dissection, mobile atheromas and thrombi, and extent and severity of calcification of the entire aorta can be determined with TEE.
  - Coronary arteries
    - The position of and flow into the ostia of the coronaries can be viewed with TEE.
- **Limitations of TEE.**
  - Patient issues with passing TEE probe
    - Esophagus issues are critical to be aware of. Dysphagia, varices, and esophageal/oral masses are not uncommon. As the TEE probe is placed blindly, knowing the esophageal anatomy prior to probe

      placement is critical. An esophagogastroduodenoscopy (EGD) may
      be necessary prior to TEE to ensure the safety of the procedure.
- ○ Very small patients may require a pediatric probe.
- ○ Severe thrombocytopenia (typically less than ~50,000) or coagu-
    lopathy (typically an INR greater than ~5) greatly increases the
    risk of passing the TEE probe.
- Patient issues with sedation
  - ○ Very obese patients or patients with sleep apnea may have dif-
      ficulty maintaining a patent airway. Screening patients for these
      potential issues and utilizing anesthesiology services when
      appropriate can avoid adverse events.
  - ○ Carefully administering sedatives, particularly in elderly and low
      body weight patients, is important in addition to being diligent
      with monitoring patients and quickly administering reversal
      agents when oversedation occurs.
  - ○ Metabolic abnormalities (such as severe hyperkalemia) may make
      sedation unsafe.
- Ventricular function
  - ○ Although a gross estimation of left and right ventricular size and
      function can been obtained from TEE, particularly in the transgas-
      tric view, specific wall motion abnormalities are typically much
      easier to discern by TTE.
  - ○ Apical abnormalities, including apical thrombi, are very difficult
      to see with TEE.
- Valve gradients
  - ○ With the exception of the mitral valve, which can be thoroughly
      assessed by TEE, the angles of interrogation obtained with TEE
      on the other 3 valves typically underestimate blood flow velocity
      values, and therefore underestimate gradients.

CARDIAC RADIONUCLIDE IMAGING[3]

Cardiac radionuclide imaging (RNI) refers to single-photon emission computed
tomography myocardial perfusion imaging and positron emission tomography
myocardial perfusion imaging. RNI uses IV radionuclides (e.g., thallium, techne-
tium) that are taken up by cardiac tissues in rough proportion to perfusion and,
thus, is primarily used to evaluate for the presence and significance of coronary
artery disease and for the determination of left ventricular size and function.
- Utility of cardiac radionuclide imaging:
  - Evaluation of chest pain of uncertain origin
    - ○ Symptomatic patients with an intermediate or high pre-test prob-
        ability for CAD are most appropriate for stress RNI. Chest pain
        with borderline elevated or equivocal troponin elevations can
        undergo RNI.
    - ○ Patients with probable unstable angina (e.g., negative troponins)
        and ongoing chest pain may be evaluated for CAD with rest RNI.

- ○ Patients with definite acute coronary syndromes should *not* undergo RNI.
- ○ Patients with positive troponins where there is a low suspicion of an acute coronary syndrome being the source of the cardiac enzyme elevation may undergo stress RNI.
- Determination of the functional significance of coronary artery stenosis or collateral vessels seen on angiography or the success of reperfusion interventions
  - ○ Although more invasive techniques, such as fractional flow reserve or intravascular ultrasound, are often used to determine the physiologic significance of a coronary stenosis, stress RNI can also be helpful in estimating the degree of myocardial ischemia related to a coronary stenosis and the relief of ischemia achieved with an intervention.
- Guidance of revascularization decisions and estimating prognosis after an acute MI
  - ○ RNI can show the extent of the perfusion abnormality due to acute MI, scarring due to previous infarcts, and residual reversible ischemia. For safety reasons, the stress portion of the test needs to be submaximal and performed more than 48 hours after peak troponin.
  - ○ Post-MI stress RNI is probably only appropriate when a conservative management strategy of the MI has been selected (e.g., no coronary angiography) or when patients present late post-MI and without symptoms of active ischemia.
  - ○ Myocardial viability testing may be useful in the post-MI setting to determine need for revascularization. Revascularization of nonviable myocardium is unlikely to be beneficial.
- Investigation of the etiology for ventricular arrhythmias or syncope (with an intermediate or high pre-test probability for CAD)
- Evaluating new-onset left ventricular systolic dysfunction
  - ○ In a patient without angina but with systolic dysfunction, an ischemic evaluation for the etiology of the systolic dysfunction is warranted (e.g., to determine if the cardiomyopathy is ischemic or nonischemic). In patients with intermediate or high pre-test probability for CAD, an invasive work-up with coronary angiography is preferred.
    - Stress RNI may be acceptable in the setting of:
      - Very low pre-test probability for CAD
      - Strong patient preference for noninvasive evaluation
      - Relative contraindications (e.g., renal dysfunction increasing risk of contrast angiography)
- Ventricular size and function
  - ○ Rest RNI may be used to serially evaluate LV or RV size and function (e.g., to monitor tolerance of cardiotoxic medications such as anthracyclines, to monitor the effect of valvular heart lesions, etc.). In multiple-gated acquisition (MUGA) scans (also called radionuclide ventriculogram, RVG), multiple images are taken of short, sequential portions of each cardiac cycle, guided by ECG,

for 5 to 10 minutes. Computer analysis then generates an average blood pool for each portion of the cardiac cycle and allows for calculation of ventricular volumes in systole and diastole. An ejection fraction is then calculated from the volumes.
  - Limited by irregularity in heart rate (VPDs, atrial fibrillation)
- Given the radioactivity required by the test, RNI is used for this purpose most often when TTE windows are limited (due to obesity, lung disease, etc.), although the accuracy and reproducibility of MUGA scans are superior to TTE and thus may be useful when it is important to detect very small changes in ejection fraction.

- Preoperative risk stratification
  - There is a dearth of evidence of benefit to pre-operative angiography and revascularization, preoperative stress RNI is only indicated in the following:
    - Symptomatic patients, where stress RNI would otherwise be indicated regardless of preoperative status.
    - Asymptomatic patients with at least 1 clinical risk factor and poor functional capacity for whom an intermediate- or high-risk procedure is planned. Risk factors are:
      - History of ischemic heart disease
      - Heart failure
      - Cerebrovascular disease
      - Insulin-dependent diabetes mellitus
      - Renal insufficiency (serum creatinine >2.0)

- **Limitations of cardiac radionuclide imaging**
  - Patient issues
    - Morbid obesity
      - Because of the amount of tissue the radiation has to penetrate, larger doses of radiation are required in these patients.
      - Use of prone imaging and technetium can improve the accuracy of the test, although the incidence of false positives will always be higher in morbidly obese patients than in nonobese patients.
      - RNI is less limited by obesity than TTE.
    - Image acquisition time
      - Although tests are continually becoming faster, a patient must be able to sit or lie for several minutes to obtain the images, which may not be possible in certain patients (due to pulmonary effusions, back pain, etc.).
  - Irregular rhythms
    - RNI is acquired with ECG gating whenever possible (e.g., using the ECG to trigger imaging separate phases of cardiac contraction). Therefore, in the case of an irregular rhythm, assessment of left ventricular size and function is markedly limited.
  - Attenuation by other structures
    - Attenuation of myocardial activity by surrounding soft tissue structures (e.g., hiatal hernia, liver mass, breasts) can cause

false positives. Breast tissue in women and the diaphragm and abdominal contents in both sexes (although more common in men) can cause attenuation of myocardial activity and make stress RNI more difficult (or even impossible) to interpret.

CARDIAC COMPUTERIZED TOMOGRAPHY (CT)[4]

Cardiac CT emerged in the 1990s as an option for imaging coronary arteries, defining cardiac structures and morphology, and coronary calcium scoring. CT is recognized as having a number of potential uses and advantages over existing technology. However, the radiation exposure, cost, and lack of existing data supporting their effect on patient outcomes make some clinical applications (particularly screening for coronary artery disease) of cardiac CT remain controversial. However, in particular circumstances, cardiac CT can be invaluable in guiding the clinical care of patients.

- Utility of cardiac CT.
  - Coronary artery calcification
    - Calcium scoring requires no IV contrast dye and limited scanning time and radiation. It has been advocated as a screening tool for identifying coronary atherosclerosis in low- or intermediate-risk patients to guide prevention measures, such as statin use. Although associated with prognosis in multiple studies, whether testing adds information that can affect patient management and impact patient outcomes has not been demonstrated.
  - Coronary artery stenoses
    - Cardiac CT with angiography can identify coronary stenoses (particularly soft plaques) and is most appropriate in the setting of a patient with ischemic symptoms and an intermediate pre-test probability of CAD.
    - Cardiac CT with angiography can also be used in patients with equivocal or uninterpretable stress tests as an alternative to invasive coronary angiography.
    - Evaluation of coronary arteries in patients with new onset heart failure is appropriate to assess etiology of the systolic dysfunction, particularly if the suspicion of CAD is low.
  - Complex congenital heart disease including anomalies of coronary circulation, great vessels, and cardiac chambers and valves
  - Cardiac structures
    - Contrast CT is frequently used by electrophysiologists to evaluate the highly variable anatomy of the pulmonary veins and left atrium in conjunction with left atrial mapping and ablation for atrial fibrillation.
    - Cardiac CT can identify abnormal cardiac, pericardial, and thoracic masses, including intracardiac thrombi.
    - Given the radiation risk, this is most appropriate when echo images are insufficient.

- Aortic abnormalities
  - Cardiac CT with angiography is often the test of choice (along with TEE) for identifying and defining aortic aneurysms, dissection, ulcers, and atheromas.
- **Limitations of Cardiac CT**
  - Patient issues
    - Very obese patients (BMI >40 kg/m^2), inability to raise arms above head, and the inability to hold breath and hold still are contraindications to cardiac CT.
  - Extensive coronary calcification and metal
    - Stenoses resulting from soft plaques are more easily defined as excessive calcium can cause shadowing and artifact.
    - Coronary stents and grafts with metal clip artifacts will cause shadowing and limit visualization, which makes CT challenging when trying to identify in-stent restenosis or ostial bypass graft stenosis.
  - Irregular and tachycardic rhythms (including frequent premature beats)
    - Due to the need for ECG gating, coronary CT angiography requires a regular slow rhythm (<70 bpm) to obtain readable images.
  - Cardiac and valvular function
    - Ventricular and valvular function can be assessed, although cardiac CT is typically inferior to other imaging tests in this regard.
    - Radiation
    - IV contrast dye and risk for acute kidney injury

CARDIAC MAGNETIC RESONANCE IMAGING (CMR)[5]

CMR is primarily used to evaluate myocardial viability and cardiac structure and function, although it can also be useful in the evaluation of ischemic heart disease with vasodilator stress perfusion imaging and dobutamine stress function imaging. CMR is available in specialized centers and typically is not available on an urgent basis.

- Utility of CMR.
  - Ventricular morphology and function
    - CMR can reliably define LV and RV volumes and ejection fractions, which is most helpful in complex congenital heart disease when TTE windows are distorted.
    - CMR may be able to aid in the diagnosis and management of specific cardiomyopathies, in particular infiltrative cardiomyopathies (e.g., amyloid, sarcoidosis), hypertrophic cardiomyopathies, noncompaction, and arrhythmogenic right ventricular cardiomyopathy.
    - Myocardial viability can be assessed; regions of poor viability may be identified.
    - In combination with perfusion imaging, CMR can be used in the evaluation of patients with ischemic symptoms and an intermediate pre-test probability for CAD.

- Quantification of blood flow
  - Valvular disease can be readily defined with CMR, including regurgitant volumes and gradients across all four valves.
  - Shunts (e.g., ASD, VSD, PDA, PAPVR) can be quantified, which can help guide operative management.
- Cardiac and extracardiac structures
- Cardiac masses (including distinguishing thrombus from soft tissue), and the pericardium (including evaluating for constriction), pulmonary veins, and aorta can be well defined with CMR.
- **Limitations of CMR.**
  - Patient factors
    - Morbid obesity prevents some patients from fitting in the scanner.
    - CMR takes several minutes in an enclosed space and may not be an option for claustrophobic or uncooperative patients.
  - Metal
    - Although MRI-compatible devices are forthcoming, most pacemakers, defibrillators, and extracardiac metal prostheses make CMR unsafe.
  - Spatial resolution
    - Very small structures (<1 cm) may not be seen on CMR. Cardiac CT and TEE have much higher resolution for these small structures.

7 ■ CARDIAC CATHETERIZATION AND ANGIOGRAPHY

INTRODUCTION

Cardiac catheterization is most widely used to diagnose the anatomic and physiologic severity of atherosclerosis. There are number of other diagnostic and therapeutic indications in adults.

INDICATIONS

Asymptomatic or stable angina. Class I indications for performing catheterization with stable angina include patient who demonstrate:

- Canadian Cardiovascular Society (CCS) Class III and IV angina, considered disabling despite medical therapy
- High-risk criteria on noninvasive testing, no matter the severity of angina
- Sudden cardiac death or serious ventricular arrhythmia
- Signs of symptoms of heart failure
- Clinical characteristics that indicate a high likelihood of Coronary Artery Disease (CAD)

Class IIa indications include patients with reduced EF (45%) and CCS class I or II angina, and demonstrable ischemia on noninvasive testing.

Unstable Angina (UA)/Non-ST Segment Elevation Myocardial Infarction (NSTEMI) (see Chapter 12: Acute Coronary Syndromes, pp. 80). An early invasive strategy is indicated when these patients have (Class I):

- Refractory angina or hemodynamic or electrical instability
- An elevated risk of clinical events

Complete guidelines on UA/NSTEMI management can be found at http://content.onlinejacc.org/misc/guidelines.dtl.

ST Elevation Myocardial Infarction (STEMI) (see Chapter 12). Primary Percutaneous Coronary Intervention (PCI) is preferred over fibrinolytic therapy unless there is an unacceptable delay.

Pre-operative risk stratification for non-cardiac surgery. Diagnostic angiography is indicated for patients with high-risk findings on noninvasive testing. See chapter on preoperative risk stratification.

Pre-operative evaluation for cardiac surgery. There is some debate as to whether all patients being considered for cardiac surgery require preoperative catheterization. While noninvasive information can quantify the degree of valvular disease and confirm ventricular function and the status of pulmonary vasculature, an invasive evaluation of the coronary arteries is often necessary.

Patients with congestive heart failure (CHF). Cardiac catheterization is indicated in patients with CHF due to systolic dysfunction with angina or regional wall motion abnormalities ± scintigraphic evidence or reversible myocardial ischemia, prior to transplantation, or secondary to complications of an MI.

- **Other conditions.**
  - Aortic diseases where presence of CAD will affect management (dissection, aneurysm)
  - Hypertrophic cardiomyopathy with angina
  - Cardiac transplant donors
  - Asymptomatic patients with Kawasaki's disease with coronary aneurysms on echocardiography
  - Recurrent ischemia after PCI or CABG
  - Quantification and detection of intracardiac shunts (ASD, VSD)

CONTRAINDICATIONS

- Absolute:
  - Refusal of a mentally competent patient to consent
- Relative:
  - Uncontrolled ventricular irritability
  - Uncorrected hypokalemia or digitalis toxicity
  - Uncorrected hypertension
  - Intercurrent febrile illness
  - Anticoagulated state for elective cases
  - Severe allergy to radiographic contrast agent
  - Severe renal insufficiency and/or anuria (unless dialysis is planned)

TECHNIQUES

- Left heart catheterization
  - **Femoral approach (Judkins Technique).** The majority of cases still use the percutaneous femoral artery approach. Both groins are generally prepared, although the right groin is most often used. For this reason, femoral and distal pulses are palpated bilaterally and auscultated for the presence of bruit, and anatomic landmarks are identified. Local anesthesia is given and a single-wall puncture is performed (see Chapter on Seldinger Technique), after which a guide wire is introduced through the needle and moved freely up the aorta (confirmed with fluoroscopy). Vascular access may also be guided by ultrasonography.
  - **Arm approach.** The radial or brachial artery approach can be used for left heart catheterization. A modified Allen's test is performed prior to radial catheterization to ensure palmar arch patency. The radial approach can be more challenging than routine transfemoral access but reduces access site complications. Brachial artery catheterization may be complicated by thrombosis. Because the supply to the forearm

is supplied exclusively by this artery, this complication may require surgical or endovascular therapy to avoid limb-threatening ischemia.
- **Right heart catheterization** (see Appendix A: Bedside Procedures, Right Heart Catheterization).
  - Generally the Seldinger technique is used to obtain venous access. A pulmonary arterial catheter is then advanced from the access site to the right atrium while monitoring pressure. If the femoral vein is used, fluoroscopic guidance is necessary. Advancement of the catheter from the right ventricle to the pulmonary arteries can be challenging from the femoral approach. The internal jugular, subclavian, or brachial veins are alternative sites for venous access.

ANGIOGRAPHY

At present, cardiac catheterization remains the gold standard for the diagnosis of coronary artery disease. Once the coronary ostia and/or surgical grafts have been cannulated, a number of different angiographic views are used to visualize coronary anatomy (see **Figures 7-1** and **7-2**). These views are summarized in **Table 7-1**.

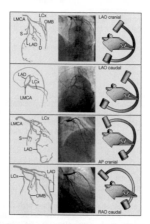

FIGURE 7-1. Angiographic views of the left coronary artery.
Adapted from *Braunwald's Heart Disease*, Volume 1, Popma J, Chapter 21: Coronary Arteriography, page 414, Copyright Elsevier 2012.

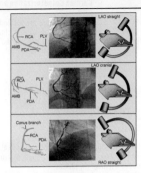

FIGURE 7-2. Angiographic views of the right coronary artery.
Adapted from *Braunwald's Heart Disease*, Volume 1, Popma J, Chapter 21: Coronary Arteriography, pp. 414, Copyright Elsevier 2012.

TABLE 7-1. Angiographic Views

View	RAO°	LAO°	Cranial°	Caudal°	Anatomy
RAO-Caudal	0–10	–	–	15–20	Left main bifurcation, proximal LAD, and proximal to mid LCx
RAO-Straight	30	–	–	–	Mid RCA and PDA
RAO-Cranial	0–10	–	25–40	–	Mid and distal LAD, clear origins of septal and diagonals, distal RCA or distal LCx
LAO-Cranial	–	60	15–30	–	Elongates left main and proximal LAD (take during maximal inspiration to pull diaphragm down and improve x-ray penetration)
LAO-Cranial	–	20	20	–	PDA/PL bifurcation and distal vessel
LAO-Straight	–	30	–	–	Initial view for RCA, shows origin and main vessel to PDA/PL bifurcation
LAO-Caudal	–	40–60	–	20	"Spider view," left main, proximal LAD, proximal LCx (improves with maximal inspiration)
PA	0	0	0	0	Left main ostium
Left Lateral	0	90	0	0	Proximal LCx, proximal and distal LAD, anastomosis of the LIMA to LAD graft

Catheterization and angiographic techniques are not limited to the coronary arteries. The pulmonary arteries, vena cavae, cardiac chambers, ascending aorta, subclavian arteries, internal mammary arteries, and saphenous vein bypass grafts are frequently visualized during cardiac catheterization.

COMPLICATIONS

Complications of catheterization include, but are not limited to:
- Death (<0.1%)
- Myocardial infarction (<0.1%)
- Stroke (0.1–0.4%)
- Emergency bypass surgery
- Cardiac perforation (0.3%)
- Major arrhythmia requiring defibrillation or pacing (0.4%)
- Local vascular injury requiring surgery or transfusion (0.4%)
- Contrast-induced nephropathy (0.4%)
- Allergic reactions (anaphylaxis)

8 ■ THE ELECTROPHYSIOLOGY STUDY

INTRODUCTION

Diagnostic electrophysiology (EP) studies are a tool the electrophysiologist uses to assess:

- Sinus node function
- Properties of the conduction system, including AV node and His-Purkinje system function
- Presence of substrate for arrhythmia
  - Accessory AV pathways (AV reentrant tachycardia)
  - Dual AV nodal physiology (AV nodal reentrant tachycardia)
  - Scar that may mediate atrial or ventricular reentrant tachycardias
- Inducibility of tachyarrhythmias
  - To prognosticate the risk of malignant ventricular arrhythmias
  - To study a clinical arrhythmia, usually for the purposes of locating a site for radiofrequency energy ablation (Cryoablation and other sources of energy are also used.)

The EP study is a type of cardiac catheterization. Unlike the more typical catheterization with hollow catheters for angiography and hemodynamics, EP catheters are insulated wires with exposed electrodes for recording electrograms and for pacing. Catheters are usually advanced through hemostatic sheaths placed in the femoral vein. Antecubital arm veins, subclavian veins, or internal jugular veins can also sometimes be used. Arterial access can be used to reach the left ventricle via the retrograde aortic approach.

In the typical EP study, multipolar electrodes are placed at strategic sites to provide information about timing. Usual catheter positions are:

- High right atrium (near the sinus node)
- The His bundle region (the high septal side of the tricuspid annulus)
  - A correctly placed His bundle catheter records an atrial electrogram, an His bundle electrogram, and a ventricular electrogram.
- The coronary sinus (CS). Since the CS runs in the left AV groove (parallel to the left circumflex artery), the electrodes on a CS catheter record both left atrial and left ventricular electrograms (accessed from the venous side of the circulation, without the need for arterial puncture or anticoagulation).
- The RV apex or base.
- A "mapping" or ablation catheter can rove throughout any of the chambers to record electrograms from sites of interest.
  - The right atrium, ventricle, and right ventricular outflow tract can be reached by venous access.

- Reaching the left heart requires either:
  - Arterial access for the retrograde aortic approach to the left ventricle (typically not used to reach the left atrium)
  - Transseptal puncture to reach the left atrium and/or left ventricle

The EP study consists of:
- Observations of the relative timing of electrograms (including the surface ECG) during sinus rhythm and during arrhythmias.
- Examination of the response to pacing:
  - "Burst pacing" and incrementally faster rates.
  - Atrial or ventricular extrastimuli (or double or triple extrastimuli).
  - Different site of stimulation for burst pacing or extrastimuli may yield different patterns of activation or of arrhythmia inducibility.
- "Mapping" tachyarrhythmias. Mapping traditionally requires construction of a mental map of an arrhythmia or substrate in coordination with fluoroscopic images of catheter location and the electrograms recorded. There are now computer-facilitated "electroanatomical mapping" systems (CARTO; EnSite NavX) that can generate 3-D maps based on positioning sensor—a highly accurate triangulation system akin to global positioning systems (GPS), using either magnetic or voltage fields to locate the catheter on the map.
  - To assess the mechanism (reentry vs. focal): **Activation mapping** tracks the electrical wave throughout the cycle.
  - To assess whether an isthmus of electrically active myocardium may be critical to reentrant arrhythmias: A special technique of pacing *during* a tachyarrhythmia to assess the interaction of a paced wavefront with a reentrant circuit is **entrainment mapping**.
  - To seek the earliest activation (the focus, or site of origin) of a focal arrhythmia: Use activation mapping and/or **pace mapping**, which compares the activation pattern of the arrhythmia to the activation pattern (e.g., the QRS complex) during pacing from different sites. For focal arrhythmias, the identical activation of arrhythmia compared with pacing suggests that the pacing site is the site of origin of the arrhythmia.
    - Less accurate in reentrant arrhythmias, though it still may be used.
  - **Substrate mapping.** Mapping during sinus rhythm to assess the nature of the myocardium. Typically utilized for VT, especially when the VT itself is too poorly hemodynamically tolerated by the patient for extended periods required for other mapping.
    - Mapping the substrate may reveal zones of scar, particularly the border zone of a scar that might contain a reentrant isthmus. Ablation across border zones may eliminate tachycardia without extended mapping during VT, though the success rate is reduced compared with detailed mapping during tachycardia.

RECORDED ELECTROGRAMS (FIGURE 8-1)

- The surface electrocardiogram is an essential component of the EP study.
  - Typically, all electrograms are shown at more rapid sweep speeds than the standard ECG. This may disorient the novice, causing the surface ECG to be overlooked.
- The backbone tracing of the EP study is the bipolar electrogram, the potential recorded between two (usually) closely spaced electrodes.
  - Used mainly to study the timing of activation of the myocardium underlying the electrodes, in comparison to the other bipolar electrograms and the surface ECG.
- Unipolar electrograms are recorded from a mapping electrode and an indifferent electrode placed at a relatively distant site, or with Wilson's Central Terminal as the indifferent electrode.
  - In addition to timing, the unipolar electrogram can give information concerning directionality of the wavefront of depolarization.
    - ○ As the wave travels toward the electrode, a positive deflection is seen, and a negative deflection is the result of the wavefront traveling away from the electrode.
    - ○ Absence of a positive deflection (a "Q-wave") suggests that the electrode is directly over the site of origin of a focal arrhythmia.

BRADYCARDIAS

An EP study can assess the health of the sinus node, the AV node, and the conduction system (often called the His-Purkinje system).

- Sinus node function
  - In addition to the sinus rate, and the response to a beta-adrenergic agonist, the sinus node can be assessed by the **sinus node recovery time (SNRT)**, the time after pacing the atrium that it takes for a sinus impulse to occur.
    - ○ Highly dependent on the autonomic state, so the **corrected sinus node recovery time (CSNRT)** is usually used.
      - CSNRT is the SNRT minus the underlying sinus cycle length
        - Normal is less than 550 ms.
        - An abnormal value reflects sinus node dysfunction, though is not in itself an indication for permanent pacing.
- The sinoatrial conduction time (SACT) assesses the communication between the sinus node and the surrounding atrium. It is frequently not assessed in an EP study.
- AV node function is highly variable with autonomic activity; can be assessed by atria pacing and paced atrial extrastimuli. Some means of assessment are:
  - The cycle length at which AV Wenckebach block occurs

- The AV nodal effective refractory period (AVN ERP)—the coupling interval of the longest paced atrial extrastimulus that does not conduct through the AV node
  - Related to the pacing cycle length before the extrastimulus (the "drive cycle length")
- Retrograde AV nodal function can be assessed with ventricular pacing.
  - Retrograde conduction may not occur, even with good anterograde AV node function. Similarly, retrograde (V-A) Wenckebach is not well correlated with anterograde conduction.
- His-Purkinje system function:
  - The surface ECG demonstrates bundle branch blocks and fascicular blocks.
  - His-Purkinje function is also assessed by the HV time:
    - Time measured from the His electrogram (the His catheter properly placed to show atial, His, and ventricular electrograms) to the earliest ventricular signal (often seen on the surface ECG)
    - Normal HV time: 35–55 ms
      - Longer HV is consistent with His-Purkinje system delay.
        - Markedly prolonged (>100 ms) HV may assist in the decision to implant a pacemaker in the symptomatic patient.
      - An abnormally short HV can only occur if:
        - There is ventricular pre-excitation via a manifest accessory pathway, or
        - The His catheter is placed too far in the ventricle; the presumed His electrogram is actually recorded from the right bundle branch.
    - A "split His" in which the His electrogram is two components separated in time.
    - Infra-Hisian block, in which an atrial impulse proceeds through AV node and a His electrogram is recorded, but the impulse is not conducted to the ventricle. Infra-Hisian block is distinctly abnormal, since His-Purkinje conduction is very fast and the refractory period of the AV node is usually much longer than that of the His bundle.

TACHYCARDIAS

Tachycardias and their substrates are studied with electrophysiologic techniques. In the past, the inducibility of VT was an important reason for electrophysiology study, since inducibility was a component of the assessment for implantable cardioverter-defibrillators (ICDs). Since most decisions concerning ICDs have become clinical, based on previous events of VT/VF or, for primary prevention of sudden death, on the LV ejection fraction, EP studies solely to assess the inducibility of VT are now relatively rare. Currently EP studies are focused on the study of an inducible rhythm to understand its physiology and (usually) to map a site for ablation to achieve a cure. In addition to pacing maneuvers, infusion of a beta-adrenergic agonist (e.g., isoproterenol) can assist in inducing tachycardia.

- Atrial arrhythmias (atrial tachycardia, atrial flutter, atrial fibrillation) can be induced by rapid atrial pacing or atrial extrastimuli and then mapped as described above. The variability of atrial fibrillation limits traditional mapping.
- Paroxysmal SVTs (AVNRT, AVRT):
  - SVTs may be induced by rapid pacing or by extrastimuli from either the atrium or the ventricle.
  - The presence of the substrate for SVT can be examined, even in sinus rhythm.
    - Accessory pathways (or "bypass tracts"). With rare exceptions, accessory pathways do not have the *decremental* conduction properties (slower conduction with rapid stimulation) that the AV node expresses. Accessory pathway conduction is usually more rapid and its conduction speed is invariable until its refractory period is met.
      - Manifest accessory pathways associated with the Wolff-Parkinson-White syndrome produce ventricular pre-excitation seen in sinus rhythm on the ECG (delta wave) and a short (or even negative) HV interval. Manifest pathways almost always conduct retrogradely as well. Therefore, they may serve as a substrate for orthodromic or antidromic AVRT.
      - Concealed accessory pathways only conduct in the retrograde (V to A) conduction, and they can only mediate *orthodromic* AVRT.

      Both concealed and manifest pathways alter retrograde atrial activation, so ventricular pacing can reveal the presence of an accessory pathway by the abnormal atrial activation and by the lack of decremental conduction.
    - Dual AV nodal physiology is the substrate for AV node reentrant tachycardia (AVNRT). Dual AV node physiology is established by the observation of a change from fast pathway (normal AV) conduction to the slow pathway. Since the refractory period of the fast pathway is long, shorten the coupling interval of an atrial extrastulus until slow pathway conduction (lengthened AH time). The "jump" to slow pathway conduction with decreasing the coupling interval of an extrastiumli results in a "jump" of the AH time by 50 ms or more (with a change in coupling interval of 10 ms or less. Atrial extrastimuli usually is initiated by atrial extrastimuli.
- Ventricular tachycardia is initiated by ventricular pacing or ventricular extrastimuli. Mapping techniques can then be used to study the arrhythmia.

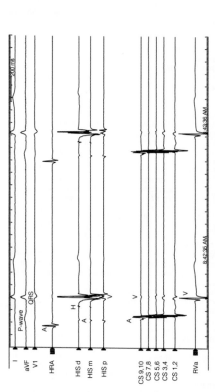

FIGURE 8-1. Electrograms recorded in normal sinus rhythm in an electrophysiology study for supraventricular tachycardia. Shown are surface leads I, aVF, & V1. Displayed intracardiac electrograms are recorded from the high right atrium (HRA), His bundle region (HIS), Coronary sinus (CS), and right ventricular apex (RVA). Electrograms are labelled as A (atrial electrogram), H (His bundle electrogram), or V (ventricular electrogram).

9 ■ PERIOPERATIVE CARDIAC EVALUATION

GOALS OF EVALUATION

The goals of perioperative cardiac risk stratification are to identify populations at risk for cardiovascular mortality and morbidity and to mitigate these risks in the perioperative setting. It should be noted that risk stratification and management can delineate and possibly reduce risk, but will not eliminate risk.

Volume shifts, blood loss, increases in myocardial oxygen demand, and other physiologic derangements during surgery and in the post-operative setting constitute a period of increased risk for cardiovascular events. Patients with underlying vascular disease (e.g., peripheral arterial disease, stroke, heart failure) are at increased risk because of a higher prevalence of associated coronary disease and/or impaired ventricular function.

The approach to risk stratification utilizes three elements: 1) patient-specific factors, 2) functional capacity, and 3) surgery-specific risk. The history, physical examination, and ECG should be targeted to assess these elements.

PATIENT FACTORS[6]

Major predictors that require intensive management and may lead to delay in or cancellation of the operative procedure unless emergent:

- Unstable coronary syndromes including unstable or severe angina or recent MI
  - Recent MI (rate of death or MI about 2% but higher <3 months). American College of Cardiology defines recent MI as between 7–30 days.
- Decompensated heart failure including NYHA functional class IV or worsening or new-onset HF
- Significant arrhythmias including high-grade AV block, ventricular arrhythmias with underlying structural heart disease, supraventricular arrhythmias with ventricular rate > 100 bpm at rest, symptomatic bradycardia
- Severe valvular heart disease, including severe aortic stenosis or symptomatic mitral stenosis

Other clinical predictors that warrant careful assessment of current status:

- History of ischemic heart disease
- History of cerebrovascular disease
- History of compensated heart failure or prior heart failure
- Diabetes mellitus
- Renal insufficiency

FUNCTIONAL CAPACITY

The history can be utilized to estimate the patient's current functional status to estimate the current physiologic stress that is tolerated. Functional status can be expressed in metabolic equivalents (1 MET is defined as 3.5 mL O_2 uptake/kg per min, which is the resting oxygen uptake in a sitting position). Perioperative cardiac and long-term risk is increased among patients who cannot achieve at least a 4-MET demand. Those patients should be risk stratified further as should patients whose status cannot be determined because a competing illness precludes activity (e.g., peripheral vascular disease, arthritis, prior stroke). Examples of various activities and their MET equivalent are shown in **Table 9-1**.

SURGICAL RISK FOR NONCARDIAC PROCEDURES (TABLE 9-2)

Risk indices. It should be noted due to the nature of the populations from which these criteria were derived, risk indices may underestimate risk in certain populations such as patients with vascular disease or aortic stenosis and provide poor discriminatory function in low risk categories. Goldman Criteria, Eagle Criteria, and Detsky modified risk criteria, and the Revised Cardiac Risk

TABLE 9-1. Metabolic Equivalents Associated with Various Activities.

Can You Complete the Following Activities without Symptoms?	Met Value
Dress without stopping because of symptoms?	2.00
Do moderate work around the house like vacuum, sweep floors, or carry groceries?	2.50
Walk down a flight of stairs unassisted and without stopping?	3.00
Do heavy work around the house like strip and make the bed, hang out washing, or wash the car?	3.25
Do moderate gardening like week or rake the leaves?	4.25
Push an electric or petrol mower on level ground?	4.50
Participate in moderate activities like walk at a normal pace (4km/h) or play golf and carry the clubs?	4.75
Walk briskly around an oval?	5.00
Do outdoor work like split wood or dig in the garden?	5.50
Carry an 8-kg weight (e.g., load of wet washing) up 8 steps?	6.00
Carry at least 10 kg (e.g., a suitcase) up 8 steps?	7.00
Carry objects that weigh at least 35kg (e.g., 11-year-old child)?	7.50
Participate in vigorous activities like swimming (crawl), joging(8km/h), cycling(17km/h), singles tennis?	9.00
MET = metabolic equivalent.	

Source: Elsevier. Reprinted from Am J Cardiol, Volumne 77, Issue 14, Rankin SL, Briffa TG, Morton, AR, and Hung J, A specific activity questionnaire to measure the functional capacity off cardiac patients, pp. 1220-3, Copyright 1996 1996 Jun 1;77(14):1220-3.

TABLE 9-2. Surgical Risk for Non-cardiac Procedures

High Risk (>5)	Intermediate Risk (<5%)	Low Risk (<1%)
Emergent operations, especially in the elderly or with significant comorbidity	Carotid endarterectomy	Endoscopic procedures
Major vascular surgery	Head and neck operations	Superficial procedures
Prolonged surgical procedures with large fluid shifts or blood loss	Intraperitoneal and intrathoracic operations	Cataracts
	Orthopedic operations	Breast operation
	Prostate operation	

Index (RCRI) have been utilized to predict risk. It is advisable to use the RCRI for patients undergoing nonemergent surgery, given greater predictive value.

Revised Goldman cardiac risk index (RCRI).[7] Six independent predictors of major cardiac complications:
(1) High-risk type of surgery
(2) History of ischemic heart disease (history of MI or a positive exercise test, current complaint of chest pain considered to be secondary to myocardial ischemia, use of nitrate therapy, or ECG with pathological Q waves; do not count prior coronary revascularization procedure unless one of the other criteria for ischemic heart disease is present)
(3) History of HF
(4) History of cerebrovascular disease
(5) Diabetes mellitus requiring treatment with insulin
(6) Preoperative serum creatinine >2.0 mg/dL (177 μmol/L)

Estimated rates of cardiac death, nonfatal myocardial infarction, and nonfatal cardiac arrest:
- No risk factors—0.4% (95% CI: 0.1–0.8)
- 1 risk factor—1.0% (95% CI: 0.5–1.4)
- 2 risk factors—2.4% (95% CI: 1.3–3.5)
- 3+ risk factors—5.4% (95% CI: 2.8–7.9)

Estimated rates of cardiac death, nonfatal MI, cardiac arrest or ventricular fibrillation, pulmonary edema, and complete heart block:
- No risk factors—0.4 to 1.0 % versus <1 % with beta blockers
- 1–2 risk factors—2.2 to 6.6 % versus 0.8 to 1.6 % with beta blockers
- 3+ risk factors—>9 % versus >3 % with beta blockers

In some cases, noninvasive testing helps refine risk among those deemed at intermediate risk or for whom risk cannot be well defined after initial clinical evaluation (Figure 9-1). The negative predictive value of stress testing exceeds 90% while the positive predictive value is quite variable (≈20%). Exercise stress testing is preferred but pharmacologic testing (e.g., adenosine, dipyridamole, or dobutamine) can be used for those who cannot exercise.

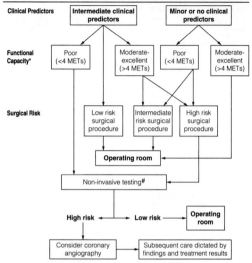

*MET = Metabolic equivalents. 1-4 METs: Daily activities, walking 1-2 blocks on level ground at 2-3 mph, light house work. 4-10 METs: Climbing stairs or hill, running short distance, heavy house work, bowling, dancing, golf, tennis, swimming, skiing

#Assessment of LV function, exercise or pharmacologic stress testing, or ambulatory ECG monitoring

FIGURE 9-1. Suggested approach to perioperative cardiac evaluation.

Recommendations (Figure 9-2):
- Despite increased risk, patients are usually best served proceeding directly for emergent or urgent surgery since further risk stratification is of likely small benefit.
- Unstable patients (active coronary ischemia, heart failure, arrhythmia, symptomatic valvular heart disease) should be stabilized.
  - In a patient with unstable cardiac disease who requires urgent surgery, it may be advisable to stabilize the patient prior to surgery but additional testing is likely of limited benefit unless the surgery

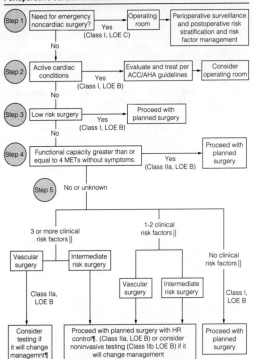

FIGURE 9-2. ACC/AHA guidelines for perioperative cardiac evaluation.

‖ Clinical risk factors include ischemic heart disease, compensated or prior heart failure, diabetes mellitus, renal insufficiency, and cerebrovascular disease.

¶ Consider perioperative beta blockade for populations in which this has been shown to reduce cardiac morbidity/mortality. ACC/AHA indicates American College of Cardiology/American Heart Association; HR, heart rate; LOE, level of evidence; and MET, metabolic equivalent.

Source: Elsevier. Reprinted from J Am Coll Cardiol, 2009; 54:13-118 with permission.

will be modified or cancelled based on the results and/or need for administration of anticoagulants or antiplatelet agents.

- Patients without active cardiac symptoms undergoing low-risk surgery and those with good functional capacity (MET level ≥4) require no pre-operative testing apart from an ECG.
- Patients with poor or unknown functional capacity, or symptoms compatible with cardiac disease who are undergoing intermediate risk or vascular surgery are managed according to the number of patient risk factors.
  - For patients with 1–2 patient risk factors, proceed with surgery, unless testing will alter management.
  - For patients with 3 or more patient risk factors scheduled to undergo intermediate risk surgery, it is reasonable to proceed without noninvasive testing, unless that testing will alter management.
  - In patients with 3 or more risk factors undergoing open vascular surgery, noninvasive testing is suggested if it will alter management

GENERAL PRINCIPLES

Primary prevention is the effort to modify risk factors to prevent the occurrence of any of the following manifestations of atherosclerotic disease:
- Coronary heart disease (CHD), which includes myocardial infarction, angina pectoris, heart failure, and coronary death
- Cerebrovascular disease which includes stroke and transient ischemic attack
- Aortic atherosclerosis, thoracic or abdominal aortic aneurysm, carotid artery disease.
- Peripheral arterial disease manifested by intermittent claudication or critical limb ischemia

Secondary prevention refers to the prevention of a subsequent episode once an individual has already experienced a cardiovascular event. It is well established that atherosclerotic disease in one of the above vascular distributions increases the risk of disease in the others, and as such patients with any form of atherosclerotic disease or diabetes mellitus are considered CHD risk equivalent and are subject to secondary prevention goals of treatment.

RISK ASSESSMENT

At the heart of primary prevention lies risk assessment. In order to effectively identify those patients who are at significant risk of developing cardiovascular disease, several methods of risk assessment have been devised. The 2002 Update of the AHA Guidelines for Primary Prevention of Cardiovascular Disease recommends that risk assessment in adults should begin at age 20, AND all adults 40 years of age or older, or those with 2 or more risk factors should have their 10-year risk of coronary heart disease (CHD) assessed at least every 5 years.

METHODS OF RISK ASSESSMENT

Framingham Risk Score:
- This risk assessment tool is used to estimate 10-year risk of developing CHD. It was derived from the Framingham Heart Study and was intended to estimate risk in adults aged 20 and older who do not have heart disease or diabetes.
- Risk factors include age, gender, total cholesterol, HDL cholesterol, smoking status, systolic blood pressure, and current treatment for hypertension.

- The calculated score is used to group patients into three risk categories: low risk (<10% CHD risk at 10 years), intermediate risk (10–20% risk at 10 years), or high risk (>20% risk at 10 years).
- An online risk calculator is available at http://hp2010.nhlbihin.net/atpiii/calculator.asp?usertype=prof

PROCAM risk scores:

- PROCAM is available in two forms and is used to estimate the 10-year risk of developing a coronary event.
  - The PROCAM Quick Check does not require lab testing, and risk factors include age, gender, diabetes, smoking status, family history of MI in first-degree relative when younger than age 60, systolic blood pressure, weight, body height, and current treatment for hypertension.
  - The PROCAM Health Check includes age, gender, diabetes, smoking status, family history, systolic blood pressure, LDL, HDL, and triglyceride levels.
- An online risk calculator is available at http://www.chd-taskforce.com/procam_interactive.html

Reynolds Risk Score:

- This risk assessment tool is used to estimate 10-year risk of developing CHD. Two versions exist—one validated from a group of men and another developed for women. An advantage of this tool over the Framingham Score is that the additional variables reclassify a majority of intermediate-risk patients into either high or low risk.
- This score includes the same variables as the Framingham tool, as well as high-sensitivity CRP level, parental history of MI before age 60, and hemoglobin A1c in patients with diabetes.
- An online risk calculator is available at http://www.reynoldsriskscore.org

SCORE:

- This risk assessment tool is used in European clinical practice to estimate 10-year risk of CHD in addition to the 10-year risk of any fatal CVD event.
- Risk factors include age, gender, systolic blood pressure, total cholesterol, HDL cholesterol, and smoking status.
- An online risk calculator is available at http://www.heartscore.org/Pages/welcome.aspx

Special Note: The 2011 Updated AHA Guidelines for the Prevention of CVD in Women recommend classification of CVD risk be divided into three levels of risk: high risk, at risk, and ideal cardiovascular heath.

RISK FACTOR MODIFICATION

BLOOD PRESSURE MANAGEMENT

General principles:

- The Seventh Report of the Joint National Committee on Prevention, Detection, Evaluation, and Treatment of High Blood Pressure (JNC 7)[8] categorizes hypertension based on elevated blood pressure readings obtained on at least 2 separate occasions.

- Normal blood pressure: SBP < 120 mmHg and DBP < 80 mmHg
- Pre-hypertension: SBP 120–139 mmHg or DBP 80–89 mmHg
- Stage 1 Hypertension: SBP 140–159 mmHg or DBP 90–99 mmHg
- Stage 2 Hypertension: SBP ≥ 160 mmHg or DBP ≥ 100 mmHg

- The risk of cardiovascular disease begins at 115/75 mmHg and doubles with each increment of 20/10 mmHg. Many clinical trials and meta-analyses have shown that the CVD–risk reduction benefit from blood pressure treatment is due to the amount of blood pressure reduction, rather than the mechanism of action of any particular drug.
- Treating hypertension has been shown to cause regression of left ventricular hypertrophy, a surrogate risk marker for MI, CHD, and sudden death. It also decreases incidence of stroke by 30–40%, MI by 20–25%, and CHF by more than 50%, and it decreases CHD mortality.
- All patients should be screened for secondary causes of hypertension including sleep apnea, medication induced, hyperaldosteronism, pheochromocytoma, aortic coarctation, thyroid or parathyroid disease, Cushing's syndrome, and chronic steroid use.
- Most patients with hypertension will require at least 2 antihypertensive agents to achieve their goal blood pressure.
- All patients should be counseled on lifestyle modification.

Goals of treatment:

- *Primary prevention:* Blood pressure goal < 140/90 mmHg, < 130/85 if patient has chronic kidney disease or congestive heart failure.
- *Secondary prevention:* Blood pressure goal < 140/90 mmHg, < 130/80mmHg if patient has diabetes or chronic kidney disease.

Therapies:

- Aldosterone antagonists.
  - **Spironolactone** is a potassium sparing diuretic that acts as an aldosterone receptor antagonist.
    - Dose for hypertension is 25–50 mg/day.
    - Requires serial monitoring of potassium and creatinine. Discontinue use if Cr > 4 mg/dL or K > 5 mEq/L.
    - Up to 20% of men who receive spironolactone develop gynecomastia.
  - **Eplerenone** is a selective aldosterone receptor antagonist that lacks the hormonal side effects of spironolactone.
    - Dose for hypertension is 50 mg/day, may increase to 50 mg twice daily.
    - Interacts with CYP3A4 system.
    - Requires serial monitoring of creatinine and potassium, cannot use if K > 5.5 or CrCl < 30mL/min.
    - The following additional contraindications apply to patients with hypertension: type 2 diabetes mellitus with microalbuminuria; serum creatinine > 2.0 mg/dL in males or > 1.8 mg/dL in females; Cl_{cr} < 50 mL/minute.

- **Angiotensin converting enzyme (ACE) inhibitors.** Inhibits the conversion of angiotensin I to angiotensin II, decreasing afterload. Bradykinin buildup as a result of ACE inhibitor action is postulated as the etiology of the side effect of cough.
  - Should be used as first-line therapy in patients with CHF, history of STEMI, or anterior NSTEMI, depressed ejection fraction ($\leq 40\%$), diabetes, or proteinuria.
  - There is no additional benefit to be gained from the combination of ACE inhibitor and ARB.
  - Contraindicated during pregnancy. Use with caution in women of childbearing age.
- **Angiotensin receptor blockers.** Function as selective angiotensin I receptor antagonists.
  - Use if patients are intolerant of ACE inhibitors due to cough or angioedema (use with caution). In patients who cannot tolerate ACE inhibitors, data from clinical trials suggest that ARBs are as effective for secondary prevention of CHD.
  - The LIFE trial[9] suggests that ARBs can be used instead of ACE inhibitors in patients with severe hypertension with ECG evidence of left ventricular hypertrophy.
  - Contraindicated during pregnancy. Use with caution in women of childbearing age.
- **Beta-blockers.** Inhibit beta-1 adrenergic receptors in the myocardium decreasing myocardial contractility and heart rate, thereby reducing myocardial oxygen demand in increasing oxygen supply.
  - All patients should receive a beta-blocker post-myocardial infarction, in the absence of contraindications.
  - Beta-blockers are useful to decrease symptoms in patients with angina.
- **Calcium channel blockers.** Inhibit myocardial and smooth muscle contractility, improving blood flow to the myocardium and decreasing oxygen demand.
  - Dihydropyridines (amlodipine, nicardipine, felodipine) versus non-dihydropyridines (diltiazem and verapamil)
  - Diltiazem and verapamil are useful in patients with atrial fibrillation for rate control.
  - Patients with angina and preserved ejection fraction, or persistent symptoms despite beta-blocker and nitrate therapy, can benefit from the addition of a calcium channel blocker.
- **Diuretics.**
  - Thiazide diuretics such as chlorthalidone and hydrochlorothiazide (HCTZ) are recommended as a first-line agent by JNC 7 for the treatment of hypertension, though this may change in the upcoming Eighth Report of the Joint National Committee on Prevention, Detection, Evaluation, and Treatment of High Blood Pressure (JNC 8) guidelines.
  - There is sufficient data from ALLHAT to support the benefit of chlorthalidone, and it should be utilized before HCTZ.

- Loop or thiazide diuretics may be used as needed to treat hypertension but neither has been shown to have morbidity or mortality benefit in patients following MI.
- **Others therapies** such as alpha-1 blockers, central alpha-2 agonists, direct vasodilators, and direct renin inhibitors are available and should be used as second- and third-line agents due to a paucity of outcomes data when compared to the therapies described earlier.

INITIAL DRUG THERAPY AND COMPELLING INDICATIONS FOR SPECIFIC ANTI-HYPERTENSIVES: FROM JNC VII EXPRESS

LIPID MANAGEMENT

General principles:
- Statins and niacin are the only medications that have been shown to effectively decrease cardiovascular events and mortality in secondary prevention trials. The benefit of statins is mitigated in primary prevention and limited to reduction in cardiovascular events, not mortality.
- Observational studies suggest that high intake of omega-3 fatty acids reduces the risk of death from CHD, but there is little evidence that supplementation can reduce the progression of atherosclerosis or decrease cardiovascular events.
- All patients should be counseled on diet and lifestyle modification.

Goals of treatment:
- Primary prevention:
  - LDL < 160 if ≤ 1 Framingham risk factor
  - LDL < 130 if 2 or more risk factors AND 10-year risk <2 0%
  - LDL < 100 if 2+ RF AND 10-year risk ≥ 20% or patient with diabetes
- Secondary prevention
  - LDL < 100 mg/dL versus < 70 mg/dL for very high-risk individuals
  - If triglycerides are ≥ 200 mg/dL, then non-HDL should be < 130 mg/dL.

Therapies:
- **Statins.** Inhibit HMG Co-A reductase, the rate-limiting step in cholesterol biosynthesis. While it is likely that some of the benefit from this class of medications comes from lipid lowering and regression of atherosclerosis, benefit is seen prior to plaque regression. Therefore, pleiotropic effects of statins such as antithrombotic or anti-inflammatory properties are also thought to be of importance.
  - Lowers LDL 18–55%, raises HDL 5–15%, decreases triglycerides 7–30%.
  - Side effects include myopathy and elevated liver enzymes.
  - If patients cannot tolerate a statin because of myopathy, try a less potent drug such as pravastatin or simvastatin at a low dose.
  - The additional benefit of high-dose statin therapy to bring LDL levels down < 70 mg/dL comes at a risk of increased LFT abnormalities and myalgias.

- Use with caution in patients on cyclosporine, macrolide antibiotics, antifungal agents, and CYP450 inhibitors.
- **Ezetimibe.** Inhibits the absorption of cholesterol in the small intestine at the brush border.
  - Lowers LDL levels up to 17%, but its long-term effects on hard outcomes as either monotherapy or in addition to a statin remain to be proven.
  - May be of use in avoiding high doses of statins, but the ARBITER 6-HALTS trial showed that niacin was superior to ezetimibe in this situation.
- **Fibrates.** Inhibits triglyceride synthesis and increases catabolism of lipoproteins.
  - Lowers LDL 5–20%, raises HDL 10–20%, decreases triglycerides 20–50%.
  - Trials primarily show CVD benefit to patients with high triglycerides, and meta-analyses suggest no benefit or a trend toward increased non-CVD mortality.
  - Use with caution in patients on statins because of a significantly increased risk of muscle injury in patients on dual therapy.
  - Use with caution in patients on warfarin as INR levels can increase significantly when on both medications.
- **Niacin.** Decreases the production of LDL and VLDL in the liver, increases lipolysis, decreases triglyceride esterification.
  - Lowers LDL 5–25%, raises HDL 15–35%, decreases triglycerides 20–50%.
  - Side effects of facial flushing, pruritus, and nausea are poorly tolerated by many though can be mitigated through the use of extended-release preparations, and nighttime dosing.
  - Can lead to hyperglycemia and hyperuricemia; use with caution in patients with diabetes and gout.
- **Bile acid sequestrants.** Binds intestinal bile acids and leads to excretion in feces rather than enteric reabsorption.
  - Lowers LDL 15–30%, raises HDL 3–5%; has no effect on, and can increase triglyceride levels.
  - Use is limited by gastrointestinal side effects of distress and constipation.
  - Use with caution in patients on warfarin and digoxin as absorption can be impaired.
  - Contraindications include dysbetalipoproteinemia, and elevated triglycerides.

SMOKING CESSATION

General principles:

The 5 As of intervention:
(1) **A**sk about tobacco use at every visit.
(2) **A**dvise the patient to quit.
(3) **A**ssess the patient's willingness to quit.

    (4) **A**ssist the patient to develop a quit plan.

    (5) **A**rrange for follow-up.

The 5 Rs of motivation:

    (1) **R**elevance: How is quitting personally relevant to the patient?

    (2) **R**isks: What are the perceived short- and long-term risks of continued use?

    (3) **R**ewards: What are the benefits to quitting?

    (4) **R**oadblocks: What is stopping the patient from quitting?

    (5) **R**epetition: Repeat these steps at every visit to provide information and motivation.

Generate a quit plan with STAR:

- **S**et a quit date within 2 weeks.
- **T**ell family and friends.
- **A**nticipate challenges to quitting.
- **R**emove tobacco products from environment.

Goals of treatment:

- Complete cessation of tobacco use, and no exposure to environmental tobacco smoke is recommended for both primary and secondary prevention of CVD.

Therapies:

- **Nicotine replacement therapy (NRT)**
  - Nicotine receptor agonists are available in a variety of formulations:
    - Patch: 21 mg/24 h for 4 weeks, 14 mg/24 h for 2 weeks, 7 mg/24 h for 2 weeks
    - Gum: if smoking 1–24 cigarettes/day, replace with 2 mg gum; if 25 or more, 4 mg gum up to 12 weeks
    - Lozenge: if first cigarette less than 30 minutes from waking up 4 mg/day; if first cigarette is after 30 minutes 2 mg/day for 12 weeks
    - Inhaler: 6–16 cartridges/day for up to 6 months
    - Nasal spray 8–40 doses/day for 3–6 months
  - Considerations: All forms of NRT are associated with a 50% increased rate of smoking cessation when compared to placebo. The transdermal patch provides durable and more consistent dosing compared to nasal and oral delivery methods which provide quick bursts of nicotine and are useful for acute cravings. The combined use of one or more forms of nicotine replacement therapy is beneficial to prevent withdrawal and treat cravings.
  - Contraindications/cautions: While there is little data testing the safety of nicotine replacement therapy in patients with acute coronary syndromes it appears to be safe. Nicotine delivered via NRT has no effect on platelet activation, and minimal effect on heart rate and blood pressure.
- **Buproprion SR.** Functions as a weak inhibitor of norepinephrine and dopamine re-uptake. Also thought to be dopaminergic and/or noradrenergic.
  - Dose: 150 mg every morning for 3 days then 150 mg twice daily, start 1–2 weeks prior to quitting; duration 7–12 weeks, or up to 6 months.

- Considerations: useful in tobacco users with depressed mood. Also good for patients who are concerned about weight gain as it has been shown in a randomized clinical trial to be associated with statistically less weight gain at 2 years when compared to placebo.
- Contraindications/cautions: Avoid in patients with bipolar, seizure, or eating disorders. Use of monoamine oxidase (MAO) inhibitors in the past 14 days.
- **Varenicline:** Partial neuronal α_4 β_2 nicotinic receptor agonist. Also binds to the serotonin 5HT3 receptor.
  - Dose: 0.5 mg daily for days 5–7 before quit date, 0.5 mg two times per day for days 1–4 before quit date, 1 mg twice daily starting on quit date; duration: 3–6 months.
  - Considerations: There is a black box warning on this medication that there is increased risk of suicidal thoughts and aggressive and erratic behavior in patients treated with varenicline. Patients on this medication should be observed for the development of neuropsychiatric symptoms.
  - Contraindications/cautions: Monitor for changes in mood, behavior, psychiatric symptoms, and suicidal ideation.
  - The FDA issued a safety communication indicating that an increased rate of cardiovascular events including MI (2% [n = 7] versus 0.9% [n = 3]) in a randomized trial of 700 patients treated with varenicline or placebo. This finding is currently being investigated.

SECTION II

CARDIOVASCULAR SYNDROMES

11 ■ ISCHEMIC HEART DISEASE AND STABLE ANGINA

ISCHEMIC HEART DISEASE

Ischemic heart disease (IHD) is a spectrum of conditions resulting in obstruction of blood flow through the coronary blood vessels to the myocardium. It is most commonly caused by the obstruction of the coronary arteries from atherosclerosis. The major risk factors for atherosclerotic IHD are hypertension, hyperlipidemia, diabetes, smoking, obesity, and advanced age. The clinical manifestations of IHD are diverse and include asymptomatic coronary disease, chronic stable angina, unstable angina, non-ST elevation myocardial infarction (NSTEMI), ST elevation myocardial infarction (STEMI), silent ischemia, and sudden cardiac death. Apart from atherosclerosis, IHD can result from coronary anomalies, spontaneous dissection, coronary vasospasm, myocardial bridging, radiation arteriopathy, and systemic vasculidities.

- IHD is the most frequent cause of death in the United States, causing 1 in every 5 deaths. IHD is also the leading cause of death worldwide.
- 13.2 million Americans have IHD.
- Lifetime risk of developing IHD after age 40 is 32% for females and 49% for men.
- In 2006, the economic cost of IHD in the United States was estimated at US$142 billion.

ANGINA

Definition:
- Typical angina is defined as a discomfort in chest or surrounding areas that reflects the myocardial ischemia that results when blood supply does not meet the metabolic demands of the myocardium.
  - *Location:* Usually substernal but may occur in left precordium
  - *Radiation:* Usually to left arm and neck but may also radiate to shoulders, jaw, right arm, and epigastrium
  - *Duration:* 5–20 minutes
  - *Severity:* Mild to severe
  - *Quality:* "Sharp," "squeezing," "crushing," "heaviness," "constricting," "burning;" anginal equivalent symptoms without pain in diabetics and elderly may include dyspnea, fatigue, faintness, etc.
  - *Exacerbating factors:* Physical exertion, emotional stress, exposure to cold, post-prandial, fever, anemia, thyrotoxicosis
  - *Relieving factors:* Relieved within minutes with rest or use of nitroglycerin

- *Note:* Several populations frequently exhibit atypical chest complaints related to myocardial ischemia. These include women, elderly patients, those with psychiatric disorders, and those with neuropathy.

Differential diagnosis:
- *Cardiovascular:* aortic dissection, pericarditis, myocarditis, myocardial infarction, mitral valve prolapse, arrhythmia.
- *Pulmonary:* pulmonary embolism, severe pulmonary hypertension, pleuritis from infection or vasculitis, pneumothorax
- *Gastrointestinal:* gastroesophageal reflux, esophagitis, esophageal spasm and nutcracker esophagus, esophageal motility disorders, biliary colic, pancreatitis, peptic ulcer disease
- *Musculoskeletal:* costochondritis, cervical radiculitis, musculoskeletal trauma
- *Other:* herpes zoster infection, psychiatric disorder

CLASSIFICATION OF ANGINA

- Chronic stable angina (pattern of angina is stable and predictable; no evidence of infarction, only ischemia)
- Prinzmetal's or variant angina
- Unstable angina (anginal pains are worsening in frequency, intensity, or are occurring at rest; no evidence of infarction, only ischemia); (see Chapter 12, Acute Coronary Syndromes, pp. 80)

CHRONIC STABLE ANGINA

Signs and symptoms:
- Typical angina presents as an exertional substernal chest pain that resolves with rest and has stable duration and frequency.
- Wide ranges of character including "squeezing," "crushing," "pressure," "burning sensation," etc.
- Duration is usually 10–20 minutes and resolves with rest or nitroglycerin.
- Stable angina does not last for hours! Consider unstable angina/acute MI or noncardiac causes for prolonged episodes of chest pain.
- Associated symptoms: may include shortness of breath, sweating, nausea, fatigue, syncope.

Physical examination:
- Physical examination may be unremarkable in chronic stable angina.
- During an anginal episode listen for: S3, S4, and rales (transient LV dysfunction from ischemia) and apical systolic murmur (transient papillary muscle dysfunction).

Pathophysiology:
- Supply ≠ demand:
  - Increased myocardial O_2 demand, for example: physical exertion, emotional stress, fever, hyperthyroidism, tachyarrhythmia, sympathomimetic use, aortic stenosis

- Decreased myocardial O_2 supply, for example: anemia, coronary vasospasm, severe coronary obstruction, hypoxemia, aortic stenosis, sympathomimetic use, hyperviscosity.

Canadian Cardiovascular Society Functional Classification of stable angina:

- Class I: Angina with strenuous or prolonged activity only. No angina with ordinary physical activity, such as climbing stairs. No limitation of ordinary activity.
- Class II: Angina with moderate activity like walking more than 2 blocks or climbing more than one flight of stairs at normal speed. Slight limitation of ordinary activity.
- Class III: Angina with mild activity like walking less than 2 blocks or with climbing one flight of stairs. Marked limitation of regular physical activity.
- Class IV: Angina with any physical activity resulting in inability to carry out any physical activity without discomfort.

Diagnostic testing:

- Resting EKG:
  - 50% of patients with chronic stable angina have a normal resting EKG.
  - Common EKG findings: Nonspecific ST-T wave abnormality with or without Q waves.
  - During episode angina, EKG abnormal in up to 50% of cases including ST segment changes and/or T wave abnormalities.
- Noninvasive stress testing:
  - Indicated in patients with intermediate pre-test probability.
  - When the intent of stress testing is to assess a diagnosis of myocardial ischemia, determine the amount of myocardium at risk, or determine whether chest symptoms are correlated with myocardial ischemia, the patient should exercise—if possible—to a workload that at least represents the degree of activity that brought on the symptoms.
    - It may be prudent to reduce or eliminate beta blockade so an adequate study can be obtained.
  - When the intent of stress testing is to assess the adequacy of medical therapy and to determine if ischemia or symptoms are occurring on treatment, it is advisable to continue medications at the prescribed doses.
- Diagnostic coronary angiography:
  - Indicated to diagnose coronary artery disease in those who have survived sudden cardiac death: when the findings of noninvasive imaging are uncertain or high risk, when a patient cannot undergo stress testing due to disability or morbid obesity, or when there is high pretest probability of left main or multi-vessel disease.
  - In patients undergoing angiography for stable angina, 15% do not have angiographically significant coronary obstruction (>70% stenosis).
  - Patients who have failed medical therapy with lifestyle-limiting symptoms (see later section regarding revascularization, pp. 77).

Risk stratification:

- Various factors are associated with reduced survival in patients with CAD with stable angina:
  - Advanced age
  - Abnormal left ventricular function
  - Extensive and/or severe CAD (left main or multi-vessel disease)
  - Comorbidities such as severe pulmonary, renal dysfunction, uncontrolled diabetes, peripheral vascular disease
- Echocardiography *is not* necessary for risk stratification in patients with normal EKG and no signs of valvular dysfunction or heart failure. Echocardiography *is* indicated in patients with stable angina if EKG is abnormal or there are findings suggestive of prior myocardial infarction, CHF, or valvular dysfunction.

Treatment:

Medical management:

- Initial treatment should include (ABCDE):
  - **A**spirin and anti-anginal therapy
  - **B**eta blockade and blood pressure control
  - **C**igarette smoking cessation and cholesterol control
  - **D**iet and diabetes control
  - **E**ducation and exercise
- Specific pharmacotherapy:
  - Aspirin
    - Indicated in all patients unless contraindicated
    - Shown to reduce MI, stroke, and death in patients with CAD
    - 81–162 mg/day comparable to 325 mg/day dose
  - Beta blockade
    - Indicated in patients with or without prior MI and angina
    - Reduces the frequency of angina
    - Reduces mortality and re-infarction in post-MI group
    - Reduces mortality in patients with CAD and heart failure
  - ACE inhibition
    - Indicated in patients with CAD who have DM and/or LV dysfunction
  - Nitrates
    - Sublingual NTG tablets or buccal spray for immediate relief of an anginal episode
    - Long-acting nitrates are indicated as initial therapy for reduction of symptoms when beta-blocker is contraindicated or in combination with beta-blocker when treatment with beta-blocker is inadequate in controlling symptoms
  - Calcium channel blockers
    - Indicated as initial therapy for reduction of symptoms when beta-blocker is contraindicated or in combination with beta-blockers when treatment with beta-blocker is inadequate in controlling symptoms

- Ranolazine
  - Approved in 2006 for use in stable angina patients who are already on beta-blocker, calcium channel blocker, and nitrate without adequate control of anginal symptoms
  - Mechanism unclear—possible effect on reducing ischemia through reduction in calcium overload in the ischemic patient via inhibition of late sodium current
  - Started at 500 mg twice daily and may be increased to a maximum dose of 1000 mg twice daily.
  - May increase QT interval; contraindicated in patients with preexisting prolonged QT, patients on other QT-prolonging drugs, and in patients with hepatic failure

Revascularization therapy (PCI and CABG):
- CABG
  - Indicated for patients with significant LM disease or triple vessel disease (greatest survival benefit if there is LV dysfunction and/or proximal LAD stenosis that is treated with a left internal mammary graft [LIMA]).
- PCI
  - Considered if significant symptoms persist despite optimal medical therapy
  - Indicated with single or double vessel disease if there is large area of viable myocardium at risk, high-risk criteria on noninvasive testing, or in patients who have survived sudden cardiac death or who have sustained ventricular tachycardia

Alternative therapies
- Trans-myocardial laser revascularization (TMR)—role unclear
- Enhanced external counter-pulsation (EECP)
  - Observational studies have reported reduction in anginal frequency and improvement in exercise tolerance in patients with refractory angina.
  - Postulated to decrease myocardial O_2 demand, enhance collateral flow, and improve endothelia function
  - Therapy over 7 weeks with 35 1-hour treatments
- Spinal cord stimulation
  - Neuro-modulation via a specially designed electrode inserted into the epidural space.
  - Observational studies have reported successful rates up to 80% in reducing severity and frequency of angina.
  - Reserved for patients with refractory angina when all other measures have been exhausted.
- The following therapies have not been shown to be beneficial in treating CAD patients.
  - Initiation of HRT in postmenopausal patients to reduce CV risk
  - Vitamins C and E supplementation
  - Chelation therapy

- Garlic
- Acupuncture
- Coenzyme Q

PRINZMETAL'S VARIANT ANGINA

Definition:
- A syndrome of ischemic anginal chest pain occurring at rest or with exertion, accompanied by ST elevation (sometimes depression), not caused by fixed coronary obstruction
- A normal coronary angiogram does not rule out vasospastic or printmetal's angina.

Pathophysiology:
- Transient increase in coronary vasomotor tone causing vasospasm
- Precise mechanisms not established yet and may be related to endothelial cell dysfunction

Clinical presentation:
- Presents in younger patients who may not have classic CV risk factors
- Usually intense chest pain at rest, between midnight and early morning
- CP occurs in clusters
- May be associated with acute MI, VT, VF, and death

EKG:
- Episodic ST elevation (sometimes depression) with chest pain episodes
- Transient conduction disturbances like AV blocks during CP
- May result in Q wave MI

Exercise stress testing:
- Variable response to exercise testing ranging from normal response to ST depression or elevation (from exercise-induced vasospasm)
- Normal exercise testing does not exclude variant angina

Coronary angiography:
- Demonstration of spasm of a proximal coronary artery segment resulting in myocardial ischemia is hallmark of variant angina.
- Areas of spasm may or may not be related to underlying fixed coronary stenosis.
- RCA is the most common site for spasm.
- Spasm in different segments of coronary arteries may be demonstrated at different times.
- Vasospasm may be induced with Ergonovine Provocation Test, which is an ergot alkaloid with direct vasoconstrictive effects (administered IV 0.05–0.40 mg). Provides a sensitive and specific test to induce vasospasm and support the diagnosis, but may cause prolonged vasospasm resulting in acute MI. This test is seldom used currently in catheterization laboratories and the diagnosis of variant angina is usually made clinically if spasm is not present on diagnostic coronary angiography at baseline.

Treatment:
- Cornerstone of treatment is calcium channel blockers with or without long-acting nitrates to promote coronary vasodilatation. The effects of calcium channel blocker and nitrates are additive.
- Sublingual nitroglycerin may be used to abort acute anginal episodes similar to classic angina.
- Nonselective beta blockers may be detrimental because of unopposed alpha receptor–mediated coronary vasoconstriction and prolongation of duration of vasospasm and angina.
- PCI usually not helpful as spasm may occur at various sites in the coronary arteries. However, recurrent spasm at the site of a fixed stenosis that does not respond to maximal medical therapy may be treated with PCI.

Prognosis:
- Overall the prognosis is good and frequency of anginal episodes gradually decreases over time.
- Patients with Prinzmetal's angina who developed serious arrhythmias during anginal episodes have higher risk of sudden cardiac death.

12 ■ ACUTE CORONARY SYNDROMES

INTRODUCTION

Acute coronary syndromes (ACS) generally stem from plaque rupture and subsequent thrombosis of the ulcerated plaque, distal embolization of atherothrombotic debris, and/or microvascular dysfunction.

- Acute coronary syndromes are a spectrum of disease where unstable angina (UA) represents an accelerating tempo or severity of ischemic complaints before there is evidence of frank infarction.
- Non-ST segment elevation MI (NSTEMI) occurs when there is partial occlusion of the vessel and myocardial damage related to ischemia and/or embolization of atherothrombotic debris.
- ST-elevation MI occurs when there is complete occlusion of the vessel.
- While atherothrombosis is the predominant cause of ACS, ACS can occur in the setting of coronary dissection, vasospasm, and embolization.

SIGNS AND SYMPTOMS

- Typically characterized by one or more of the following, but may be asymptomatic or atypical symptoms:
  - Rest angina lasting > 20 minutes
  - New-onset angina that is at least CCS III intensity
  - Accelerated angina that is getting more intense with lesser activity and more prolonged

PHYSICAL EXAMINATION

- Vital signs—look for hypotension, tachycardia, tachypnea, hypoxia
- Mitral regurgitation murmur from papillary muscle dysfunction
- S3 and S4
- Congestive Heart Failure—higher Killip Class with worse prognosis:
  - *Killip Classification*: Class I—no signs of heart failure; Class II—S3- elevated JVP, rales < ½ of posterior lung fields; Class III—overt pulmonary edema; Class IV—cardiogenic shock

DIAGNOSTIC TESTING

- EKG:
  - Should be done on initial presentation and serially to assess for dynamic ST/T wave changes as indicated clinically

- • Transient ST segment elevation or depression > 0.05 mV during CP strongly suggestive of severe CAD
- • Symmetric T wave inversion > 0.2 mV across precordial leads suggest acute LAD ischemia
- • ST elevation if aVR suggests LM or three-vessel disease and an increased risk for recurrent ischemia and heart failure during hospitalization.
- • Laboratory testing:
  - • Serial CK-MB and troponin to differentiate from acute NSTEMI (troponin more sensitive than CK-MB)
  - • CBC, comprehensive metabolic profile, lipid profile

RISK STRATIFICATION FOR UA/NSTEMI

Treatment decisions are based upon patient risk. Moderate- and high-risk patients are selected for more aggressive pharmacotherapy and invasive catheterization therapy.

Risk calculators:

- • TIMI (thrombolysis in myocardial infarction) risk score (www.timi.org):
  - • 7-point risk score variables
    - ○ Age > 65 years
    - ○ Three or more risk factors for CAD
    - ○ Prior CAD with stenosis >50%
    - ○ ST segment deviation on EKG
    - ○ Two or more anginal episode in prior 24 hours
    - ○ Use of aspirin in last 7 days
    - ○ Elevated serum cardiac biomarkers
  - • Predicts risk of death, infarction, or recurrent ischemia requiring revascularization at 14 days
    - ○ TIMI Score 0–1 = 5 % risk
    - ○ TIMI Score 2 = 8% risk
    - ○ TIMI Score 3 = 13%
    - ○ TIMI Score 4 = 20%
    - ○ TIMI Score 5 = 26%
    - ○ TIMI Score 6–7 = 41%
- • GRACE (Global Registry of Acute Coronary Events) Risk Score (http://www.outcomes-umassmed.org/grace/acs_risk/acs_risk_content.html)
  - • Utilizes categories of age, heart rate, systolic blood pressure, creatinine, congestive heart failure, as well as the presence/absence of cardiac arrest at presentation, ST-segment deviation, and elevated cardiac biomarkers to predict in-hospital death and death or death/MI at 6 months

TREATMENT

- The goal of therapy in UA is to prevent progression to infarction.
- The goal of therapy in NSTEMI and STEMI is to halt infarction, reduce infarct size, and avoid the complications of MI.
- General measures:
  - Admit to telemetry bed
  - Bed rest initially, may increase ambulation if no recurrent angina for 12–24 hours
  - Supplemental oxygen if indicated (usefulness not well documented)
- Relief of chest pain:
  - Morphine
    - 1–4 mg IV, repeat as tolerated
    - Analgesic, anxiolytic, and venodilatory effects (reduces pulmonary congestion)
    - Naloxone 0.4–2.0 mg IV to reverse effects if respiratory depression
  - Nitrates
    - Initially SL or spray (0.3–0.6 mg)
    - If chest pain persists, then intravenous nitroglycerin drip at 5–10 mcg/min; rate may be increased by 10 mcg/min every 3–5 minutes until relief of symptoms or systolic BP < 100 mmHg
    - Caution if suspect right ventricular involvement in inferior MI
      - Obtain right-sided ECG (STE in V4r most specific finding)
  - Beta-blockers
    - Use in all patients unless contraindicated
    - Reduce infarct size, re-infarction, recurrent ischemia, and mortality
  - Calcium channel blockers
    - Indicated only in patients who have persistent angina despite full dose beta-blockers and nitrate therapy, contraindication to beta-blockers or in patients who have hypertension
- Antiplatelet therapy:
  - Aspirin
    - All patients should receive 182–325 mg daily
    - 50% reduction in rate of death and myocardial infarction in this patient group
    - Administered to all patients with ACS unless contraindication (allergy, ongoing life-threatening bleeding)
  - Thienopyridines
    - Inhibit platelet activation by binding to the $P2Y_{12}$ ADP receptor
    - Clopidogrel
      - Achieves approximately 30% inhibition of peak platelet aggregation depending upon assay used
      - Initial loading dose of 600 mg followed by 75 mg per day
      - Addition of clopidogrel to aspirin added 20% reduction of CV death, MI, or stroke when compared to aspirin alone in US/NSTEMI in both low- and high-risk groups

- One study (OASIS-7)[10] suggests benefit of 150 mg maintenance dose for 1 week after PCI for ACS
- Reduced hepatic metabolism to active form may reduce efficacy (CYP2C19)
  - Prasugrel
    - Activated by intestinal esterase
    - Improved outcomes compared with clopidogrel (300 mg loading dose and 75 mg daily dose) in TRITON-TIMI 38
    - Indicated for patients with ACS undergoing PCI (60 mg loading dose and 10 mg QD)
      - Contraindicated if prior history of TIA/stroke
      - Caution with age older than 75 years or weight <60 kg (may consider 5 mg maintenance dose)
  - Ticagrelor
    - Reversible ADP receptor antagonist; does not require hepatic activation
    - Ticagrelor had better mortality rates than clopidogrel (9.8% vs. 11.7%, $p < 0.001$) in the PLATO trial.
    - Approved by the FDA on July 20, 2011
    - Should be used with a maintenance dose of 75–100 mg aspirin QD
- Glycoprotein IIb/IIIa inhibition
  - >80% inhibition achieved within minutes after initiation
  - Inhibits the final common pathway in platelet aggregation
  - Greater benefit in high-risk patients with ST segment changes, diabetics, elevated troponin
  - May be started at the time of presentation or at the time of PCI
  - Increases risk for bleeding and thrombocytopenia
- Combination antiplatelet therapy in UA/NSTEMI
  - In the setting of clopidogrel pretreatment, the benefit of adding a GPI in high-risk NSTE ACS patients undergoing PCI was demonstrated in the ISAR-REACT 2 trial[11].
  - Whether the converse, clopidogrel added in the context of immediate inhibition of platelet aggregation by GPI during PCI remains unclear.
- Duration of dual antiplatelet therapy (aspirin + thienopyridine)
  - Avoidance of stent thrombosis
    - >10% mortality or major morbidity if it occurs
    - Substantial increased risk of stent thrombosis if dual antiplatelet therapy discontinued prematurely
      - Avoid discontinuation if at all possible.
      - Attempt to continue at least aspirin.
    - Uninterrupted 30 days after BMS
    - Uninterrupted for 1 year after DES
  - Secondary prevention after ACS, preferably for 1 year
    - After/if window of stent thrombosis has occurred, may start and stop medication administered for this indication
    - Controversial to continue after 1 year

- Antithrombotic therapy
  - Heparin
    - IV unfractionated heparin (UFH) is considered cornerstone of therapy for UA/ACS.
    - 33% reduction in death or MI comparing UFH +aspirin to aspirin alone.
    - 60 U/kg bolus and 12 U/kg/h infusion.
    - Frequent PTT monitoring with target PTT is 50–70 seconds.
  - Low molecular weight heparin (LMWH-enoxaparin) may be used as substitute unless the patient may require CABG surgery.
  - Bivalirudin
    - Direct thrombin inhibitor when compared with heparin + GPI was shown to reduce bleeding complications and costs with equivalent ischemic outcomes (ACUITY trial)[12] for NSTEMI, and to reduce bleeding complications and mortality in STEMI (HORIZONS-AMI)[13] patients getting PCI
  - Fondaparinux
    - Factor Xa inhibitor that reduces bleeding complications compared with heparin. Catheter thrombosis may occur in patients managed invasively so use as suggested in patients managed medically.
- Coronary angiography and revascularization for STEMI:
  - Numerous randomized trials[14] have shown superiority of PCI for STEMI (Primary PCI-PPCI) compared with fibrinolysis for patients who are candidates for reperfusion.
    - Fibrinolysis restores normal flow in 60–80% of infarct arteries and is widely available.
    - PPCI restores normal flow in >90% of arteries but is only available in selected centers.
    - PPCI is associated with reduced chances of death, recurrent MI, stroke, and intracranial bleeding compared with fibrinolysis.
      - The benefit of PPCI over fibrinolysis is time dependent and varies with patient risk.
    - STEMI patients presenting to hospitals without PPCI capability must either receive onsite fibrinolysis or must be transferred for PPCI.
      - Randomized trials support transfer for PPCI over onsite fibrinolysis but treatment times are more rapid than in routine U.S. practice where median door-to-balloon times (time for initial hospital contact to inflation of balloon in culprit artery) exceed 150 minutes.
  - Door-to-balloon times should be <90 minutes or <120 minutes if a transfer is involved.
  - Door-to-needle times (time from initial hospital contact to fibrinolysis administration)
  - Combinations fibrinolytic and PCI strategies
    - **Facilitated PCI** is a strategy of fibrinolysis and/or GPI administration immediately followed by PCI, with a planned door-to-balloon time of 90–120 minutes with the goal of improving PPCI outcomes.

This strategy has not proven beneficial and may be harmful (ASSENT-IV PCI, FINESSE Trials)[15]. With these trial designs, all patients get PPCI and some get additional fibrinolytic therapy.

- **Pharmacoinvasive therapy** is the strategy administering fibrinolysis at a non-PCI facility and then promptly and systematically transferring the patient to a PCI facility with the goal of improving outcomes with fibrinolysis with PCI. Angiography and/or PCI are performed 2–24 hours after the start of fibrinolytic therapy, regardless of whether fibrinolysis results in successful reperfusion. (TRANSFER-AMI, CARESS-in-AMI trials). With these trial designs, all patients get fibrinolytic therapy and some get PCI.
- **Rescue PCI** is PCI performed after failed fibrinolysis and is associated with improved outcomes compared with conservative therapy or repeat fibrinolytic administration.

- Coronary angiography and revascularization for UA/NSTEMI
  - The following patient groups with UA/NSTEMI should undergo coronary angiography and revascularization **(Figure 12-1)**:
    - Elevated troponin or CK-MB
    - New ST depression
    - Recurrent CP with CHF

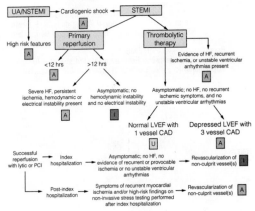

FIGURE 12-1. Acute coronary syndromes. Key for revascularization: A – appropriate, I – inappropriate, U – uncertain.
Adapted from ACCF/AHA Coronary RevascularizationGuidelines. *J Am Coll Cardiol.* 2009; 53(6):530-553.

- ○ Recurrent CP despite medical therapy
- ○ LV dysfunction (EF < 40%)
- ○ Hemodynamic instability
- ○ Sustained VT
- ○ Prior PCI within 6 months
- ○ Prior CABG
- CABG favored over PCI in patients with:
  - ○ LV dysfunction
  - ○ Severe LM or three-vessel disease
  - ○ Two vessel disease with severe proximal LAD stenosis in diabetics
- Conservative therapy and late risk stratification (**Figure 12-2**):
  - Low- to intermediate-risk UA/NSTEMI patient who does not have recurrent ischemia after medical therapy may undergo stress testing within 72 hours of presentation.
  - Patients able to exercise > 5 METS without ischemia have predicted cardiac mortality of < 1% per year and may be managed medically.
  - Patients with < 5 METS exercise capacity and evidence of ischemia on stress test have >4% annual cardiac mortality and should undergo coronary angiography
- Post-hospital discharge care:
  - Aspirin 75–325 mg daily indefinitely unless contraindicated
  - Combination of aspirin and clopidogrel 75 mg daily for 9 months post-UA/NSTEMI episode or longer if drug eluting stent has been implanted
  - Beta blocker unless contraindicated
  - Lipid lowering agents and diet therapy with LDL goal of < 70 mg/dL
  - ACE inhibitor for patients with LV dysfunctions, DM, or hypertension.

Conservative Strategy for Likely or Definite UA/NSTEMI[1]

Administer aspirin or clopidogrel if aspirin intolerant [I]

↓

Initiate anticoagulant [I]: enoxaparin or fondaparinux or unfractionated heparin (enoxaparin or fondaparinux are preferred [IIa])

↓

Start clopidogrel if not already given [I] & consider adding eptifibatide or tirofiban [IIb]

↓

Stress test and echocardiogram:
If EF ≤40%, diagnostic angiography [IIb], If stress test not low risk, angiography [I]

↓

If ejection fraction >0.4 and low risk stress test:
Continue aspirin indefinitely. Continue clopidogrel for 1 month–1 year. Discontinue eptifibatide/tirofiban. Discontinue anticoagulant therapy.

1Class I, II, recommendations are listed in brackets [ ].
2If subsequent recurrent symptoms/ischemia, heart failure, or serious arrhythmia consider diagnostic angiography3 Abciximab should not be administered to patients unless PCI planned. *Circulation* 2007; 116: e148.

FIGURE 12-2. Conservative strategy for likely or definite UA/NSTEMI.

Myocardial Infarction (MI) & Acute Coronary Syndromes (ACS)

Utility of Various Tests for Diagnosis of Acute MI/ Cardiac Ischemia

Table below details predictive values for diagnosis of Acute Myocardial Infarction if non-italicized and *Acute Cardiac Ischemia (ACI) if italicized.*

Diagnostic Test	Sensitivity	Specificity	PPV[h]	NPV[h]
12 lead ECG (liberal criteria)[a]	94-99	19-27	21	98
12 lead ECG (strict criteria)[b]	38-44	97-98	76	91
15 lead ECG (+V8,V9,V4R)	55-60[f]	97-98		
22 lead ECG (multiple AP thorax leads)	88[f]	---		
Continuous/serial ECG	39	88		
ECG stress test (ACI)			Data sources:	
CK-MB enzymes over 24 h *(ACI)*	100 *(31)*	98 *(95)*	*Circulation*	
1st CK-MB, pain onset < 4 h prior	41	88	2007;115: 402,	
1st CK-MB, pain onset > 4 h prior	63	90	2006; 114: 1761	
Serial CK-MB isoform, pain = 6 h[c]	96	94	*Ann Emerg Med*	
CK-MB at 0,1,2,3 h after ED arrival[d]	80	94	2007; 49: 125.	
Myoglobin, pain onset = 2 h prior	89	96	2001; 37: 453.,	
Myoglobin, pain onset 12-24 h prior	59	95	1992; 21: 504.	
Troponin T, pain onset 2 h prior	33	100	*Am J Med* 2006;	
Troponin T, pain onset 6 h (12-24 h) prior	78 *(93)*	99 *(99)*	119: 203.	
Stress echocardiography	90	89	*Acad Emerg*	
Sestamibi rest (technetium 99m scan) [f]	74-87	56-85	*Med* 1997;4:13.	
CT angiography multidection 64 slice	86-100%	90-100%	99% NPV	

Coronary artery calcium score: (CACS) A CACS = 0 makes presence of atherosclerotic plaque highly unlikely. A score of 0 also makes the presence of significant luminal obstruction highly unlikely (NPV[x] 95-99%). A positive score (CACS > 0) confirms the presence of coronary artery plaque. A high score (> 100) is consistent with a high risk of a cardiac event within the next 2-5 years (> 2% annual risk). Individuals with a low clinical risk (< 10% over 10 years), and high clinical risk (> 20% over 10 years) do not benefit from CACS. (AHA/ACC Class III recommendation). *Circulation* 2007 (see above)

a nonspecific ST segment or T wave changes abnormal but not diagnostic of ischemia; Or ischemia, strain, or infarction known or not known to be old.

b ST segment elevation or pathologic Q waves not known to be old.

c CK-MB isoforms collected every 30-60 minutes for at least 6 hours after symptom onset when studied. Criteria for AMI diagnosis: MB2 > 1U/L or MB2/MB1 > 1.5.

d Sensitivity/specificity if > 6 hours from pain onset. Numbers are lower if < 6 hours.

e Must have ongoing chest pain and no nitrate or β blocker administered before test.

f Sensitivity using criteria strict ECG above

g Sensitivity is higher for three vessel disease and lower if LVH noted on ECG.

h NPV - negative predictive value, PPV - positive predictive value

Unstable Angina (US)/Non ST Elevation MI (NSTEMI) Guidelines

Class I Recommendations for Anti-Ischemic Therapy if High Risk Features[1] or Continuing Ischemia

- Bed/chair rest with continuous ECG monitor
- Continuous pulse oximetry, oxygen if arterial saturation < 90%, respiratory distress, or high risk features for hypoxemia.
- <u>Aspirin</u> 162-325 mg PO (if unable to take aspirin, take clopidogrel 300 mg PO)
- <u>Nitroglycerin</u> (NTG) SL q 5 min X 3. Assess IV NTG need. See Class III cautions.
- NTG IV for 1st 48 hours for persistent ischemia, heart failure, or hypertension
- Administer β blockers (oral route) within 24 hours unless contraindicated whether or not percutaneous coronary intervention (PCI) is performed.
- If β blockers contraindicated, give nondihydropyridine <u>calcium antagonist</u> (diltiazem, verapamil) unless contraindicated (e.g. severe LV dysfunction)
- Clopidogrel or Glycoprotein IIb/IIIa inhibitor can be administered before PCI.
- Prasugrel, clopidogrel or Glycoprotein IIb/IIIa inhibitor can be administered at the time of PCI.
- For planned PCI, Clopidogrel 300-600 mg should be given ASAP, or Prasugrel 60 mg ASAP and no later than 1 hr after PCI. Clopidogrel or Prasugrel should be administered for 12 months unless bleeding complication outweighs benefit.
- <u>Anticoagulants</u> – (1) *invasive strategy*: enoxaparin, unfractionated heparin, bivalirudin, or fondaparinux, (2) *conservative strategy*: enoxaparin, unfractionated heparin, or fondaparinux/F (F preferred if ↑ risk of bleeding)
- (Inpatient) Administer <u>ACE inhibitor</u> (oral) or angiotensin receptor blocker (ARB), if ACE intolerant, within the 1st 24 hours if pulmonary congestion or ejection fraction (EF) < 40% unless contraindication.
- Discontinue nonsteroidal anti-inflammatory medicine (except aspirin).

Class IIa Recommendations for Anti-Ischemic Therapy

- Supplemental <u>oxygen</u> to all patients in the 1st 6 hours.
- <u>Morphine</u> sulfate IV if uncontrolled pain despite NTG, appropriate therapy above.
- IV <u>β blockers</u> unless contraindications (e.g. heart block, shock, asthma)
- Oral long acting nondihydropyridine <u>calcium antagonists</u> for recurrent ischemia in the absence of contraindications after β blockers and NTG fully used.
- <u>Glycoprotein IIb/IIIa</u> inhibitor IV **AND** <u>clopidogrel</u> if angiography/PCI planned.
- <u>Anticoagulants</u> –*conservative strategy*: enoxaparin or fondaparinux is preferred to unfractionated heparin unless CABG planned within 24 hours.
- An <u>ACE inhibitor</u> without heart failure if no contraindications exist. (inpatient)
- Intra-aortic balloon pump if (1) severe ischemia continues/recurs frequently despite intensive medical therapy (2) hemodynamic stability is present before or after coronary angiography or (3) mechanical complications of MI
- May omit Glycoprotein IIb/IIIa inhibitor of bivalirudin is used and clopidogrel has been administered >6 hrs prior to planned catherization or PCI

(continues)

Class IIb Recommendations for Anti-Ischemic Therapy
• Gp IIb/IIIa inhibitors if PCI NOT planned (eptifibatide or tirofiban only)
• Extended release nondihydropyridine <u>calcium antagonists</u> instead of β blockers.
• Immediate release nondihydropyridine calcium antagonists after adequate β blockade if ongoing ischemia or hypertension.
• Prasugrel may be administered prior to angiography if PCI is planned and need for CABG deemed unlikely
• NSTEMI patients undergoing PCI can receive a 600 mg clopidogrel followed by 150 mg QD x 7 days then 75 mg a day is bleeding risk is not high
• May administer Glycoprotein IIb/IIIa inhibitor to patients at high risk for ischemic events already receiving aspirin and theinopyridine

[1] See footnotes next page.   *Circulation* 2007; 116: e148.

Unstable Angina (UA)/Non ST Elevation MI (NSTEMI) Guidelines
Continued...

Class III Recommendations for Anti-Ischemic Therapy (DO NOT USE)
• <u>Do not administer nitrates if</u> systolic blood pressure < 90 mm Hg or ≥ 30 mm Hg below baseline, severe bradycardia (< 50 beats/minute), tachycardia [> 100 beats/minute] (in the absence of symptomatic heart failure, or right ventricular infarction), or if patients have used a phosphodiesterase inhibitor for erectile dysfunction in prior 24 hours (if sildenafil/*Viagra*) or prior 48 hours (if tadalafil/*Cialis*), unknown delay needed for vardenafil/*Levitra* use.
• <u>Do not administer immediate release dihydropyridine calcium antagonists</u> in absence of a β blocker.
• <u>Do not administer an IV ACE inhibitor within</u> the 1st 24 hours of UA/NSTEMI due to the increased risk of hypotension.
• <u>IV β blockers may be harmful if</u> contraindication (heart failure, low output state, or other risk factors for cardiogenic shock)
• <u>Do not give nonsteroidal anti-inflammatory</u> (except aspirin) during hospitalization.
• <u>Do not administer abciximab</u> to patients in whom PCI is not already planned.
• <u>Do not administer fibrinolytic therapy</u> to patients without acute ST segment elevation, a true posterior MI, or a presumed new left bundle branch block.
• <u>An early invasive strategy is not recommended if</u> (1) extensive comorbidity (e.g. liver failure, pulmonary failure, cancer) when the risks of revascularization and comorbidity are likely to outweigh the benefits of revascularization, (2) low likelihood of acute coronary syndrome, or (3) in patients who will not consent to revascularization.
• <u>Do not administer Prasugrel</u> to patients with prior history of stroke and/or TIA
• <u>Do not administer Glycoprotein IIb/IIIa inhibitor</u> to patients at low risk for ischemic events already receiving aspirin and clopidogrel

[1] High Risk Features: Recurrent angina, ischemia related ECG changes (≥ 0.05 mV ST segment depression or bundle branch block) at rest or with low level activity, ischemia (associated with heart failure, S_3 gallop, or new or worsening mitral regurgitation), hemodynamic instability, serious ventricular arrhythmia, or depressed left ventricular function (EF < 0.4)

Circulation 2007; 116: e148.

AHA/ACC Guidelines for Invasive vs. Conservative therapy in UA/NSTEMI (Primarily Cardiologist's Decision)

Conservative	• Low Risk Score (e.g. TIMI [www.timi.org], GRACE [www.outcomes-umassmed.org/grace/]), • Physician or patient preference in the absence of high risk factors
Invasive	• Recurrent angina/ischemia at rest of with low level activity despite intensive medical therapy, • Elevated cardiac biomarkers (e.g. TnT or TnI) • New or presumably new ST depression • Signs/symptoms of heart failure or new/worse mitral regurgitation • High risk findings on non-invasive tests • Sustained ventricular tachycardia or hemodynamic instability • Prior CABG or percutaneous coronary intervention (PCI) • High risk score (e.g. TIMI, or GRACE) • Reduced left ventricular function (e.g. ejection fraction < 40%)

Conservative Strategy for Likely or Definite UA/NSTEMI[1]

Administer aspirin or clopidogrel if aspirin intolerant [I]

↓

Initiate anticoagulant [I]: enoxaparin or fondaparinux or unfractionated heparin (enoxaparin or fondaparinux are preferred [IIa])

↓

Start clopidogrel if not already given [I] & consider adding eptifibatide or tirofiban [IIb]

↓

Stress test and echocardiogram:
If EF ≤ 40%, diagnostic angiography [IIb], If stress test not low risk, angiography [I]

↓

If ejection fraction > 0.4 and low risk stress test:
Continue aspirin indefinitely. Continue clopidogrel for 1 month - 1 year.
Discontinue eptifibatide/tirofiban. Discontinue anticoagulant therapy.

[1] Class I, II, recommendations are listed in brackets [ ] (See explanation page 2
[2] If subsequent recurrent symptoms/ischemia, heart failure, or serious arrhythmia consider diagnostic angiography [3] Abciximab should not be administered to patients unless PCI planned. *Circulation* 2007; 116: e148.

Initial Invasive Strategy for Likely or Definite UA/NSTEMI[1]

Administer aspirin or clopidogrel if aspirin intolerant [I]

↓

Start anticoagulant[I]: enoxaparin, fondaparinux, bivalirudin or unfractionated heparin

↓

Prior to angioplasty start one [I] of clopidogrel or IV GP IIb/IIIa inhibitor[2] or both [IIa].
Consider both agents if delay to angioplasty, high risk, early recurrent ischemia.

↓

Diagnostic angiography

[1] Class I, II, recommendations are listed in brackets [ ]. See explanation page 2.
[2] GP IIb/IIb inhibitors may not be necessary if patient received at least 300 mg clopidogrel at least 6 hours earlier and bivalirudin selected as anticoagulant.
Circulation 2007; 116: e148.

ACC/AHA Recommendations for ST Elevation Myocardial Infarction (STEMI)
Class I Recommendations for STEMI [1]

- **ECG**: If possible, perform & interpret ≤ 10 minutes from ED arrival. If ECG is not diagnostic and high suspicion for STEMI, repeat ECG or perform continuous 12 lead ST monitoring. If inferior MI, obtain right sided ECG for RV infarction.
- **Radiography**: Obtain CXR - do not delay reperfusion unless contraindication possible (e.g. aortic dissection). High quality CXR, transthoracic or trans-esophageal echo, contrast chest CT, or MRI is used to differentiate STEMI from aortic dissection if diagnosis unclear.
- **Oxygen**: Administer supplemental oxygen if oxygen saturation < 90%.
- **Aspirin** (162-325 mg) chewed if not yet taken. Nonenteric is preferred.
- **β blockers** (oral): Administer if no contraindications regardless of concomitant fibrinolytic therapy or performance of percutaneous coronary intervention/PCI.
- **Prasugrel** (60 mg) or **Clopidogrel** (300-600 mg PO) should be given ASAP before primary PCI
- **Clopidogrel** (300-600 mg PO followed by 75 mg QD) is the theinopyridine of choice in STEMI treated with fibrinolysis
- If CABG, discontinue clopidogrel 5 days or more or prasugrel 7 days or more.
- **NTG**: If ongoing ischemic pain, administer SL nitroglycerin (NTG) q 5 min X 3. IV NTG is indicated for ongoing pain, hypertension, or pulmonary congestion.
- **Morphine** IV repeated at 5-15 min. intervals is the analgesic of choice for STEMI.
- **Anticoagulation with PCI in STEMI**- Supportive anticoagulation choices for primary PCI among patients who have received aspirin and a theinopyridine include unfractionated heparin or bivalirudin.
- If enoxaparin is used and last dose <8 hrs, give no additional. Otherwise, administer additional 0.3 mg/kg IV
- If fondaparinux given prior to PCI, administer supplemental intravenous anticoagulant with anti-IIa activity
- **Anticoagulation options – post fibrinolytics**: Administer ≥ 48 hours up to 8 days if undergo fibrinolysis. Use enoxaparin or fondaparinux if administered > 48 hours.
  - **IV heparin** dose if reperfusion with alteplase, reteplase, or tenecteplase: bolus 60 U/kg (max 4000 U) then 12 U/kg/hour (max 1000/hour) adjusted to maintain aPTT at 1.5-2 times control. UFH should be administered IV if treated with nonselective fibrinolytic agents and high risk for systemic emboli (large or anterior MI, Afib, prior embolus, or LV thrombus. Monitor platelet count daily.
  - **Enoxaparin** dose (if creatinine < 2.5 mg/dl in male or < 2 mg/dl in female): If < 75 years old, 30 mg IV, then 15 min later 1 mg/kg SQ q 12h. (some experts administer 0.5 - 0.75 mg/kg IV pre PCI; *New Engl J Med* 2006; 355: 1006.). If ≥ 75 years, no IV bolus, administer 0.75 mg/kg SQ q 12h. At any age, if creatinine clearance is < 30 ml/min, administer 1 mg/kg SQ q 24 hours. Administer maintenance dose ≤ 8 days.
  - **Fondaparinux** dose (if creatinine is < 3 mg/dl): 2.5 mg IV, then 2.5 mg SQ q 24 hours. Continue during hospitalization up to 8 days. (Due to risk of catheter thrombosis, do not use as sole anticoagulant to support PCI).
- **Anticoagulation – PCI completed**: See guidelines (www.acc.org)

(continues)

Class I Recommendations continued![1]

- <u>Reperfusion choice:</u>(PCI and fibrinolysis): All require rapid evaluation for reperfusion (i.e. PCI ≤ 90 min. or fibrinolysis ≤ 30 min. of arrival). PCI preferred if skilled PCI lab available (esp. ≤ 90 min. of arrival), high risk STEMI (shock, Killip III/IV), fibrinolysis contraindications, or arrive > 3 h after onset. Fibrinolysis may be preferred if early presenter (< 3 h after onset) esp. if PCI unavailable (or has long transport), difficult vascular access or arrival to PCI time is > 90 min.

- <u>Fibrinolysis:</u> STEMI patients at site without PCI available or cannot transfer in ≤90 min. should undergo thrombolysis unless contraindicated. Class I indications –symptoms < 12 hours and ST elevation > 0.1 mV in ≥ 2 contiguous precordial or 2 adjacent limb leads. Perform exam to look for stroke or cognitive deficit pre-administration. Assess for contraindications (page 35). If intracranial bleed (ICH) risk is ≥ 4%, perform PCI - not fibrinolysis. Treat neurologic deterioration as ICH until CT. Consider neurology, neurosurgical consult, FFP, protamine, platelets.

- <u>PCI:</u> Perform in STEMI or MI with new LBBB if can undergo PCI within 12 hours onset (90 min arrival). Primary PCI if < 75 y with STEMI or LBBB and shock within 36 h of MI, & suitable for revascularization. Diagnostic coronary angiography/PCI is performed if (1) PCI candidate, (2) cardiac shock if revascularization candidate and < 75 years old (Class IIa if ≥ 75 years old), (3) candidate for VSD or severe MR repair. (4) persistent electrical instability.

- <u>Insulin:</u> An insulin infusion to normalize blood glucose is recommended for patients with STEMI and complicated courses.

- <u>Intra-aortic balloon pump</u> counterpulsation is recommended for STEMI with cardiogenic shock not quickly reversed with medications to stabilize.

- <u>ACE:</u> (inpatient) Administer ACE inhibitor (oral) within 1st 24 hours of STEMI if anterior MI, pulmonary congestion, or LVEF < 0.4 unless hypotension is present (SBP < 100 mm Hg or ≥ 30 mm Hg below) or contraindicated (e.g. allergy).

- <u>ARB:</u> Administer an angiotensin receptor blocker (ARB) to STEMI patients who are intolerant of ACE inhibitors and who have heart failure or LVEF < 0.4.

Class IIa Recommendations for STEMI[1]

- <u>Radiography:</u> Portable echo is reasonable for clarifying STEMI diagnosis and risk stratify patients who present to the ED, especially if LBBB or pacemaker present, or suspicion of posterior STEMI with anterior ST depression.

- <u>Oxygen:</u> Supplemental O₂ to all uncomplicated STEMI patients in the 1st 6 hours

- <u>Clopidogrel</u> – Administer 300 mg PO if < 75 years old if STEMI regardless of whether or not receive reperfusion therapy. (See CABG caution Class I). Long term (> 1 year), administer 75 mg PO daily for > 1 year if STEMI.

- <u>β blockers</u> It is reasonable to administer IV β blockers to patients at the time of presentation of STEMI who are hypertensive without contraindications (heart failure, low output state, increased risk for cardiogenic shock, or other relative contraindications including PR interval > 0.24 seconds, 2nd or 3rd degree heart block, active asthma, or reactive airway disease).

- <u>CCB:</u> It is reasonable to administer calcium channel blockers/CCB (verapamil or diltiazem) if β blockers are contraindicated due to ongoing ischemia, atrial fibrillation /flutter after STEMI in the absence of CHF, LV dysfunction or AV block.

[1]More comprehensive/detailed recommendations are cited within article and online
  Circulation 2008; 117; 296 ; JACC 2008; 51: 210 (update 2004 guidelines - JACC 2004; 44: 671.)

(continues)

Class IIa STEMI recommendations continued

- <u>Glycoprotein IIa/IIIb inhibitors</u> – Decision to use these agents generally involves cardiologist with consideration of type of intervention.
- <u>Anticoagulation</u>: If STEMI and no reperfusion+ no contraindications continue LMWH (enoxaparin/ or fondaparinux) for ≥ 48 h up to 8 days (Class I dosing)
- <u>Primary PCI</u> if ≥ 75 years with ST elevation or LBBB and develop shock post-fibrinolysis and suitable for revascularization, or hemodynamic/ electrical instability, or persistent ischemia or failed fibrinolysis (ST elevation < 50% resolved 90 min after initiation in lead showing worst elevation with moderate or large area of myocardium at risk [ant. MI, inferior MI with RV involved, or precordial ST depression]).
- <u>Fibrinolytics</u> - If no contraindications exist, fibrinolytics are reasonable to give (1) if symptoms began within prior 12 hours and 12 lead ECG shows a true posterior MI or (2) STEMI patients with symptoms onset within prior 12-24 hours if continuing ischemic symptoms are present and there is ST elevation > 0.1 mV in a least 2 contiguous precordial leads or at least 2 adjacent limb leads.
- <u>Insulin</u>: During the 1st 24-48 hours of STEMI in patients with hyperglycemia, it is reasonable to administer an insulin infusion to normalize glucose even in patients with uncomplicated courses. After the acute phase of a STEMI, individualize hyperglycemia control with oral agents or insulin.
- <u>Magnesium (Mg)</u>: Correct deficits esp. if patients receiving diuretics before onset of STEMI. Treat torsade de pointes VT assoc. with prolonged QT with 1-2 g Mg.
- <u>ACE</u>: An ACE inhibitor (oral) administered within the 1st 24 hours of STEMI can be useful in absence of Class I recommendations or contraindications.
- <u>Pharmacoinvasive Strategy</u> for high risk patients (Transfer to PCI capable facility after administration of fibrinolysis at non-PCI capable facility). Consider administration of anticoagulant and antiplatelet medication before and during transfer. High risk is 1 or more of: extensive ST elevation, new LBBB, prior MI, CHF, LVEF <40% in inferior MI, Anterior MI if 2 mm or more ST elevation).

Class IIb Recommendations for STEMI

- <u>Combination abciximab and half dose reteplase</u> (or tenecteplase) may be considered for prevention of reinfarct and other STEMI if anterior MI, age < 75 years, and no risk factors for bleeding. This combination also may be considered if anterior MI and age < 75 years if early angiography and PCI is planned.
- <u>Glycoprotein IIb/IIIa inhibitor</u>: Upstream (prior to catheterization laboratory) is of unclear benefit
- <u>UFH</u>: It may be reasonable to give UFH IV to patients receiving streptokinase.
- <u>LMWH</u>: Low molecular weight heparin (LMWH) is alternative to UFH as ancillary therapy for patients < 75 years old receiving fibrinolytics if creatinine < 2.5 mg/dl in men (< 2 mg/dl in women). Enoxaparin (30 mg IV bolus + 1 mg/kg SC q 12 hours until discharge) combined with full dose tenecteplase is most studied
- <u>PCI Angiography</u> – No Class I or IIa indications and moderate to high risk patient
- <u>Pharmacoinvasive Strategy</u> for non-high risk patients (Transfer to PCI capable facility after administration of fibrinolysis at non-PCI capable facility). Consider administration of anticoagulant and antiplatelet medication before and during transfer

+More comprehensive/detailed recommendations are cited.   Circulation 2008; 117; 296.

(continues)

Class III Recommendations for STEMI (DO NOT USE)

- <u>NTG:</u> Do Not administer NTG if SBP < 90 mm Hg or ≥ 30 mm Hg below baseline, severe bradycardia (< 50 beats per min), tachycardia (unless related to heart failure), suspected RV infarction, or to patients with recent phosphodiesterase inhibitor use for erectile dysfunction (e.g. sildenafil/*Viagra* use in prior 24 hours, tadalafil/*Cialis* use in prior 48 hours, unknown delay for vardenafil/*Levitra* use).

- <u>ACE:</u> An IV ACE inhibitor should not be administered within the 1st 24 hours of STEMI except in the setting of refractory hypertension.

- β blockers Do Not administer if signs of CHF, cardiogenic shock risk, low output state, or other relative contraindications (PR > 0.24 sec, 2nd, 3rd degree heart block, active asthma or reactive airway disease).

- <u>Heparin:</u> Do Not use low molecular weight heparin as an alternative to UFH in patients > 75 years old receiving fibrinolytics or in patients < 75 years receiving fibrinolytics with renal dysfunction–creatinine > 2.5 mg/dl in men (> 2 in women).

- <u>Antithrombins:</u> if heparin induced thrombocytopenia, consider bivalirudin as an alternative to heparin used in conjunction with streptokinase. Give 0.25 mg/kg IV bolus, followed by 0.5 mg/kg/hour X 12 hours, then 0.25 mg/kg/hour X 36 hours. Reduce the infusion rate if PTT is above 75 seconds within the 1st 12 hours.

- <u>PCI</u> – Do Not perform in asymptomatic patients > 12 hours after onset of STEMI if hemodynamically and electrically stable. Do not perform PCI without on site cardiac surgery capability or proven plan for rapid transport to cardiac surgery unless appropriate hemodynamic support, capability for rapid transfer. Full dose fibrinolytic therapy followed by immediate PCI may be harmful.

- <u>Fibrinolytics</u> – See recommendations page 98. If ICH occurs, optimize BP and blood glucose, reduce ICP with mannitol, intubation/hyperventilation and consider need for neurosurgery.

- Do not perform <u>coronary angiography</u> in patients with extensive comorbidity in whom risk of revascularization outweighs the benefits.

- <u>Combination therapy</u> with abciximab and half dose reteplase (or tenecteplase) should not be given if > 75 years old.

- <u>CCB:</u> Diltiazem and verapamil are contraindicated in STEMI associated with LV dysfunction or CHF. Nifedipine (immediate release) is contraindicated in STEMI due to reflex tachycardia, sympathetic activation, hypotension.

- <u>Nonsteroidal anti-</u>inflammatory – Do not take during STEMI admit (aspirin is OK)

- Do not administer prasugrel to STEMI patients with prior history of TIA and/or stroke

[1]Rescue PCI , post fibrinolysis PCI, and CABG indications are detailed in cited article and online
Circulation 2008; 117;296.

Absolute Contraindications to Thrombolytic Use	
Prior CNS bleed,	Active internal bleeding (not menses)
CNS structural lesion or neoplasm	Significant head trauma past 3 months
Ischemic stroke in past 3 months	Suspected aortic dissection, pericarditis
Relative Contraindications or Cautions to Thrombolytic Use	
Chronic, severe, poorly controlled HTN	Recent internal bleeding (< 2-4 weeks)
SBP > 180 or DBP > 110 on arrival	Noncompressible vessel puncture
Stroke (< 3-6 mo old), dementia, other	Pregnancy or active peptic ulcer
intracranial pathology not noted above	Current anticoagulants (esp. high INR)
Traumatic or prolonged (> 10 min) CPR	For streptokinase (Streptase): prior
Major surgery < 3 weeks ago	exposure or prior allergic reaction to SK

J Am Coll Cardiol 2004; 44: e1.

AHA/ACC Recommendations for Thrombolytic Therapy in Acute MI

Class	Recommendation (See STEMI PCI Recommendations 1st)
I	• Onset ≤ 12 hours **AND** (1) ST elevation > 0.1 mV in ≥ 2 contiguous leads **or** (2) new left bundle branch block
II a	• Onset ≤ 12 hours and true posterior MI • STEMI symptoms onset 12-24 hours prior with continuing ischemic symptoms and ST elevation > 0.1 mV in ≥ 2 contiguous leads
III	• ST elevation + time to therapy > 24 h **Or** ST segment depression only (unless true posterior MI is present)

Cardiol Clin 2006; 24: 37.

Thrombolytics in STEMI - See Above for Indications/Contraindications

Agent	Dose
reteplase (r-PA, Retavase)	• 10 units IV over 2 min, repeat dose in 30 min
tenecteplase (TNK-ase)	• Single IV bolus over 5 seconds; if < 60 kg (30 mg), 60-69 kg (35 mg), 70-79 kg (40 mg), 80-89 kg (45 mg), ≥ 90 kg (50 mg)
alteplase, (t-PA, rtPA, Activase)	• 15 mg bolus + 0.75 mg/kg (max 50 mg) over 30 min + 0.50 mg/kg (max. 35 mg) over 60 min + heparin 60 U/kg bolus + 12 U/kg/h. PTT goal is 1.5-2.0 X control.
streptokinase (Streptase)	• 1.5 million U. IV over 1 hour

Cardiol Clin 2006; 24: 37

Indications for Transcutaneous Patches/Pacing in Acute MI

Hemodynamically unstable bradycardia (< 50 beats/minute)

Mobitz type II 2nd degree AV block, or 3rd degree heart block

Bilateral BBB, Alternating BBB or RBBB and alternating LBBB

Left anterior fascicular block or newly acquired or age-indeterminate LBBB

RBBB or LBBB and 1st degree AV block

In ED, place pads on all, only pace if unstable.   *Circulation 2000: 102: (suppl).*

Select Parenteral Cardiovascular Medications & AHA/ACC Guidelines
[*Circulation* 2008; 117:296; 2002; 106: 1896; *JACC* 2004;44:e1] (www.acc.org)

Abciximab (ReoPro)	• PCI – 0.25 mg/kg IV pre PCI, + 0.125 mcg/kg/min (maximum of 10 mcg/min) X 12 h after PCI ***Class I – UA/NSTEMI* –**for 12-24 hours if PCI planned next 24 hours ***Class IIa – STEMI*** reasonable to use as early as possible pre-PCI ***Class IIb – STEMI*** combination with half dose reteplase or half dose tenecteplase may be considered for prevention of reinfarct and other STEMI circumstances (per cardiology recommendation) ***Class III – UA/NSTEMI*** – patients in whom PCI is not planned
ACE inhibitors (e.g. benazepril, captopril, enalapril, fosinopril, lisinopril quinapril, ramipril, trandolapril)	***Class I* –** (1) 1st 24 h of acute MI with ST elevation in > 2 ant precordial leads or CHF without ↓ BP or contraindication (2) UA/NSTEMI – hypertension despite NTG & β blocker if LV systolic dysfunction or CHF and in patients with diabetes. ***Class IIa* –** all other within 24 h of suspected MI. All post acute coronary syndrome patients. ***Class IIb* –** after MI recovery with normal or mildly abnormal LV function.
Adenosine (Adenocard)	• SVT – 6 mg IV. Repeat 12 mg IV q 2 min X 2 doses. Avoid if: 2nd/3rd degree AV block, sick sinus syndrome, on dipyridamole
Alteplase (t-PA)	• See thrombolytics page 98
Amiodarone (Cordarone)	• VF/pulseless VT – 300 mg IVP • Recurrent VF/Pulseless VT – 150 mg IVP • Ventricular arrhythmias – 150 mg IV over 10 minutes, then 1 mg/min X 6 h (360 mg), then 0.5 mg/min X 18 h (540 mg) ***Class I Cardiac arrest* –** preferred anti-arrhythmic for VF/VT during cardiac arrest and post VT/VF cardiac arrest ***Class I Polymorphic VT* –** in absence of abnormal repolarization related to long QT syndromes ***Class I STEMI* –** (1) sustained monomorphic VT not associated with angina, pulmonary edema or hypotension. As alternate to above regimen may administer 150 mg (or 5 mg/kg) over 10 minutes and repeat same dose q10-15 minutes. Do not exceed 2.2 g in 24 hours.(2) AF in patients with hemodynamic compromise that does not respond to electrical cardioversion

(continues)

	Class IIa – (1) monomorphic VT that is hemodynamically unstable, refractory to countershock or recurrent despite alternate medication administration (2) Atrial fibrillation/flutter with normal cardiac function (3) VT/pulseless VT refractory to electric shock (3) repetitive monomorphic VT in setting of coronary artery disease (3) incessant VT **Class IIb** – *(1) monomorphic VT with impaired cardiac function (2) polymorphic VT (3)VT storm (4) Atrial fibrillation/flutter- impaired cardiac function/underlying WPW*
Argatroban (formerly *Acova*) *Use if heparin induced thrombocytopenia*	• UA/STEMI for PCI – 350 mcg/kg IV over 3–5 minutes plus 25 mcg/kg/min. Check activated clotting time (ACT) 5–10 min. after bolus complete. Therapeutic ACT is 300–450 sec. If ACT < 300 sec., administer 2nd bolus of 150 mcg/kg and ↑ infusion to 30 mcg/kg/min and recheck ACT in 5–10 minutes. If ACT > 450 sec., ↓ infusion to 15 mcg/kg/min and recheck ACT in 5–10 minutes. May take with aspirin. • Dosing for prophylaxis and treatment of HIT/HITTS is substantially lower (2 mcg/kg/min with titration till aPTT is 1.5-3.0 times patient's baseline) • Dose adjustment is necessary for moderate hepatic impairment (0.5 mcg/kg/min)
Aspirin	• Acute MI – 162 – 325 mg PO **Class I** – *STEMI/UA/NSTEMI* – *begin immediately* *If allergy, choose clopidogrel over ticlopidine, dipyridamole*
Atenolol (*Tenormin*)	• Acute MI –50 mg/day PO increased to 50 mg PO BID as tolerated. 5 mg IV over 5 minutes, repeat in 10 minutes, **Class I** – *STEMI/UA/NSTEMI* – *Oral administration within 12 hr of MI or ongoing, recurrent pain.* **Class IIa STEMI** – *IV administration if no contraindications.* **Class IIb** – *STEMI* –*moderate LV failure (bibasilar rales without low cardiac output) or other relative contraindications to β blockers, provided patients can be monitored closely.* **Class III STEMI/UA/NSTEMI – DO NOT use** - *severe LV failure, ↓ HR,or other contraindications*

(continues)

Atropine	• <u>Asystole</u> – 1 mg IV, repeat q 3-5 minutes (Max 0.04 mg/kg) • <u>Bradycardia</u> 0.5 – 1.0 mg IV q 3-5 minutes (Max 0.04 mg/kg) ET dose is 2-3 mg diluted in 10 ml NS. ***Class I – Acute MI –*** *(1) sinus bradycardia with low cardiac output & hypoperfusion, or frequent PVCs at onset of acute MI (2) inferior MI with type I 2nd or 3rd AV block & ↓BP, ischemic pain or ventricular arrhythmias (3) sustained ↓ HR/BP after nitroglycerin (4) nausea and vomiting associated with morphine (5) asystole* ***Class IIa – Acute MI –*** *symptomatic inferior infarction and type I 2nd or 3rd degree heart block at AV node (narrow QRS or known BBB)* ***Class IIb - Acute MI –*** *(1) administration with morphine in the presence of bradycardia (2) asymptomatic with inferior infarction and type I 2nd or 3rd degree heart block at the AV node (3) 2nd or 3rd degree AV block of uncertain mechanism when pacing unavailable* ***Class III - Acute MI - DO NOT use –*** *sinus bradycardia > 40 without hypoperfusion or frequent PVCs (2) type II AV block or 3rd degree AV block with new wide QRS complex presumed due to MI*
Bivalirudin *(Angiomax)*	• **Indication:** a direct thrombin inhibitor used if unstable angina and undergoing PCI (if heparin allergy/thrombocytopenia). This agent is an alternative to heparin in STEMI and UA/NSTEMI if heparin induced thrombocytopenia • **STEMI** - HERO-2 dosing recommended by ACC/AHA. Bolus 0.25 mg/kg then 0.5 mg/kg/hour for 12 hours, then 0.25 mg/kg/hour for 36 hours. Reduce infusion if PTT is > 75 seconds within the 1st 12 hours. • Alternate **UA/NSTEMI/PCI** dosing: (1) 0.75 mg/kg IV bolus pre-procedure1 mg/kg IV bolus prior to PCI, then 1.75 mg/kg/hour during procedure up to 4 hours after procedure (with IIb/IIIa agent).
Bumetanide	• *(Bumex)* 0.5-1.0 mg IV/IM; 1mg *Bumex* ~ 40 mg *Lasix*
Clopidogrel *(Plavix)*	• 300 mg PO loading dose, then 75 mg PO daily ***Class I – UA/NSTEM/STEMI*** *(1) all patients unable to take aspirin (2) add to aspirin whether or not undergo fibrinolysis (Caution - withhold 5-7 days if elective CABG is planned).* ***Class IIa STEMI*** *- If < 75 years old, 300 mg PO X 1 (see caution)*
Dalteparin *(Fragmin)*	• UA/NSTEMI – 120 units/kg SC q 12 h. Max dose 10,000 units
Digoxin *(Lanoxin)*	• <u>Rapid Afib</u> - 0.25 mg IV q 2 hours up to 1.5 mg. ***Class Ib*** *- Afib - if congestive heart failure* ***Class IIb*** *- Afib - rate control if no congestive heart failure*

PCI – procedural coronary intervention, MI – myocardial infarction, UA – unstable angina, NSTEMI – nonST elevation MI, STEMI – ST elevation MI

(continues)

Diltiazem (Cardizem)	• 20 mg (0.25 mg/kg) IV over 2 min. Repeat 25 mg (0.35 mg/kg) IV 15 min after 1st dose prn. Drip at 5-15 mg/h prn **Class I – UA/NSTEMI** –continuing or recurring ischemia when β blockers are contraindicated & no contraindications. **Class I – Atrial Fib/flutter/SVT**– preserved LV function – rate control **Class IIa– UA/NSTEMI** – oral long acting agents if recurrent ischemia in absence of contraindications & β blockers/nitrates are fully used. **Class IIb – Atrial Fib/flutter** – if CHF; **Class IIb– U/IINSTEMI** – (1) extended release form of non-dihydropyridine calcium antagonist (diltiazem, verapamil) instead of β blocker Or (2) immediate release dihydropyridine calcium antagonist (nifedipine) in presence of a β blocker. **Class III – Atrial fibrillation/flutter – DO NOT USE** if preexistation - WPW
Dobutamine (Dobutrex)	• 2-20 mcg/kg/min IV; 250 mg in 250 ml NS or D5W = 1 mg/ml
Dopamine (Intropin)	• 2-50 mcg/kg/min IV, Mix 400 mg in 250 ml D5W = 1.6 mg/ml. • 1-5 mcg/kg/min (renal), 5-10 mcg/kg/min (cardiac), > 10 mcg/kg/min (vasoconstriction), > 40 consider norepinephrine
Dofetilide (Tikosyn)	• <u>AF</u> -Specialized dose based on creatinine, body size, and age. **Class I** – cardioversion if AF of < or > 7 days duration. May be more effective for atrial flutter than for atrial fibrillation.
Enoxaparin (Lovenox)	• <u>STEMI</u> – (if creatinine [Cr] < 2.5 mg/dl if male, < 2 mg/dl if female). Age < 75 years, 30 mg IV, then 15 min later 1 mg/kg SC q 12 h. If ≥ 75 years, no IV bolus, administer 0.75 mg/kg SC q 12h. If Cr clearance < 30 ml/min, 1 mg/kg SC q 24 hours. (Some experts administer 0.5 - .75 mg/kg IV pre PCI) • <u>UA/NSTEMI/PCI</u> – 1 mg/kg SC q 12 hours (with aspirin) and continued ≥ 2 days until clinically stable. Max single dose is 150 mg SC. Overdose associated with severe bleed may be reversed by slow infusion of protamine sulfate IV (page 105). See heparin for specific AHA/ACC recommendations
Epinephrine (Adrenalin)	• <u>Cardiac arrest</u> – 1 mg IV q 3-5 min. (10 ml of 1:10,000 followed by 20 ml NS flush). ET dose: 2-2.5 mg • <u>Shock</u> – 2 –10 mcg/min. IV infusion. Mix 1 mg in 500 ml NS and infuse at 1-5 ml/min.
Eptifibatide (Integrilin)	• <u>UA/NSTEMI</u> – 180 mcg/kg IV, + 2 mcg/kg/min X 72-96 h. If serum creatinine (Cr) > 2 mg/dl or Cr clearance < 50 ml/min, bolus same amount and decrease infusion to 1 mcg/kg/min. • <u>PCI</u> above dosing or alternate dosing –of 135 mcg/kg/min IV, plus 0.5mcg/kg/min X 20-24 hours **Class I – UA/NSTEMI** –high risk, troponin positive pre PCI **Class IIa – UA/NSTEMI/STEMI** – administered pre PCI **Class IIb – UA/NSTEMI** – if conservative (nonPCI) strategy

PCI – procedural coronary intervention, MI – myocardial infarction, UA – unstable angina, NSTEMI – nonST elevation MI, STEMI – ST elevation MI

(continues)

Esmolol (Brevibloc)	• SVT/AF/Flutter/(Torsades with normal baseline QT) - Load 500 mcg/kg IV over 1 min, then 50 mcg/kg/min X 4 min. If no response, 500 mcg/kg IV over 1 min, then 100 mcg/kg/min X 4 min. Continue to repeat 500 mcg/kg over 1 min prn while increasing infusion by 50 mcg/kg/min until desired effect achieved or max. of 300 mcg/kg/min. Once adequate response, do not change rate > 25 mcg/kg/min or rebolus. *Class I – Afib – rate control*
Flecainide (Tambocor)	• AF – 200-300 mg PO OR 1.5-3 mg/kg IV over 10-20 minutes (IV formulation not available in the U.S) *Class I – AF – cardioversion of AF of up to 7 days duration.* *Class IIb – AF – cardioversion of AF of > 7 days duration.* Oral dosing is up to 91% effective for cardioversion at 8 hours. Frequent side effects (IV or PO) include atrial flutter with rapid ventricular rate, bradycardia (after cardioversion), hypotension, and mild neurologic side effects. Avoid if known organic heart disease (esp. if abnormal ventricular function).
Fondaparinux (Arixtra)	• STEMI & NSTEMI – 2.5 mg SC daily until hospital discharge or up to 8 days total. Do not use as sole PCI anticoagulant. • DVT/PE – 5 mg SC daily (if < 50 kg), 7.5 mg SC daily (50-100 kg), 10 mg SC daily (if > 100 kg). *Class I – STEMI – (if creatinine < 3 mg/dl), 2.5 mg IV, then 2.5 mg SC q 24hours.* *Class I – UA/NSTEMI – may use as anticoagulant for conservative or invasive strategies (see page 93)*
Furosemide	• (Lasix) 0.5-2.0 mg/kg IV
Group IIb/IIIa Inhibitors	see Abciximab (ReoPro), Eptifibatide (Integrilin) and Tirofiban (Aggrastat)
Heparin *Unfractionated* See enoxaparin & dalteparin for low molecular heparin options	• UA/NSTEMI/PCI/PE/DVT- 80 U/kg IV + 18 U/kg/h,titrate to PTT • MI/alteplase use – 60 U/kg IV (max 4,000 U), + 12 U/kg/h [max 1000 U/h] (PTT goal 50-70 sec or 1.5-2.0 X control) • In patients at risk for heparin induced thrombocytopenia consider fondaparinux, bivalirudin or argatroban as an alternative (see page 99, 100, 103). Consult cardiology. *Class I – STEMI – Patients undergoing PCI or surgical revascularization (unfractionated heparin/UFH). Administer UFH IV if undergoing reperfusion with alteplase, reteplase, or tenecteplase. If receiving nonselective fibrinolytic, administer UFH IV if at high risk for systemic emboli (large or anterior MI, atrial fibrillation, prior embolism, or known LV thrombus).* *Class I –UA/NSTEMI – add to aspirin and clopidogrel* *Class IIa STEMI - If no reperfusion, no contraindication continue UFH or LMWH for at least 48 hours or until patient ambulatory.* *Class IIa –UA/NSTEMI - Lovenox is preferred over unfractionated heparin in UA/NSTEMI in absence of renal failure unless CABG planned in24 hours.*

(continues)

	Class IIb – STEMI – It may be reasonable to give UFH IV to patients receiving streptokinase. LMWH may be considered an acceptable alternative. See indications/contraindications page 38 *Class IIb UA/NSTEMI* – SC use if non-selective thrombolytics given & low risk for emboli until walking.
Ibutilide *(Corvert)*	• <u>AF</u> – If > 60 kg, 1 mg IV over 10 minutes. If < 60 kg, 0.01 mg/kg IV over 10 minutes. May repeat initial dose for either weight 10 minutes after completion of either infusion. *Class I* – AF cardioversion of up to 7 days duration. *Class IIb* – AF cardioversion if present > 7 days. 4% risk of torsades de pointes (esp. if female) usually within 1st hour but occasionally up to 4 hours after use. Avoid if low ejection fraction, CHF, prolonged QT interval, current use of Ia or III anti-arrhythmics. Ensure K, Mg are normal prior to use.
Isoproterenol *(Isuprel)*	• <u>Bradycardia</u> – 2 – 10 mcg/min IV (if atropine, dopamine have failed and no pacer) *Class indeterminate – polymorphic VT as temporizing measure*
Lidocaine	• <u>Vfib/Pulseless Vtach</u> - 1.0-1.5 mg/kg IV (2-4 mg/kg ET) may repeat 0.5-0.75 mg/kg IV over 3-5 minutes (Max 3 mg/kg) • <u>Vtach – monomorphic, stable, normal cardiac function</u> 1.0-1.5 mg/kg IV q 5-10 min.; <u>Vtach - impaired cardiac function</u> – 0.5 – 0.75 mg/kg IV q 5-10 minutes. (Max 3 mg/kg) • If conversion with lidocaine infuse 1-4 mg/min IV *Class IIa* – for 24-48 hours after ventricular fibrillation/tachycardia *Class IIb* – sustained monomorphic ventricular tachycardia (VT) not associated with angina hypotension or CHF. *Class III* – prophylaxis with thrombolytics, isolated PVC's, couplets, accelerated idioventricular rhythm, nonsustained VT *Class Indeterminate* – (1) pulseless Vfib/Vtach, (2) monomorphic ventricular tachycardia with impaired cardiac function.
Magnesium	• <u>Torsades/Various tachyarrhythmias</u> - 2 g IV over 15 minutes *Class I* – no class I recommendations *Class IIa* – Treating ↓K, ↓Mg, or torsades de pointes (indeterminate)
Metoprolol *(Lopressor)*	• <u>Acute MI</u> – 25-50 mg PO q6h OR 5 mg IV q 5 min X 3, then 50 mg PO q 12 h X 24 hours, then ↑ to 100 mg q 12 h or 50 mg q 6 h as tolerated • <u>Afib</u>- 2.5-5.0 mg IV (over 2 min) q 5 min, up to 3 doses *Class I – STEMI/UA/NSTEMI* – <12 h of MI or with ongoing, recurrent pain. Class I STEMI – orally administered. *Class I – Afib* – if no congestive heart failure *Class IIa – STEMI* – IV administration if no contraindication *Class IIb – Afib* – if congestive heart failure *Class III* – heart failure, bradycardia or other contraindication
Nitroglycerin	• <u>MI/CHF/UA/NSTEMI</u> – Initiate at 10-20 mcg/min IV. Increase 5-20 mcg/min q 3-5 min until desired effect. One study found high dose (200-400 mcg/min) IV effective if pulmonary edema, systolic BP > 160 or MAP > 120. Ann Emerg Med 2007; 144

(continues)

	Class I *– (1) 1st 24 – 48 hours in acute MI with CHF, large anterior infarct, persistent ischemia or hypertension. (2) continued use (> 48 h) if recurrent angina, or persistent pulmonary congestion.* ***Class IIb*** *– (1) 1st 24-48 hours after MI without ↓BP, ↑HR or ↓HR (2) continued use (> 48 h) if large or complicated infarction* ***Class III - DO NOT USE*** *– systolic BP < 90 mm Hg or ≥ 30 mm Hg below baseline, or HR < 50, or within 24 hours of sildenafil (Viagra), 48 hours of tadalafil/Cialis use with unknown delay needed for vardenafil*
Norepinephrine *(Levophed)*	• <u>Shock</u> – 0.5-1 mcg/min, ↑1-2 mcg/min q 3-5 min until desired effect. Usual maintenance dose is 2-4 mcg/min, occasionally 8-30 mcg/min is required. Use central line if possible.
Prasugrel *(Effient)*	• 60 mg PO loading dose, then 10 mg PO QD • Caution if >75 years or <=60 kg (consider using 5 mg PO QD maintenance dose) • Contraindicated if prior TIA/Stroke • Indication acute coronary syndrome (ACS) patients undergoing PCI • Withhold 7 or more days if elective CABG is planned
Procainamide	• <u>Afib/Flutter,Wide complex tachycardia</u> - 30 mg/min IV (max total dose 17 mg/kg) until (1) ↓BP, (2) QRS complex increases 50%, (3) arrhythmia stops or (4) total 17 mg/kg • <u>VF/pulseless VT</u> –50 mg/min IV (up to max dose 17 mg/min) ***Class IIa*** *- stable SVT/Atrial fib/flutter/ventricular tachycardia.* ***Class IIb*** *– VT/shock refractory VF, polymorphic VT, or Supraventricular tachycardia in WPW*
Propafenone *(Rythmol)*	• <u>AF</u> – 600 mg PO **OR** 1.5-2 mg/kg IV over 10-20 minutes. ***Class I*** *– AF cardioversion if present up to 7 days.* ***Class IIb*** *– AF cardioversion if present > 7 days.* *Adverse effects include rapid atrial flutter, ventricular tachycardia, intraventricular conduction disturbances, hypotension, and bradycardia (after cardioversion). Avoid in patients with heart failure, severe obstructive lung disease, and use cautiously in patients with organic heart disease.*
Protamine sulfate	• 1 mg protamine neutralizes 100 units unfractionated heparin, 100 anti-Xa units of dalteparin or tinzaparin, OR 1 mg of enoxaparin *(Lovenox)*. If aPTT is still elevated 2-4 hours after initial protamine dose, give 0.5 mg protamine for each 100 anti-Xa units of dalteparin or tinzaparin OR each 1 mg of enoxaparin. Administer by slow IV injection of 1% solution over > 10 minutes. Maximum dose is 50 mg. • Observe for anaphylaxis/hypotension if given too rapidly. Increased risk of allergic reaction if prior exposure (e.g. insulin), fish allergy, vasectomy (anti-protamine antibodies) . • Protamine reverses anti-thrombin activity but only partially reverses anti-Xa activity.

PCI – procedural coronary intervention, MI – myocardial infarction, UA – unstable angina, NSTEMI – nonST elevation MI, STEMI – ST elevation MI

(continues)

Reteplase	(r-PA, Retavase) see thrombolytics page 98
Sodium Nitroprusside	• 0.1 mcg/kg/min IV titrated up q 3-5 minutes to desired effect up to maximum of 10 mcg/kg/min
Sotalol (Betapace, Betapace AF)	Maintenance of sinus rhythm in Afib: 80 – 320 mg PO bid. **Class IIa – Afib/flutter** – pre-electric cardioversion to prevent recurrence of Afib/flutter. **Class III** – DO not use to cardiovert atrial fibrillation/flutter. Note: there is high incidence of torsades if > 320 mg/day administered, female, or heart failure.
Streptokinase	(Streptase) see thrombolytics page 98
Tenecteplase	(TNKase) see thrombolytics page 98
Thrombolytics	• See page 98
Ticagrelor (Brilinta)	• 180 mg PO loading dose and then 90 mg PO BID • Indication acute coronary syndromes (ACS) • Should utilize aspirin dose 75 mg to 100 mg PO QD • Withhold 5 days before elective CABG
Tirofiban (Aggrastat)	• UA/NTESMI/PCI – 0.4 mcg/kg/min X 30 min, then 0.1 mcg/kg/min X 48-108 hours or until 24 hours after procedure. **Class I – UA/NSTEMI** –high risk, troponin positive pre PCI **Class IIa – UA/NSTEMI/STEMI** – administered pre PCI **Class IIb – UA/NSTEMI** – if conservative (nonPCI) strategy
Vasopressin	• Vfib/Pulseless Vtach – 40 units IV. No repeat dose. • Asystole – 40 units IV q 3 min X 2. May follow with epi prn.
Verapamil (Calan)	• SVT – 2.5-5.0 mg IV over 2 minutes. May repeat 5-10 mg IV over 2 minutes, 15-30 minutes after 1st dose • Afib – 0.075 – 0.15 mg/kg IV over 2 min. **Class I – Afib** – no congestive heart failure **Class IIb – Afib** – congestive heart failure
Vernakalant (Cardiome)	• Atrial fibrillation - 3 mg/kg IV over 10 min. If arrhythmia does not terminate after 15 minutes, administer 2 mg/kg IV. As of publication date, not yet FDA approved.

PCI – procedural coronary intervention, MI – myocardial infarction, UA – unstable angina, NSTEMI – nonST elevation MI, STEMI – ST elevation MI

13 ■ HEART FAILURE

ACUTE DECOMPENSATED HEART FAILURE

Acute decompensated heart failure (ADHF) is the sudden development of signs and symptoms of insufficient cardiac output. ADHF accounts for a substantial number of inpatient hospitalizations and is associated with significant morbidity, necessitating rapid diagnosis and expeditious management.

- **Pathophysiology of ADHF.** Cardiogenic pulmonary edema occurs when pulmonary capillary pressure exceeds the forces that maintain fluid within the vascular space, including serum oncotic pressure and interstitial hydrostatic pressure.
  - Increased pulmonary capillary pressure is most commonly caused by LV failure of any cause or valvular disease, especially mitral stenosis. Rare causes include atrial myxoma and pulmonary veno-occlusive disease.
  - Accumulation of fluid in the pulmonary interstitium is followed by alveolar flooding and impairment of gas exchange.
- ADHF can occur in patients with known myocardial dysfunction, as well as in patients without structural or functional LV impairment. Factors resulting in decompensation:
  - Cardiac causes: Acute myocardial ischemia, new or progressive (atrial or ventricular) arrhythmia, acute or progressive valvular dysfunction, exposure to myocardial toxins.
  - Additionally, various noncardiac factors can exacerbate heart failure: Infection, renal failure, hypertension, thyroid disease, post-operative status, peripartum status, and iatrogenic hypervolemia.
  - In patients with chronic compensated HF, medication noncompliance and dietary indiscretion (increased Na intake/increased fluid intake) are important factors.
  - Acute right-sided HF may result from pulmonary venous thromboembolism.
- **Diagnosis of ADHF.**
  - Clinical presentation:
    - Clinical manifestations of pulmonary edema can occur rapidly:
      - Dyspnea, anxiety, restlessness, and expectoration of pink frothy fluid
  - Physical signs:
    - Decreased peripheral perfusion, pulmonary congestion, use of accessory respiratory muscles, and wheezing
  - Electrocardiography and laboratory studies:
    - Abnormalities in the ECG are common and can include supraventricular and ventricular arrhythmias, conduction delays, and nonspecific ST-T changes.

- Serum levels of *B-type natriuretic peptide* (BNP) are elevated in patients with asymptomatic LV dysfunction as well as symptomatic heart failure. A serum BNP < 100 pg/mL has good negative predictive value and usually excludes ADHF as primary diagnosis.[16]
- Serial cardiac enzymes should be obtained to evaluate ongoing myocardial ischemia.
- Laboratory abnormalities may also include elevated BUN and creatinine, hyponatremia, anemia, and elevated serum levels of hepatic enzymes.
  - Imaging:
    - A chest x-ray (CXR) is useful in identifying cardiomegaly, interstitial and perihilar vascular engorgement, Kerley B lines, and pleural effusions.
    - The radiographic abnormalities may follow the development of symptoms by several hours; CXR resolution may be out of phase with clinical improvement.

- **Therapy for ADHF.**
  - Initial Management
    - Continuous pulse oximetry and telemetry, frequent assessment of vital signs. Reliable intravenous access needs to be maintained.
    - Supplemental oxygen should be administered to increase arterial oxygen content to greater than 60mm Hg. Mechanical ventilation is indicated if oxygenation is inadequate by noninvasive means or if hypercapnia coexists.
      - Placing the patient in a sitting position improves pulmonary function.
      - Strict bedrest, pain control, and relief of anxiety can decrease cardiac workload.
      - Correcting precipitating factors, as possible, is critical. Successful resolution of pulmonary edema can often be accomplished only by correction of the underlying process.
  - Medications. Nitrates, loop diuretics, and morphine sulfate are first-line agents in the pharmacologic management of acute HF. Additional therapies include nitroprusside or nesiritide, and inotropic support (dobutamine or milrinone) in the setting of refractory pulmonary edema.
    - **Nitrates**
      - As a potent vasodilator, *nitroglycerin* (NTG) affects both venous and arterial vascular beds. The main purpose of its use in ADHF is to relieve pulmonary and systemic venous congestion.
      - Nitroglycerin (NTG) is the preferred vasodilator for treatment of HF in the setting of acute coronary syndromes. Intravenous administration is preferred for its rapid titration.
      - IV NTG can be started at 5–10 mcg/min and increased every few minutes until dyspnea is relieved or limiting hypotension occurs, to a maximum of 300 mcg/min.

- **Loop diuretics**
  - Furosemide is a direct venodilator and diuretic. Furosemide decreases pulmonary congestion within minutes of IV administration, long preceding its diuretic activity.
  - An initial dose of 20–80 mg IV should be administered and can be titrated based on response to a maximum of 200 mg in subsequent doses. Patients who already take furosemide will likely need higher doses to achieve the same effect.
- **Morphine sulfate**
  - Morphine sulfate functions as an anxiolytic, in addition to dilating the pulmonary and systemic vasculature.
  - Morphine, 2–5 mg IV, can be administered and repeated every 10–25 minutes until an effect is seen.
- **Additional therapies**
  - *Nitroprusside* is a potent vasodilator that can prove useful in ADHF resulting from acute valvular regurgitation or severe hypertension. Pulmonary arterial catheterization and continuous direct arterial pressure monitoring should be considered to guide titration.
  - Recombinant BNP (*nesiritide*) is administered as an IV bolus followed by continuous infusion. It reduces intracardiac filling pressures through vasodilation and results in a net increase in cardiac output. With concurrent loop diuretic use, nesiritide produces natriuresis and diuresis.
  - Inotropic agents, such as *dobutamine* or *milrinone*, may be helpful after initial treatment of ADHF in patients with concomitant hypotension or shock.
- **Special considerations**
  - *Pulmonary artery catheterization* is useful in cases in which a prompt response to therapy does not occur. The pulmonary artery catheter differentiates between cardiogenic and noncardiogenic causes of pulmonary edema via measurement of central hemodynamics and cardiac output and can guide subsequent therapy.
  - *Acute hemodialysis* and *ultrafiltration* may be effective, especially in the patient with significant renal dysfunction and diuretic resistance.

CHRONIC HEART FAILURE AND CARDIOMYOPATHY

- **General principles**
  - *Definition:* Chronic HF is a syndrome defined by the inability of the heart to maintain an output necessary to meet metabolic demands at normal intracardiac pressures.
  - *Epidemiology:* The current estimated prevalence of HF is 5 million cases in the United States; incidence is estimated at 550,000 cases per year.[17]
  - Five-year mortality following a new diagnosis of heart failure approaches 50%.

- *Classification.* Several schema for the classification of chronic HF exist:
  - *Functional*: HF can be associated with poor myocardial contraction (*systolic dysfunction*), abnormal ventricular relaxation and filling (*diastolic dysfunction*), or both.
  - *Etiologic*: *Ischemic* (the most common cause of cardiomyopathy in the United States) versus *non-ischemic* (including hypertensive, valvular, peripartum, viral/toxic, and other causes of HF).
  - *Anatomic*: *Right-sided* versus *left-sided* heart failure can often be distinguished by symptomatology.
  - *Severity*: HF can be classified according to New York Heart Association (NYHA) status or metabolic capacity.
- **Pathophysiology**
  - HF manifests as end-organ hypoperfusion (due to a insufficient cardiac output and decreased cardiac reserve) and pulmonary and systemic venous congestion.
  - Compensatory adaptations occur, including:
    - Increased left ventricular (LV) volume (dilatation) and mass (hypertrophy)
    - Increased systemic vascular resistance (SVR) secondary to enhanced activity of the sympathetic nervous system and elevated levels of circulating catecholamines
    - Activation of the renin-angiotensin-aldosterone and vasopressin (antidiuretic hormone) systems
- **Diagnosis**
  - Clinical Presentation: Presentation with HF can vary depending on multiple factors: rapidity of cardiac decompensation, underlying etiology, age, and comorbidities.
  - History: Patients often complain of fatigue, exercise intolerance/exertional dyspnea, orthopnea, or paroxysmal nocturnal dyspnea. Presyncope, palpitations, and angina may be present, especially with accompanying arrhythmia.
  - Physical examination: Signs of chronic pulmonary and systemic venous congestion may be present, including lung crackles, edema, elevated jugular venous pressure, pleural and pericardial effusions, hepatic congestion, and ascites. Third and fourth heart sounds are common.
  - Laboratory studies
    - BNP is synthesized by right and left ventricular myocytes and released in response to stretch, volume overload, and elevated filling pressures. BNP levels correlate with the severity of HF and predict overall survival.
    - Similar laboratory and ECG abnormalities found in acute heart failure (elevated levels of BUN and creatinine, hyponatremia, anemia, serum hepatic enzymes) may be present in patients with chronic HF.
    - Imaging
      - Radiographic abnormalities include cardiomegaly and evidence of pulmonary vascular redistribution.

- Upon diagnosis, ventricular function should assessed—either via transthoracic echocardiography, radionuclide ventriculography, or cardiac catheterization with left ventriculography.

- **Treatment**
  - Goals of therapy:
    - Improve long-term survival.
    - Reduce symptoms.
    - Increase functional capacity.
    - Reduce hospitalizations.
    - Prevent deleterious cardiac remodeling.
  - Behavioral recommendations:
    - Exercise training is recommended in stable HF patients. It should be initiated gradually under monitored conditions in an outpatient setting. Target durations should be 20–45 minutes a day for 3–5 days a week for a total of 8–12 weeks.
    - Patients in exercise training programs have reported increased exercise capacity, decreased symptoms, increased quality of life, and have been found to have a decreased hospitalization rate. The survival effects of long-term exercise training are not well defined.
    - Weight loss and fluid restriction should be recommended when appropriate.
  - Medications: Pharmacotherapy involves the antagonism of neurohormones that are increased in patients with chronic HF. Vasodilator therapy and beta-adrenergic blockade are the pillars of therapy for patients with chronic HF. Diuretics are reserved for symptomatic relief and volume overload. Most patients require multiple medications to control symptoms and prolong survival.
    - **Beta-adrenergic receptor antagonists** (beta-blockers) are critical components of HF pharmacotherapy.
      - Large randomized trials have documented the beneficial effects of beta-blockers on survival in patients with NYHA class II–IV symptoms.[18,19,20,21]
      - Improvement in LVEF, exercise tolerance, and functional class are common after the institution of a beta-adrenergic antagonist. Usually 2–3 months of therapy are required to see significant beneficial effects on LV function, but suppression of arrhythmia and decreased risk of sudden cardiac death occur earlier.
      - Beta-blockers should be initiated at a low dose and titrated with careful attention to blood pressure and heart rate. Patients can experience transient volume retention and worsening HF symptoms that respond to an increase in diuretics.
      - Different beta-blockers have unique properties and the beneficial effect in HF may not be a class effect. Therefore, it is recommended that agents with proven effects on patient survival in large clinical trials be used preferentially. These agents include *carvedilol, bisoprolol,* and *metoprolol succinate.*

○ **Vasodilator therapy** is another critical component of HF management. Arterial vasoconstriction (afterload) and venous vasoconstriction (preload) occur in patients with HF as a result of activation of the renin-angiotensin-aldosterone axis and adrenergic nervous system. These medications should be cautiously used in patients with fixed cardiac output (e.g., aortic stenosis [AS] or hypertrophic cardiomyopathy [HCM]) or with diastolic dysfunction. Oral vasodilators should be initiated in patients with symptomatic chronic HF and in those patients who are discontinuing parenteral vasodilators therapy. When treatment with oral vasodilators is being initiated in hypotensive patients, it is prudent to use agents with a short half-life.

■ **Angiotensin-converting enzyme (ACE) inhibitors** attenuate vasoconstriction, vital organ hypoperfusion, hyponatremia, hypokalemia, and fluid retention attributed to activation of the renin-angiotensin system. Treatment with ACE-inhibitors decreases afterload while increasing cardiac output.

　▫ Large clinical trials have shown that ACE-inhibitors improve survival and symptoms in patients with HF and depressed EF.[22] ACE inhibitors may prevent the development of symptoms in patients with asymptomatic LV dysfunction and in those at high risk of developing structural heart disease (coronary artery disease, diabetes mellitus, HTN). One study suggests that higher doses of ACE-inhibitors decrease morbidity without improving overall survival.[23] Absence of an initial beneficial response to treatment with an ACE-inhibitor does not preclude long-term benefit.

　▫ Most ACE-inhibitors are excreted by the kidneys, requiring cautious dose titration in patients with renal insufficiency. Acute renal insufficiency can occur in patients with bilateral renal artery stenosis. Additional side effects include rash, angioedema, dysgeusia, increases in serum creatinine, proteinuria, hyperkalemia, leukopenia, and cough.

　▫ Because of hyperkalemia, potassium supplements and salt substitutes and potassium-sparing diuretics should be avoided.

　▫ *ACE-inhibitors are contraindicated in pregnancy*

■ **Angiotensin II–receptor blockers** (ARBs) inhibit the renin-angiotensin system via specific blockade of the angiotensin II receptor. Unlike ACE-inhibitors, there is no increase in bradykinin levels, which may be responsible for ACE-inhibitor associated cough.

　▫ ARBs reduce mortality and morbidity in HF patients who are not receiving an ACE-inhibitor.[24,25,26]

　▫ ARBs should be considered in patients who are intolerant to ACE-inhibitors due to cough or angioedema.

　▫ As with ACE-inhibitors, caution must be exercised when ARBs are used in patients with renal insufficiency and bilateral renal artery stenosis, because hyperkalemia and acute renal failure can develop. Renal function and potassium levels should be periodically monitored.

- *ARBs are contraindicated in pregnancy.*

- **Hydralazine** is a potent direct arteriodilator. In combination with nitrates, hydralazine improves survival in HF.[27]

  - A combination of hydralazine and isosorbide dinitrate (starting dose: 37.5/20 mg 3 times daily) when added to standard therapy with beta blockers and ACE-inhibitors has been shown to reduce mortality in Black patients.[28]

  - Reflex tachycardia and increased myocardial oxygen consumption may occur, requiring careful use in patients with ischemic heart disease.

- **Nitrates** are predominantly venodilators and help relieve symptoms of venous and pulmonary congestion. Myocardial function is enhanced by decreasing ventricular filling pressures and by dilating coronary arteries.

  - Nitrate therapy may precipitate hypotension in patients with reduced preload.

○ **Parenteral vasodilators** are reserved for patients with severe HF or those who cannot take oral medications. **Nitroglycerin** and **nitroprusside**, discussed previously, are commonly used intravenous vasodilators.

- **Nesiritide** is a combined arterial and venous vasodilator.[29] It is administered as a 2 µg/kg IV bolus followed by a continuous IV infusion starting of 0.01 µg/kg/minute, and is approved for use in acute HF exacerbations and relieves symptoms early after its administration. It should not be used to improve renal function or to enhance diuresis. Hypotension is a common side effect, and it should be avoided in patients with systemic hypotension (systolic BP < 90 mmHg) or cardiogenic shock. Episodes of hypotension should prompt discontinuation of nesiritide and cautious volume expansion or pressor support if necessary.

- **Enalaprilat** is an active metabolite of the ACE-inhibitor enalapril that is available for IV administration.

● **Digoxin** is a cardiac glycoside that increases myocardial contractility and may antagonize the neurohormonal activation associated with HF.

○ Digoxin therapy results in fewer HF hospitalizations, without altering overall mortality.[30]

○ Discontinuation of digoxin in patients who are stable on a regimen of digoxin, diuretics, and an ACE-inhibitor may result in clinical deterioration.

○ Digoxin has a narrow therapeutic window, and serum levels should be followed closely, especially in patients with unstable renal function.

○ Usual daily dose is 0.125–0.25 mg and should be decreased in patients with renal insufficiency. Clinical benefits may not be related to serum levels, and toxicity can occur in the therapeutic range of 0.8–2.0 ng/mL.[31]

- **Diuretics** can lead to improvement in symptoms in HF patients. Frequent assessment of weight and careful observation of fluid intake and output is essential when initiating or changing therapy. Frequent complications include electrolyte derangement (hypokalemia, hyponatremia, and hypomagnesemia), intravascular volume depletion with contraction alkalosis, and hypotension. Therefore, electrolytes, BUN, and creatinine should be followed. Hypokalemia may be life threatening in patients who are receiving digoxin or in those with severe LV dysfunction predisposing to ventricular arrhythmia. Potassium supplementation or a potassium-sparing diuretic should be considered.
  - **Thiazide** diuretics (*hydrochlorothiazide, chlorthalidone*) can be used as initial agents in patients with normal renal function in whom only a mild diuresis is desired. Metolazone, unlike other thiazides, exerts its action at the proximal as well as the distal tubule and can be used in combination with loop diuretics in patients with a low glomerular filtration rate.
  - **Loop diuretics** (*furosemide, ethacrynic acid, bumetanide*) are used in patients who require significant diuresis and in those with decreased renal function. Use of loop diuretics may be complicated by hyperuricemia, hypocalcemia, ototoxicity, rash, and vasculitis.
- **Potassium-sparing diuretics** do not exert a potent diuretic effect when used alone, but have been shown to improve survival and decrease hospitalizations, presumably as a result of antagonism of the rennin-angiotensin-aldosterone axis.[32]
  - **Spironolactone** (25 mg daily) is an aldosterone receptor antagonist that should be considered in NYHA class III–IV patients. The potential for development of life-threatening hyperkalemia exists with the use of these agents.
    - Gynecomastia may develop in 10–20% of men treated with spironolactone.
    - Serum potassium must be monitored closely after initiation; concurrent use of ACE-inhibitors and NSAIDs, and the presence of renal insufficiency (creatinine > 2.5 mg/dL), greatly increase the risk of hyperkalemia.
  - **Eplerenone**, a selective aldosterone receptor antagonist without the hormonal side effects of spironolactone, is used in the treatment of HTN and HF, and reduces mortality in patients with HF associated with acute MI.[33]

ADVANCED THERAPEUTIC MANAGEMENT OF HF

- *Inotropic agents*: Sympathomimetic agents are potent drugs that are used in severe HF. Beneficial and adverse effects are mediated by stimulation of myocardial beta-adrenergic receptors. The most important adverse effects are related to the arrhythmogenic nature of these agents and the potential for exacerbation of myocardial ischemia. Treatment needs to be guided by careful hemodynamic and ECG monitoring. Patients with refractory HF may benefit symptomatically from continuous ambulatory administration of IV inotropes as palliative therapy or as a bridge to mechanical ventricular support or cardiac transplantation. However, this strategy may increase the risk of life-threatening arrhythmias or indwelling catheter-related infections.

- **Dopamine** should be used for stabilization of the hypotensive patient.
- **Dobutamine** is a synthetic analog of dopamine. Several studies have demonstrated increased mortality in patients treated with continuous dobutamine. This medication does not have a significant role in the treatment of HF resulting from diastolic dysfunction or a high-output state.
- **Milrinone** is a phosphodiesterase inhibitor that increases myocardial contractility and produces vasodilation by increasing intracellular cyclic adenosine monophosphate. Milrinone is currently available for clinical use and is indicated for treatment of refractory HF.[34] Hypotension may develop in patients who receive vasodilator therapy or have intravascular volume contraction, or both.
- **Implantation of a cardioverter-defibrillator (ICD)** should be considered in patients with severe symptomatic left ventricular dysfunction (ejection fraction < 35%) for the prevention of sudden cardiac death.[35] Medical optimization of standard HF agents and discontinuation of pro-arrhythmic drugs should occur prior to implantation.
- **Cardiac resynchronization therapy** ("biventricular pacing") appears to be beneficial in patients with an ejection fraction of 35% or less, NYHA class III HF and conduction abnormalities (left bundle branch block and intraventricular delay).[36] It has been demonstrated to improve quality of life and reduce the risk of death in carefully selected patients.
- **Intra-aortic balloon pump (IABP)** placement can be considered for patients in whom other therapies have failed, have transient myocardial dysfunction, or are awaiting a definitive procedure such as transplantation or ventricular assist device placement.
  - Balloon inflation is synchronized with the cardiac cycle and results in significant preload and afterload reduction, with decreased myocardial oxygen demand and improved coronary blood flow, resulting in improved cardiac output. Severe aortoiliac atherosclerosis and aortic valve insufficiency are contraindications to IABP pump placement.
- **Ventricular assist devices** require surgical implantation and are indicated for patients with severe refractory HF, intractable cardiogenic shock, and for patients whose conditions deteriorate while they await cardiac transplantation. Ventricular assist devices improve survival in patients with refractory HF who are not candidates for cardiac transplantation ("destination therapy").[37]

- **Cardiac transplantation** is an option for selected patients with severe end-stage HF, though the scarcity of organs for transplant is a limitation. Candidates considered for transplantation should be younger than 65 years (although selected older patients may also benefit), have advanced HF, have a strong psychological/social support system, have exhausted all other therapeutic options, and be free of irreversible end-organ dysfunction that would limit recovery or predispose them to post-transplantation complications.
  - Survival rates of 90% at 1 year and 70% at 5 years have been reported since the introduction of cyclosporine-based immunosuppression.
  - In general, functional capacity and quality of life improve significantly after transplantation. Post-transplant complications include acute and chronic rejection, infections, and adverse effects of immunosuppressive agents. Cardiac allograft vasculopathy (coronary artery disease/chronic rejection) and malignancy are the leading causes of death after the first post-transplant year.

14 ■ CARDIOMYOPATHY[38]

INTRODUCTION

The most common cause of heart failure and cardiomyopathy in the Unites States is coronary artery disease (CAD), accounting for approximately half of cases. The other half is due to a variety of etiologies. With a new diagnosis of cardiomyopathy, it is important to distinguish between ischemic and nonischemic etiologies, as the treatment may differ.

ISCHEMIC CARDIOMYOPATHY

Cardiomyopathy due to ischemic or flow-limiting CAD or previous myocardial infarction (MI). This term is not used for heart failure (HF) patients who have an incidental finding of nonobstructive CAD.

HF in the setting of CAD is a heterogeneous condition with several factors contributing to LV systolic dysfunction and HF symptoms. After an MI, there is loss of functioning myocytes, development of myocardial fibrosis, LV remodeling, chamber dilatation, and neurohormonal activation—all leading to progressive dysfunction of the remaining viable myocardium.

- The diagnostic approach for CAD should be individualized based on angina history, risk factors, and patient preference. Either coronary angiogram or noninvasive stress testing are acceptable.
- Patients with ischemia, viable myocardium, and suitable anatomy should be revascularized.
- Antiplatelet agents, smoking cessation, and lipid-lowering therapy are particularly important in the treatment of ischemic cardiomyopathy.
- ACE-inhibitors are indicated for all patients with CAD, regardless of EF.
- Patients with low EF (< 40%) should be treated with appropriate medical therapies for systolic HF (see Heart Failure chapter, pp. 103).
- Device therapy (ICDs and/or CRT) is indicated in patients with EF < 35% (see HF chapter).

DILATED CARDIOMYOPATHY

Dilated cardiomyopathy (DCM) represents the most common form of "nonischemic cardiomyopathy" (NICM). It is characterized by dilation of the cardiac chambers and reduction in ventricular contractile function. For the majority of patients with DCM, the etiology is idiopathic. (See **Table 14-1**.) When possible, etiology should be diagnosed, as there are potential reversible causes. The lifetime incidence of DCM is approximately 35 cases per 100,000 persons.

TABLE 14-1. Final Diagnoses in Patients with Cardiomyopathy of Initially Undetermined Origin

Final diagnosis in 1230 patients with initially unexplained cardiomyopathy	Percent%
Idiopathic	50
Myocarditis	9
Coronary disease	7
Infiltrative disease (Amyloid, sarcoid, hemochromatosis)	5
Peripartum Cardiomyopathy	4
Hypertension	4
HIV	4
Autoimmune	3
Substance abuse (Alcohol or cocaine)	3
Chemotherapy (anthracycline)	1
Other	10

Adapted from Felker GM, et al. Underlying causes and long-term survival in patients with initially unexplained cardiomyopathy. NEJM. 2000; 342:1077–1084.

- DCM may be secondary to progression of any process that affects the myocardium and dilation is directly related to neurohormonal activation.
- Dilation of the cardiac chambers and varying degrees of hypertrophy are anatomic hallmarks. **Tricuspid and mitral regurgitation (TR, MR)** are common due to the effect of chamber dilation on the valvular apparatus.
  - **Atrial and ventricular arrhythmias** are present in 30–50% of patients.
- Specific etiologies of dilated cardiomyopathy other than idiopathic include (see Table 14-1 for relative frequencies).
  - Infectious, toxic (alcohol, cocaine)
  - Chemotherapy (particularly anthracyclines)
  - Metabolic (hyper or hypothyroid, selenium deficiency, Cushing's syndrome)
  - Stress-induced or takotsubo cardiomyopathy
  - Tachycardia-induced
  - High-output heart failure
  - Autoimmune
- Diagnosis (but not etiology) is typically by echocardiography or radio-nuclide ventriculography.
  - Endomyocardial biopsy is not routinely recommended in dilated cardiomyopathy because it provides little information that affects treatment.

HYPERTROPHIC CARDIOMYOPATHY

Hypertrophic cardiomyopathy (HCM) is the most common inherited heart defect, occurring in 1 of 500 people in the United States, most of whom are unaware of their disease. This myocardial disorder is characterized by ventricular hypertrophy, small LV cavity, normal, or enhanced systolic contractility, and impaired diastolic function in the absence of other identifiable causes (e.g., hypertension).

- More than one-third of young athletes who die suddenly have probable or definite HCM, making it the leading cause of sudden cardiac death in athletes. It is most common between the ages of 10 and 35 years, and usually occurs during or shortly after periods of strenuous exertion.
- **Echo findings.** Myocardial hypertrophy is typically predominant in the ventricular septum
  - So-called "asymmetrical hypertrophy" or "asymmetric septal hypertrophy (ASH)," or LVH may involve all ventricular segments equally.
  - There is an **apical (Yamaguchi)** variant that does not result in outflow tract obstruction.
    - ECG reveals signs of hypertrophy in the apical (V_4–V_6) leads.
  - LV outflow tract obstruction may or may not be present. *Systolic anterior motion (SAM)* of the anterior leaflet of the mitral valve:
    - Is associated with MR.
    - May contribute to LV outflow tract obstruction.
- There are several associated gene mutations. One common one affects the *myosin heavy chain.*
  - Inheritance is autosomal dominant with variable penetrance.
  - In addition to hypertrophy, the phenotype includes abnormal arrangement of the myocytes within the myocardium, *myocardial disarray.*
- **Symptoms** vary but may include:
  - Dyspnea/exertional dyspnea
  - Angina (from mismatch in myocardial oxygen supply and demand)
  - Palpitations
  - Syncope
  - Cardiac failure
  - Sudden death
- **Objective findings:**
  - Forceful double or triple apical impulse
  - *Pulsus bisferiens,* a double upstroke of the peripheral pulse due to obstruction of the outflow tract (by SAM), in the midportion of systole, then continuation of the pressure upstroke with continued ventricular contraction
  - Coarse systolic outflow murmur along the left sternal border
    - Murmur is accentuated by any maneuver decreasing LV filling (preload) or increasing the LVOT pressure gradient.
      - Standing
      - Valsalva maneuver
      - Amyl nitrate (a profound arterial vasodilator) administration

- ○ Murmur is diminished by maneuvers that increase ~~decrease~~ the LVOT gradient.
  - Hand grip
  - Squatting
  - Phenylephrine (a vasoconstrictor) administration
- ECG is abnormal in more than 95% of cases, showing left ventricular hypertrophy.
- ST- and T-wave abnormalities.
- Echocardiogram findings are described earlier in this chapter.
- Holter monitor may demonstrate ventricular arrhythmias which can aid in risk stratification for sudden death.
- Brockenbrough-Braunwald-Morrow sign: decreased *pulse pressure* in the beat after a premature ventricular contraction. Most easily detected with pressure recordings from the catheterization laboratory, but may be detected on examination of the peripheral pulse.
- **Risk of sudden death** is elevated in hypertrophic obstructive cardiomyopathy, apparently due to ventricular arrhythmias related to disruptions in normal ventricular activation created by myocardial disarray (though other mechanisms, such as abnormal vasoregulation and loss of cardiac output due to obstruction, are possible).
  - Risk stratification is desirable to determine who may benefit from implantable defibrillator (ICD) therapy. In addition to a history of sudden death or sustained VT, factors that increase the risk of sudden death include:
    - ○ Septal thickness
      - < 20 mm: low risk
      - >20 mm and < 30 mm: intermediate risk
      - > 30 mm: high risk
    - ○ Syncope (not clearly explained by other causes)
    - ○ Nonsustained VT
    - ○ Family history of sudden death with hypertrophic cardiomyopathy
    - ○ Hypotensive response to exercise
  - More than 1 of the major risk factors suggests risk of death more than 4% per year, and ICD implantation should be considered.
  - Less clear risk factors:
    - ○ Young age at diagnosis
    - ○ LVOT gradient > 30 mmHg
    - ○ Diastolic dysfunction
    - ○ Myocardial ischemia
    - ○ Late gadolinium enhancement on MRI
    - ○ Genotype

RESTRICTIVE CARDIOMYOPATHY

Restrictive cardiomyopathy (RCM) is characterized by a rigid heart with poor ventricular filling. Etiology can be infiltrative (amyloidosis or sarcoidosis) or noninfiltrative (diabetic or idiopathic). Pericardial disease (constrictive pericarditis) can present in a similar fashion but carries a different prognosis and treatment options and so therefore must be excluded.

- **Cardiac amyloidosis.** Amyloid deposits in the interstitium replace normal myocardial contractile elements. Of the different types of amyloidosis, cardiac involvement is most common in primary (AL) amyloidosis and least likely in secondary (AA) amyloidosis. Other types include senile systemic amyloidosis and familial (due to transthyretin gene mutations).
  - **ECG** classically shows low voltage with poor R wave progression, while echocardiogram will show ventricular hypertrophy with a granular, sparkling appearance of the ventricular walls, significant biatrial enlargement, and restrictive diastolic filling.
  - **Prognosis** is generally poor once amyloidosis affects the heart but depends on type of amyloidosis, with AL having the worst survival of < 6 months.
- **Cardiac sarcoidosis** occurs in 5% of sarcoid patients, and is characterized by patchy scar formation around infiltrating, noncaseating granulomas. Conduction system disease is also very common, and may present with essentially any rhythm disturbance, including SCD due to ventricular arrhythmias or high-degree AV block.
- **Hemochromatosis** results from increased deposition of iron in the heart, and can manifest as either systolic or diastolic dysfunction, as well as cardiac arrhythmia. During the initial phase of the cardiomyopathy, the hemodynamic profile represents a restrictive pattern, but as the severity advances, **dilated cardiomyopathy** ensues.
  - Diagnosis is suggested by elevated serum ferritin and transferring saturation of > 50%.
  - Cardiac MRI or biopsy of accessible organ (often the liver) are also useful modalities.
  - Extracardiac manifestations are present before cardiomyopathy develops, including diabetes, liver involvement, and skin discoloration.
- **Other etiologies of restrictive cardiomyopathy** include:
  - Gaucher's and Hurler's cardiomyopathy (rare glycogen storage diseases)
  - Hypereosinophilic syndrome
  - Idiopathic restrictive
  - Diabetic cardiomyopathy
  - Carcinoid heart disease

PERIPARTUM CARDIOMYOPATHY (PPCM)

- Defined as left ventricular systolic dysfunction diagnosed in the last month of pregnancy or within 5 months postpartum.
- Incidence varies by country suggesting a hereditary predisposition. In the United States, occurs in 1 in 3000 pregnancies.
- Etiology remains unclear. Postulated mechanisms with variable evidence include **viral** triggers, hormonal triggers (secondary to a

prolactin cleavage product), or **fetal microchimerism**, in which fetal cells escape into the maternal circulation and induce an autoimmune myocarditis.

- **Risk factors** include advanced maternal age, multiparity, preeclampsia and gestational hypertension, and African American race.
- **Clinical presentation** is usually with classic signs and symptoms of heart failure, including dyspnea, orthopnea, paroxysmal nocturnal dyspnea, and lower extremity edema. These symptoms are often attributed to late pregnancy making PPCM difficult to recognize. There may be a displaced apical impulse or new mitral regurgitation murmur on physical exam.
- Arrhythmia or sudden cardiac death can also occur.
- **Diagnosis** requires an echocardiogram demonstrating a depressed LV ejection fraction and LV dilatation.
  - On ECG, left ventricular hypertrophy or ST-T abnormalities may be seen.
- **Treatment** mainstay is preload and afterload reduction.
  - Afterload reduction: Hydralazine is used in the pregnant patient and ACE-inhibitors in the postpartum patient.
  - **Beta-blockers** are also used, preferably B1-selective (e.g., metoprolol) in order to avoid peripheral vasodilatation and uterine relaxation.
  - **Digoxin** is also safe during pregnancy and can be useful in these patients, though levels should be closely monitored.
  - **Diuretics** are used for fluid retention and symptom relief.
  - **Anticoagulation** is required in patients with thromboembolism with heparin during pregnancy followed by Coumadin after delivery. Some studies suggest that those with severely reduced ejection fraction (< 35%) should also be anti-coagulated due to the high risk of thromboembolism in these patients.
- **Prognosis** overall is better than other forms of cardiomyopathy, with most recovery occurring in the first 6 months. Women should be counseled about risk of subsequent pregnancies causing further deterioration in LV function, particularly those women who do not recover their LV function. In severe cases, PPCM can result in fulminant heart failure or even death.

15 ■ VALVULAR HEART DISEASE

INTRODUCTION

Generally speaking, valves can become dysfunctional in ways, **stenosis** and/or **regurgitation**. A mild degree of regurgitation is commonly seen in healthy individuals, thus we will define valvular disease as that which is conducive to symptoms or pathologic complications, such as myopathy, if left untreated.

Although each valve has its own predisposition to certain types of pathologies, there is a general recurrence of reasons why they become regurgitant or stenotic.

- **Stenosis** typically occurs due to:
  - Calcification (*e.g.*, calcific aortic stenosis)
  - Fibrosis (*e.g.*, rheumatic mitral stenosis)
  - Commonly, a combination of calcification and fibrosis is at work
- **Regurgitation** occurs due to:
  - Destruction of the valve (*e.g.*, infectious endocarditis)
  - Intrinsic problems with the valve tissue (*e.g.*, myxomatous degeneration)
  - Problems with the supporting structure of the valve (e.g., functional mitral regurgitation due to dilated cardiomyopathy)
  - A stiffened valve fixed in the open position (*e.g.*, carcinoid involvement of the tricuspid valve)
  - Rarely, high velocity jets under a valve can create a suction phenomenon (Venturi effect) and cause regurgitation (e.g., aortic regurgitation associated with a supracristal ventricular septal defect or mitral regurgitation in hypertrophic obstructive cardiomyopathy).

Symptoms of valvular heart disease are variable depending on the severity of disease, affected valve(s), type of lesion, acuteness of the lesion, presence of concomitant coronary obstruction, and state of the underlying myocardium. Some common symptoms include:

- Fatigue
- Generalized weakness
- Lack of energy
- Dyspnea
- Exercise intolerance
- Lightheadedness
- Syncope
- Angina
- Congestive heart failure

Specific presentations for each type of valvular pathology will be touched on with more detail in the subsequent sections.

The evaluation and treatment of valvular heart disease can at times be challenging as symptoms may be insidious and patients may adapt their lifestyles gradually, not perceive their own limitations, and classic signs and symptoms may not always be easily noted on clinical exam. Thus, a high index of suspicion must be maintained and occasionally stress testing may be indicated in patients with severe "asymptomatic" valvular heart disease.

Therapy for valvular heart disease remains mainly surgical. Recent advances in catheter-based therapies are, however, making the field a rapidly evolving one. The goal of the clinician should be to identify those patients who will derive a morbidity and/or mortality benefit from intervention.

- In general, the timing should be such that the patient benefits from the intervention prior to the development of irreversible complications, such as cardiomyopathy or arrhythmias.
- Conversely, some patients with severe valvular disease may be truly asymptomatic and stable for years, thus intervening prematurely could unnecessarily put them at risk from invasive procedures and complications from having a prosthetic valve.
- As surgical techniques continue to improve, risks become lower and repairs and replacements become less invasive and more durable, there is a trend toward intervening earlier.

AORTIC STENOSIS (AS)

- Etiology:
  - Calcific: usually occurring with age
  - Congenitally bicuspid: aortic stenosis tends to present at a younger age than calcific, though significant overlap exists
  - Less frequent causes include
    - Rheumatic
    - Post-radiation
    - Anorexigenic drug induced
    - Ochronosis (stiffening of valve tissue due to deposition of phenols, e.g., homogentisic acid)
- Physiology and natural history: AS is a lesion of pure afterload excess. It leads to progressive left ventricular hypertrophy. Patients with AS appear to have a survival curve that parallels that of age-matched patients up to the point that they become symptomatic. The median life expectancy once symptoms develop is between 2 and 5 years. If the stenosis is successfully relieved immediately at the onset of symptoms, survival normalizes to that expected for age-matched subjects.
  - Physical exam findings:
    - Loud and harsh or musical murmur. Typically best heard at the right upper sternal border and radiates to the carotids. The more severe the AS, the later the murmur peaks.
    - Aortic valve excursion is limited and thus the A2 component of the second heart sound is soft.

- An opening snap is suggestive of a bicuspid valve.
- *Pulsus parvus et tardus*: Carotid upstrokes are weak and delayed.
- Gallavardin phenomenon: The musical component of the murmur may be best heard at the apex.
- Criteria for *severe AS*: It is currently recommended that AS be diagnosed by echocardiography and that invasive catheterization be reserved for cases in which there is a discrepancy between the clinical scenario and echocardiographic findings. The following echocardiographic criteria are used to define AS:
  - Valve area < 1 cm^2
  - Mean transvalvular pressure gradient > 40 mmHg
  - Peak instantaneous transvalvular gradient > 64 mmHg (peak Doppler velocity > 4 m/s)
- Symptoms/presentation: three cardinal symptoms
  - **Angina** occurs due to the increased demand of the hypertrophied myocardium as well as increased left ventricular pressures.
    - Approximately 50% of patients with AS will have concomitant significant coronary artery disease.
  - **Syncope** is classically exertional.
  - **Congestive heart failure (CHF)** is perhaps the most difficult to assess clinically.
    - Insidious onset
    - Gradually decreased activity level due to decreased exercise tolerance may mask CHF symptoms.
    - Fatigue is often attributed to aging.
- Criteria for valve replacement:
  - Symptomatic severe AS.
  - Asymptomatic severe AS with EF < 50%.
  - Reasonable in asymptomatic severe AS patients with abnormal treadmill exercise stress test, severely calcified valve or very high gradients and low surgical risk.
  - Moderate to severe AS when patient undergoing other cardiac surgery.
- Therapeutic options:
  - **Balloon aortic valvuloplasty** results in a mild reduction in the transvalvular gradient that generally deteriorates within several months. It is occasionally an option for younger patients with congenital AS but it is not a durable therapy for most adults with AS. Valvuloplasty may be considered as a temporary bridge to get a patient over a noncardiac surgical procedure or until more definitive therapy can be provided.
  - **Surgical aortic valve replacement (AVR)** remains the gold standard. The morbidity and mortality of surgical AVR has improved significantly over the years. Surgically implanted valves are either *mechanical* or *bioprosthetic*.
    - Mechanical valves are generally thought to be more durable but require lifelong anticoagulation.

- ○ Bioprosthetic valves spare the need for anticoagulation but are generally thought to be less durable (though modern bioprosthetic valves appear to be achieving better longevity than their predecessors).
- **Transcatheter aortic valve implantation (TAVI)** is a novel approach by which a valve is mounted in a stent and is deployed inside the native valve, crushing the native calcified stenotic valve open with a balloon inflation and leaving the stented valve in its position. The calcified native valve serves as a scaffolding to hold the stent in a secure and stable position. Recent data demonstrates TAVI to be a feasible procedure with significant mortality benefit in patients that are not eligible for surgical AVR. The role of TAVI in high-, intermediate-, and low-risk surgical candidates remains to be established.
- Special situations in AS:
  - ○ **Stress testing**
    - ○ *Symptomatic AS*: Stress testing is contraindicated in patients with symptomatic AS.
    - ○ *Asymptomatic AS*: It is reasonable to perform treadmill exercise stress testing in patients with severe *asymptomatic* AS in order to objectively evaluate exercise capacity as well as to objectively follow them over time.
      - Failure to increase or a decrease in blood pressure with exercise, ST segment depressions, and a reduced exercise capacity are poor prognostic findings during a stress test.
        - A drop in blood pressure or development of ST depressions should lead to immediate termination of the test.
  - ○ **Bicuspid aortic valve (BAV):** BAV is not just a valvular disease, but also a disease of the aorta. All patients with BAV should have evaluation of their aortas for coarctation and aneurysms. A lower threshold of a 4.5 cm diameter should be considered for aortic root replacement at the time of valvular surgery.
  - ○ **AS with low ejection fraction (EF):** Patients with low EF and AS occasionally pose a clinical dilemma. The diseased myocardium may not generate enough force to create a substantial gradient; thus the patient will have severe AS with low gradients. Alternatively, the patient may have a moderately stenotic valve but due to the myopathy may not be able to generate enough force to open the valve fully, thus having a reduced valve area, *pseudo-severe AS*. Patients with pseudo-severe AS are high-risk surgical candidates (due to their severe myopathy) and AVR may not alleviate their symptoms. Thus, caution must be taken when evaluating this population of patients.
    - ○ **Dobutamine echocardiography:** Stimulating contractility with dobutamine is a useful tool in distinguishing low-gradient severe AS from pseudo-severe AS. When contractility is enhanced:
      - Low-gradient severe AS patients will have an increase in the gradient and the calculated valve area will remain less than 1 cm^2.

- Pseudo-severe AS patients will have no or a small increase in the gradient and the calculated valve area will increase to more than 1 cm^2.
- Another useful bit of information obtained from dobutamine echocardiography is the presence or absence of **contractile reserve**, defined as a $\geq 20\%$ increase in stroke volume with dobutamine administration. Patients with contractile reserve have a more favorable prognosis with surgery than those without. It was previously thought that patients without contractile reserve should not be considered surgical candidates, however recent data suggest that though they have a high perioperative mortality, the ones who survive have a better prognosis than those medically treated. Thus, surgery (or possibly TAVI) should not automatically be disregarded in those without reserve.

- **Low-gradient severe AS with normal EF:** Sometimes referred to as *paradoxical low-gradient AS*. This situation is generally thought to arise in patients with an exaggerated hypertrophic response and a small LV cavity. Due to the reduced volume of the LV cavity, stroke volume is reduced despite a normal EF. Because stroke volume is low, the generated gradient is low, even in the presence of a severely narrowed valve. Paradoxical low gradient AS poses a therapeutic dilemma because replacing the valve does not result in much relief of a pressure gradient, making the intervention questionable. That said, it is likely that if the valve can be replaced with a more functional one (hopefully with a larger effective orifice area and lesser gradient), the driving force for the hypertrophic response will have been removed, allowing the ventricle the opportunity to beneficially remodel. The role of AVR and TAVI in this patient population remains an area of active investigation.

AORTIC REGURGITATION (AR) OR AORTIC INSUFFICIENCY (AI)

- Etiology: Aortic regurgitation (AR) can be a disease of the aortic valve, aorta, or a combination. The etiology and presentation of AR varies greatly depending on the rapidity with which it develops. AR is therefore generally classified as acute or chronic.
  - **Acute**
    - Infective endocarditis
    - Ascending aortic dissection
    - Trauma
  - **Chronic**
    - Bicuspid aortic valve (BAV) (with or without aortic dilatation)
    - Aortic dilatation/aortopathies
    - Myxomatous degeneration of the AV
    - Associated with AS from any cause
    - Connective tissue disorders

- ○ Collagen vascular diseases
- ○ Long-standing hypertension
- ○ Supracristal ventricular septal defect with aortic valve prolapse
- ○ Secondary phenomenon in subvalvular AS
- Physiology and natural history:
  - **Acute:** Acute severe AR generally presents with pulmonary edema and/or cardiogenic shock. The left ventricle has not had the opportunity to remodel and compensate for the regurgitant volume and therefore forward stroke volume is reduced and left ventricular end diastolic pressure is markedly increased (can equal systemic diastolic pressure if AR is severe enough). Acute severe AR is generally considered a surgical urgency/emergency.
  - **Chronic:** In chronic AR the ventricle compensates for the regurgitant volume by dilation (increased preload) and *eccentric hypertrophy*. The ventricular dilatation results in increased wall stress (increased afterload) and is compensated by eccentric hypertrophy (LaPlace's Law: Wall stress is directly proportional to radius and inversely proportional to thickness). AR is therefore a mixed hemodynamic lesion of both increased preload and afterload resulting in a combination of eccentric and concentric hypertrophy of the LV. Increased preload with a relatively normalized afterload result in an exaggerated stroke volume (to compensate for the regurgitant volume). Over time these mechanisms fail to compensate (afterload mismatch) and the diastolic pressure in the left ventricle and atrium begin to increase. Asymptomatic patients with chronic severe AR and normal LV function may remain stable for many years. However, patients with asymptomatic chronic severe AR with depressed LV function will become symptomatic at a rate of more than 25% per year. Symptomatic patients with severe AR have a mortality of greater than 10% per year.
- Physical exam findings:
  - **Acute**
    - ○ Shocky (cool and clammy) due to low effective forward stroke volume.
    - ○ Tachycardia (in order to try to maintain cardiac output with low stroke volume).
    - ○ **Short diastolic murmur** (frequently inaudible) due to rapid equalization of aortic diastolic and ventricular pressures.
    - ○ Pulse pressure will *not* be increased as there will not have been time for LV to remodel.
    - ○ Rales/pulmonary edema.
    - ○ Other findings suggestive of endocarditis or dissection.
  - **Chronic**
    - ○ Laterally displaced point of maximal impulse due to cardiomegaly.
    - ○ Diastolic decrescendo murmur best heard at the left sternal border during held-end expiration with patient leaning forward. If heard best at right sternal border, suspect aortic dilatation.

- Murmur duration, not intensity, correlates with severity.
- Systolic ejection murmur due to increased stroke volume through a functionally narrow AV annulus.
- Apical diastolic rumble due to functionally impaired opening of the anterior mitral leaflet (Austin Flint murmur).
- S3 due to volume overload.
- Wide pulse pressure (exaggerated stroke volume leads to elevated systolic pressure and regurgitation leads to a lower diastolic pressure). Wide pulse pressure results in a variety of eponymous signs, mainly of anecdotal interest. These a few:
  - Watson's water hammer (peripheral) pulse
  - Corrigan's (carotid) pulse
  - de Musset's sign: head bobbing with the pulse
  - Traube's sign (also termed "pistol shot pulse"): systolic sound over the femoral artery
  - Duroziez's sign: systolic and diastolic bruit over the femoral artery when compressed slightly with the stethoscope
  - Quincke's sign: pulsations in the capillaries of the nail bed
  - Müller's sign: pulsation of the uvula
  - Rosenbach's sign: pulsation of the liver
  - Shelly's sign: pulsation of the cervix

- Criteria for *severe* AR: These are generally divided into qualitative and quantitative. It is recommended that an integrated approach using both qualitative and quantitative measurements be used. For chronic severe AR, the LV should be enlarged. Criteria for severe acute AR may be more subtle than for chronic. AR is considered severe angiographically when it is 3–4+. The following criteria define severe AR by echocardiographic methods:
  - **Qualitative**
    - Color Doppler regurgitant jet > 60% of the LV outflow tract diameter
    - Vena contracta width > 6 mm
    - Holodiastolic flow reversal in the aorta (more specific if noted in the abdominal aorta)
    - Dense continuous wave Doppler jet
    - Presystolic opening of the AV
    - Diastolic MR
  - **Quantitative**
    - Regurgitant volume > 60 mL/beat
    - Regurgitant fraction > 50%
    - AR pressure half time < 250 ms
    - AR effective orifice area greater than 0.3 cm^2

- Symptoms/presentation depend on the rapidity of development of AR. Acute AR will present with symptoms of CHR, pulmonary edema, and/or cardiogenic shock. Severe AR in the decompensated phase will generally present with decreased exercise tolerance, congestive heart failure, and/or angina.

- Criteria to replace valve:
  - Severe symptomatic AR regardless of the EF
  - Asymptomatic severe AR with depressed EF or marked LV dilatation:
    - EF < 50%.
    - LV end diastolic dimension > 75 mm
    - LV end systolic dimension > 55 mm
  - Asymptomatic moderate to severe AR undergoing another cardiac or aortic surgery.
- Therapeutic options:
  - **Valve replacement:** The choice of mechanical or bioprosthetic valve is made by the patient and surgeon, taking into account factors such as the patient's age and candidacy or desire to take long-term anticoagulants.
  - **Vasodilator therapy:** Treatment with afterload-reducing agents (e.g., nifedipine, ACE inhibitors) with hopes of increasing effective forward stroke volume has been studied and there is no definitive data that their use delays symptom onset or development of LV dysfunction. It is therefore currently recommended to use chronic vasodilator therapy only in the following situations:
    - Symptomatic severe AR who *are not* surgical candidates
    - Symptomatic patients in order to improve hemodynamics in preparation for AVR
    - Asymptomatic patients with normal EF but evidence of LV dilatation
    - Treatment of hypertension in patients with AR
  - **Intra-aortic balloon counterpulsation devices are contraindicated in severe AR** as they will augment diastolic pressure, which in turn results in increased LV diastolic pressure.

MITRAL STENOSIS (MS)

- Etiology: The predominant etiology of mitral stenosis (MS) remains rheumatic. Calcific MS is less common. Rare causes include infiltrative diseases, anorectic drugs, or rheumatologic diseases. Occasionally masses, a membrane (cor triatriatum), vegetations, or thrombi can cause a functional obstruction of the LV inflow.
- Physiology and natural history: Impaired emptying of the LA lead to increased LA pressure, which in turn causes pulmonary hypertension and right-sided heart failure. The LV is protected in cases of pure MS. LA emptying and dissipation of the transvalvular gradient are heavily dependent on diastolic emptying time and cardiac output. Thus conditions that decrease diastolic filling time (e.g., tachycardia) or increase cardiac output (e.g., pregnancy) will lead to elevated LA pressure and may cause decompensation.
  - Rheumatic MS is a disease that progresses over decades with asymptomatic or minimally symptomatic patients having an excellent

10-year prognosis without treatment. Moderate to severe symptoms, arrhythmias (atrial fibrillation), and pulmonary hypertension are markers of more advanced disease and a worse prognosis.

- Physical exam findings:
  - Mid-diastolic rumbling murmur with presystolic accentuation. Best heard at the apex with the bell.
  - In rheumatic MS, abrupt tensing of the tented valves after opening leads to an *opening snap (OS)*. The more severe the MS and higher LA pressure the faster the OS will occur in diastole, therefore the time from aortic valve closure to OS (A2-OS time) is inversely proportional to MS severity (more severe MS has shorter A2-OS time).
  - Findings of pulmonary hypertension (loud P2, RV heave, PA tap) and right heart failure (increased JVP, hepatomegaly, edema).
  - Classic ECG with RVH and left atrial or biatrial enlargement.
- Criteria for *severe* MS:
  - Echocardiography is the gold standard as it can determine MS severity and etiology.
  - Valve area < 1 cm². Usually determined by:
    - Direct planimetry (best with 3D echocardiography)
    - Formula: Valve area = 220/pressure half time
  - Mean gradient > 10 mmHg (highly dependent on HR and output state)
- Symptoms/presentation: Symptoms typically progress slowly over decades after a prolonged latent asymptomatic period. Increased LA pressure will lead to symptoms of heart failure (dyspnea, decreased exercise tolerance, edema). Atrial fibrillation is common and may present with palpitations; a rapid ventricular response may lead to abrupt decompensation and pulmonary edema. Increased venous pressure in the lungs may lead to venous rupture and hemoptysis. Systemic emboli due to atrial fibrillation or other atrial thrombi.
- Therapeutic options:
  - **Percutaneous mitral balloon valvotomy (PMBV):** Rheumatic MS is characterized by fusion at the valve commissures and therefore certain patients are candidates for PMBV. Candidates for PMBV must have pliable leaflets without much calcium so that the valvotomy results in commissural splitting without significant MR. PMBV *should not* be performed in patients with calcific MS, LA thrombi, or moderate to severe MR. An echocardiographic score (Wilkins score) based on leaflet mobility, thickness, calcification, and subvalvular thickening is frequently used to determine candidacy for PMBV. In appropriate candidates, PMBV carries a low morbidity with a high success rate and durability.
  - **Surgical replacement** with mechanical or bioprosthetic valve choice depending on patient age, characteristics, preference, and candidacy for anticoagulation.
  - **Medical therapy** should aim at relieving heart failure symptoms (diuretics) and avoiding conditions that lead to unfavorable

hemodynamics like tachycardia (beta-blockers) or high output states (avoid anemia, caution with pregnancy).
  ○ Anticoagulation is indicatin ed patients with atrial fibrillation, known LA thrombus or systemic emboli (even if no documented arrhythmia). In cases of rheumatic MS, appropriate antibiotic prophylaxis should be given as indicated.
- Criteria for valvular intervention in MS depend on the patient's candidacy for PMBV. Patients who are candidates for PMBV are generally thought to be candidates for intervention earlier than those who are not (because of the slow rate of disease progression and higher morbidity of surgery).
  - **Percutaneous Mitral Balloon Valvotomy (PMBV)**
    ○ NYHA Class II–IV heart failure symptoms.
    ○ Asymptomatic patients with pulmonary hypertension (PASP > 50 mmHg at rest or > 60 mmHg with exercise)
  - **Surgical**
    ○ NYHA Class III or IV patients not eligible for PMBV (e.g., unfavorable anatomy, significant MR, LA thrombus)
    ○ NYHA Class III or IV when PMBV is not available
- Special situations:
  - **Atrial fibrillation/flutter:** Atrial fibrillation or flutter is common in patients with MS. Patients with rapid ventricular responses may present with palpitations or with a **rapid decompensation and pulmonary edema** (due to decreased diastolic filling time from tachycardia and loss of adequate atrial contraction). Tachycardia should be avoided. Some patients may not tolerate atrial fibrillation even when the ventricular rate is controlled, in which case efforts should be made to maintain sinus rhythm. Maintenance of sinus rhythm may be difficult in these patients and thus this may lead to consideration for intervention on the valve.
    ○ Atrial fibrillation with MS carries a **high risk of embolic events** and patients should therefore be fully anticoagulated.
  - **Symptomatic patient with "moderate" MS:** Occasionally patients will report severe limitations in exercise performance but only moderate MS on echocardiography. These patients should have exercise testing with measurement of the transmitral gradient and PASP with exercise. The tachycardic response of exercise may lead to severely elevated gradients and severe pulmonary hypertension. These patients may be treated with beta-blockers or may need intervention on their valves if the abnormalities are severe enough.

MITRAL REGURGITATION (MR)

- Etiology: As with AR, the etiology, presentation, and treatment of mitral regurgitation (MR) will vary greatly depending on the chronicity of the lesion. Acute MR should therefore be distinguished from chronic MR.

The etiology of MR may be due to leaflet problems or ventricular problems (such as dilatation or alterations in the normal ventricular geometry).

- **Acute**
  - Infective endocarditis
  - Ischemia (due to a hypokinetic or akinetic wall with tethering of the valve leaflet in the acute setting; may go on to become chronic "ischemic" or post-infarction MR)
  - Papillary muscle (typically the posteromedial) rupture as a mechanical complication of myocardial infarction
  - Acute rupture of chordae tendineae (typically in valves with myxomatous degeneration)
- **Chronic**
  - Myxomatous degeneration or mitral valve prolapse syndrome (Barlow's disease is the extreme case where there is severe bileaflet prolapse with annular dilatation)
  - Functional, due to annular dilatation (as seen in dilated cardiomyopathy)
  - Functional "ischemic" MR (typically due to inferior infarction with basal posterior akinesis and displacement of the papillary muscle as well as annular dilatation leading to tethering and incomplete coaptation of the posterior mitral leaflet). The term *papillary muscle dysfunction* is also occasionally used to describe functional ischemic MR.
  - Any cause of acute MR may cause chronic MR
  - Rheumatic
  - Congenital (cleft valve associated with cushion defects)
  - Associated with MS
  - Connective tissue diseases
  - Collagen vascular disease (lupus with Liebman-Sacks endocarditis)
  - Associated with hypertrophic cardiomyopathy (can be due to either abnormal leaflet anatomy and/or Venturi effect suctioning the anterior leaflet towards the LV outflow)
- Physiology and natural history:
  - **Acute:** In acute severe MR the left atrium (LA) has not had time to dilate and is relatively noncompliant. LA pressure therefore rises rapidly and dramatically and results in pulmonary congestion and edema. The LV has also not had time to dilate and therefore end diastolic volume is limited. Forward stroke volume (and in turn cardiac output) is limited by the volume regurgitated into the LA; cardiogenic shock may ensue. The prognosis is typically poor unless the underlying cause is addressed. Patients who are left untreated and survive will proceed to chronic MR.
  - **Chronic:** In chronic severe MR the LA dilates and becomes more compliant and LA pressure is not as increased as in the acute setting. Chronic MR is a state in which the LV sees an increased preload (from the regurgitant volume coming back to the LV in diastole), as

well as decreased afterload (as the LV can pump blood into the aorta
and the LA). Both the increased preload and decreased afterload
lead to an exaggerated ejection fraction (EF), despite the decrease
in effective forward stroke volume. Patients may develop LV dysfunction prior to having symptoms and may have irreversible LV dysfunction if surgery is postponed until the time of symptom onset. It is key
to understand that the LV may be dysfunctional despite a "normal"
EF as MR leads to an exaggerated EF (due to increased preload and
reduced afterload). Therefore, an EF of < 60% is considered abnormally low in severe MR. The natural history is variable depending on
the etiology of the MR. Patients with mitral valve prolapse without
regurgitation may live their normal lifespans without developing
MR. A relative minority of these patients will develop progressive
MR leading to severe MR. Once severe MR develops, patients may
continue to be asymptomatic for several years, but the vast majority
will have a complication or need surgery over the next 10 years. The
prognosis of functional MR is tied to the prognosis of the underlying
cardiomyopathy and is therefore generally worse than that of mitral
prolapse. In general, the prognosis of the patient with functional MR
is worse than that of a patient with a similar degree of LV dysfunction
without MR. This is, at least in part, presumably because MR leads to
continued progressive unfavorable ventricular remodeling, which in
turn leads to more MR ("MR begets MR").

- Physical exam findings:
  - **Acute:** The patient will be uncomfortable, tachycardic, tachypneic,
    and possibly frankly hypoxic.
    ○ Findings of crackles suggestive of pulmonary edema.
    ○ The skin may be cool and clammy due to poor forward flow and
      hypotension may be present.
    ○ The **murmur of acute MR may be soft, short, or even absent**
      because the rapid elevation of LA pressure will lead to loss of a
      pressure gradient between the LA and LV during systole.
  - **Chronic**
    ○ Holosystolic murmur best heard at the apex
    ○ Radiation of the murmur will depend on the direction of the MR:
      ■ Classically to the axilla
      ■ Anterior radiation in posterior leaflet prolapse
      ■ Posterior radiation (to the back) in anterior leaflet prolapse
    ○ Mid-systolic click in cases of prolapse
    ○ S3 due to volume overload
    ○ Early diastolic flow with rumbling murmur is indicative of a large
      regurgitant volume returning to the LV and is a sign of severe
      MR.
    ○ Lateral displacement of the point of maximal impact due to LV
      dilatation
    ○ Loud P2 may indicate the presence of pulmonary hypertension.
    ○ Signs of CHF (crackles, increased jugular veins, edema)

- **Criteria for _severe_ MR:** As with AR, these are generally divided into qualitative and quantitative. It is recommended that an integrated approach using both qualitative and quantitative measurements be used. For chronic severe MR the LA and LV should be dilated. Criteria for severe acute MR may be more subtle than for chronic as there is rapid loss of systolic pressure gradient between the LA and LV. MR is considered severe angiographically when it is 3–4+. The following criteria define severe MR by echocardiographic methods:
  - **Qualitative**
    - Color Doppler MR jet area > 40% LA area
    - Vena contracta width > 7 mm
    - Pulmonary vein systolic flow reversal
    - Dense, continuous-wave Doppler jet
  - **Quantitative**
    - Regurgitant volume > 60 mL/beat
    - Regurgitant fraction > 50%
    - MR effective orifice area > 0.4 cm^2
    - In ischemic MR, a lower threshold of 0.2 cm^2 is used to define it as severe.
- **Symptoms/presentation:**
  - **Acute MR:** Acute MR is generally tolerated poorly and is frequently a surgical urgency or emergency. Patients develop respiratory distress from pulmonary edema and may need intubation and mechanical ventilation. There is a tachycardic response secondary to the reduced stroke volume. Significant hypotension may develop.
  - **Chronic MR:** When MR is developed gradually over time the patient may be asymptomatic even despite the presence of severe regurgitation. As ventricular dysfunction ensues, the ability to compensate becomes impaired and patients will develop progressive symptoms of congestive heart failure. Chronic MR is a risk factor for development of atrial fibrillation, which may be the presenting symptom, typically manifesting as palpitations. Patients with mitral valve prolapse syndrome also tend to have concomitant chest pains and palpitations, independently of the severity of MR. Premature atrial and ventricular contractions are common in these patients.
- **Treatment and criteria for valve replacement or repair:** Surgical advances have greatly improved the morbidity and mortality of mitral valve surgery. That, combined with the fact that patients may have irreversible LV dysfunction at the time of symptom onset has led toward a trend to operate sooner on patients with MR. Repair, as opposed to replacement, has lower perioperative and long-term morbidity and mortality with excellent long-term results. This has led to repair being the preferred option whenever possible. The role of surgery is better established for patients with disease due to primary valve dysfunction, such as myxomatous degeneration or endocarditis, than it is for patients with functional MR due to ventricular problems. In patients with ischemic MR, a combination of revascularization and annuloplasty

is generally employed. Patients with functional MR due to dilated cardiomyopathy appear to have improved symptoms and quality of life with surgery, but no mortality benefit. Patients with atrial fibrillation may undergo a concomitant MAZE procedure at the time of their valvular surgery. Patients with severe LV dysfunction (regardless of the etiology of the MR) have a worse prognosis and higher perioperative mortality, therefore the indications for surgery in this population are more conservative than in those with normal or mild LV dysfunction. The following are indications for surgery for MR:

- Symptomatic acute severe MR
- Symptomatic chronic severe MR with EF > 30%
- Asymptomatic patient with EF < 60% or LV end systolic diameter > 40 mm when expected repair success rate is 90% or greater
- Asymptomatic chronic severe MR with normal EF with new onset atrial fibrillation or pulmonary hypertension (> 50 mmHg at rest or > 60 mmHg with exercise)
- Reasonable to consider repair in patients with severe LV dysfunction (EF < 30%, end systolic diameter > 55 mm) with NYHA class III–IV symptoms despite maximal medical therapy (including biventricular pacing).

- **Nonsurgical therapeutic options:**
  - **Acute MR:** Acute MR is frequently a surgical urgency or emergency. Afterload reduction with nitroprusside may reduce the regurgitant volume and increase forward flow. An intra-aortic balloon counterpulsation device may be placed for further afterload reduction and hemodynamic support. These measures generally serve as a bridge to surgical treatment. Cardiac output in acute MR is dependent on heart rate due to a decreased stroke volume, therefore treating tachycardia may lead to a drop in cardiac output.
  - **Chronic MR:** No medical therapy is currently known to prevent disease progression in MR. The roles of beta-blockers and ACE-inhibitors in prevention of ventricular dysfunction are being studied. Patients with LV dysfunction should be treated for their cardiomyopathy with standard therapy including ACE-inhibitors and beta-blockers and considered for ventricular resynchronization therapy with biventricular pacemakers when appropriate.
  - **Percutaneous therapy:** The role, feasibility, and efficacy of multiple percutaneous approaches to treat MR is actively being investigated. These include procedures such as clipping together of the mitral leaflets, devices aimed at reducing the annular diameter (typically placed in the coronary sinus), and devices aimed at altering the geometry of the ventricle such as balloons inflated within the pericardium.
- **Special situations:**
  - **Asymptomatic severe MR:** Patients may not endorse symptoms of MR due to a gradual adjustment in their lifestyles with a progressively more sedentary lifestyle (typically attributed to aging). Careful history taking is key. Treadmill exercise stress testing may be used

to objectively gauge the patient's functional capacity. The addition of echocardiography should be considered in order to assess for the presence of exercise-induced pulmonary hypertension (> 60 mmHg with exercise).

- **Symptomatic patient with mild to moderate MR:** Identifying severe MR may occasionally be challenging, particularly in cases of eccentric regurgitant jets. Thus, if the physical exam findings (e.g., an early diastolic flow murmur is present) or the patient's symptoms are more severe than the observed valve lesion, further testing should be performed with transesophageal echocardiography, left ventricular angiography, or cardiac MRI. If the MR severity is still discordant with the symptoms, then alternative diagnoses such as concomitant CAD should be considered.

TRICUSPID REGURGITATION

- Etiology: Mild tricuspid regurgitation (TR) is present in the majority of the population. Pathologic degrees of TR are most frequently due to right ventricular and annular dilatation and right ventricular failure (most commonly secondary to LV failure or pulmonary hypertension). Diseases that primarily involve the valve include:
  - Endocarditis (most commonly in IV drug users)
  - Carcinoid (fixed valve in open position may cause concomitant stenosis)
  - Iatrogenic (e.g., pacemaker leads, trauma from biopsies)
  - Trauma (blunt chest trauma may lead to rupture and avulsion of the anterior tricuspid leaflet)
  - Tricuspid prolapse is infrequently described but may be present in conditions such as Marfan's syndrome.
- Physiology and natural history: Severe TR leads to volume overload of the RV and RV dilatation. In the absence of pulmonary hypertension, severe TR may be well tolerated for many years. Patients with severe TR and pulmonary hypertension typically develop right-sided congestion due to elevated RA and central venous pressure, resulting in peripheral edema or anasarca, and may develop cardiac cirrhosis.
- Physical exam findings:
  - Holosystolic murmur best heard at the left lower sternal border that increases with inspiration
  - Dilated jugular veins with prominent V-wave
  - Hepatomegaly with a pulsatile liver
  - Peripheral edema due to right-sided heart failure
- Criteria for *severe* TR: The following echocardiographic findings suggest severe TR:
  - TR jet area > 10 cm^2
  - TR vena contracta > 0.7 cm
  - Hepatic vein Doppler systolic flow reversal

- Dilated RA and RV
- Dense, triangular shaped, early peaking Doppler jet (indicative of rapid pressure equalization between RV and RA)
- Symptoms/presentation: Symptomatic patients will usually develop progressive edema or anasarca. Signs of hepatic dysfunction such as jaundice, encephalopathy, or coagulopathy may develop. The forward output of the RV may be impaired, particularly in the setting of pulmonary hypertension, and may limit cardiac output, leading to fatigue and exercise intolerance.
- Criteria to repair or replace valve: The role, outcomes, and durability of isolated tricuspid valve surgery is less well established than that of aortic or mitral valve surgery. Annuloplasty rings are preferred to replacement and when valve surgery is required. Bioprosthetic valves are preferred because mechanical valves have a higher risk of thrombosis (presumably due to low pressures in the right-sided chambers). Indications for surgery include:
  - Severe TR at the time of mitral surgery
  - Severe symptomatic primary TR
- Therapeutic options: Medical treatment generally consists of diuretics and treatment of concomitant left-sided heart failure or pulmonary hypertension with afterload-reducing agents and pulmonary vasodilators as indicated.

Tricuspid stenosis, pulmonic stenosis, and pulmonic regurgitation: These conditions are less frequently encountered by the general cardiologist.

- Tricuspid and pulmonic stenosis are generally congenital in etiology.
- Carcinoid syndrome leads to the tricuspid and pulmonic valves being fixed in an open position leading to varying degrees of combined stenosis and regurgitation.
- Pulmonic regurgitation is typically congenital (or following interventions for congenital disease), or may be seen in the presence of pulmonary hypertension.

16 ■ INFECTIOUS ENDOCARDITIS[39,40]

Infective endocarditis (IE) is infection of endothelium of the heart, typically on a valve leaflet. The primary lesion is a **vegetation**—organized thrombus colonized by microbial pathogens. The bacteria are relatively protected within the vegetation, making sterilization of the vegetation difficult. Cure of IE usually requires a long course of parenteral antibiotics. Removal of infected foreign bodies is usually required to achieve cure.

- Acute bacterial endocarditis (ABE) progresses over days, caused by aggressive organisms (e.g., *Staphylococcus aureus*).
  - Subacute bacterial endocarditis (SBE) is typically caused by less virulent organisms such as viridans streptococci
  - Prosthetic valve endocarditis (PVE) is infection of a replacement valve (bioprosthetic or mechanical).
    - Infection of other endocardial foreign bodies (e.g., pacemaker, ICD leads) has implications similar to PVE.

Pathogenesis of Infective Endocarditis

IE most commonly occurs in the setting of an existing valvular lesion or other predisposition. Potential predispositions include:

- Prosthetic heart valve
- Previous IE
- Congenital heart disease
- Mitral regurgitation (with or without mitral valve prolapse)
- Patent ductus arteriosus
- Ventricular septal defect
- Aortic coarctation
- Mitral stenosis
- Tricuspid valve disease
- Pulmonic valve disease

Typically, these lesions are disruptions of the valvular (or other) endothelium, prompting platelet activation and deposition of fibrin and platelets to form a noninfective thrombus, which then may be colonized during an episode of bacteremia. Bacteremia leading to IE is more likely in several settings:

- IV drug abuse
- Poor dentition
- Immunosuppression, including HIV
- Pregnancy and the puerperium
- Hemodialysis
- Indwelling central venous lines, especially if they reach the right atrium

ORGANISMS MOST COMMONLY CAUSING ENDOCARDITIS

- Streptococci
  - Alpha-hemolytic (viridans) streptococci are historically among the most common pathogen, though the proportion has been decreasing. There are multiple viridans *Streptococcus* species (with frequently changing names and classification)
    - *S. sanquis*
    - *S. mitis*
    - *S. oralis*
    - *S. gordonii*
  - Group D streptococci
    - *S. bovis* is highly associated with colon cancer and other GI lesions.
  - *Enterococcus faecalis*
    - May be associated with urinary tract disease
    - Common in drug addicts
  - *S. pneumoniae* (pneumococcus) usually affects the aortic valve.
  - Beta-homylitc streptococci are rare cause of IE.
- Staphylococci
  - *S. aureus* is most common cause of acute bacterial endocarditis
    - High mortality and morbidity
      - Embolic complications
      - Valve destruction
      - Local invasion
        - Abscess may affect the conduction system with progressive AV block.
  - *S. epidermidis* is a rare cause of native valve endocarditis, but it causes 40–50% of prosthetic valve endocarditis.
- Gram-negative bacteria are a relatively small contributor to IE
  - The HACEK group:
    - *Heamophilus*
    - *Actinobacillus*
    - *Cardiobacterium hominis*
    - *Eikenella corrodens*
    - *Kingella kingae*
  - Other Gram-negative bacteria are rare but more likely in prosthetic valve endocarditis. Most common are:
    - *Pseudomonas*
    - *Serratia*
    - *Enterobacter*
- Yeasts/Fungi
  - Mostly Candida and Aspergillus, often with prosthetic valves
- Other
  - Coxiella burnetti, the organism of Q fever
  - Bartonella
  - Chlamydia

- Culture-negative endocarditis
  - Most commonly culture negative due to suppressive anitbiotics
  - Slow-growing organisms such as HACEK
  - Difficult-to-culture organisms
    - Coxiella, Chlamydia, Mycoplasma, Bartonella, Legionella
    - Anaerobes
    - Aspergillus
  - Non-IE fever
    - Rheumatic fever, tuberculosis, malignancy
  - Non-infectious endocarditis
    - Libman-Sacks (anti-phospholipid antibody syndrome, systemic lupus erythematosus)

PRESENTATION AND CLINICAL MANIFESTATIONS

- **Signs and symptoms of infection**
  - Fevers, rigors, sweats, fatigue, malaise, weight loss
    - Symptoms may persist over many weeks in SBE.
  - New murmurs of valvular incompetence should raise suspicion.
  - Laboratory tests
    - Leukocytosis is common but lacks sensitvity and specificity.
    - Erythrocyte sedimentation rate (ESR), C-reactive protein (CRP) are usually elevated, but not diagnostic.
    - Blood cultures are the most important of tests, since bacteremia is nearly constant.
      - Previous antibiotic therapy may confound culturing.
      - As always, avoid skin contamination when drawing cultures.
      - Draw aerobic and anaerobic cultures.
    - Echo (ECG), transthoracic (TTE), and transesophageal (TEE) cardiograms have assumed an important role in diagnosis.
      - Valve lesions and valvular function can be assessed.
      - The composition of a lesion cannot be determined. A lesion must be regarded in the clinical context.
    - ECG is not diagnostic. However progressive conduction system disease (prolongation of the PR interval, development of a bundle branch, or fascicular block or AV block) in a patient with suspected endocarditis suggests abscess formation and extension in the myocardium. Surgery may be required.
- **Vascular lesions** of IE should always be sought in the physical examination of a patient with prolonged or unexplained fevers.
  - Petechiae
  - Splinter hemorrhages of the nails
  - Osler's nodes: on the pads of the fingers. Painful/tender, nodular.
  - Janeway lesions: ethyematous maculi on the palms and soles, not painful, not hemorrhagic. Blanch with pressure.

- Ocular lesions:
    - Roth spots: hemorrhagic retinal microinfarctions
    - Conjuctival and retinal hemorrhages
- **Complications**
    - Heart failure, often due to severe valve damage and sometimes requiring urgent surgery
    - Embolism to an extremity, coronary artery, brain, spleen, gut, eye
    - Destruction of conduction system
        - Progressive conduction system failure (even new PR prolongation) is suggestive of perivalvular abscess.
        - TEE is helpful to assess for abscess.
        - Surgery is often required
    - Central nervous system
        - Embolism/CVA
        - Toxic mental status changes
        - Meningitis/cerebritis
    - Mycotic aneurysm, may lead to hemorrhage

MODIFIED DUKE CRITERIA FOR DIAGNOSIS FOR INFECTIOUS ENDOCARDITIS[39]

- Major criteria
    - Microbiologic
        - Typical organism isolated from two separate blood cultures
            - *Viridans* streptococci, *S. bovis*, HACEK organisms, *S. aureus*
            - Community-acquired *enterococcus* without primary focus
        - Persistently isolated blood culture with appropriate organism
        - Single culture or phase 1 IgG Ab titer > 1:800 for *Coxiella burnetti*
    - Endocardial lesions
        - Discrete echogenic, oscillating intracardiac mass at site of endocardial injury, or
        - Periannular abscess, or
        - New dehiscence of a prosthetic valve.
- Minor criteria
    - Predisposing cardiac condition or injection drug use
        - Previous endocarditis, aortic valve disease, rheumatic heart disease, prosthetic valve, coarctation of the aorta, complex cyanotic congenital heart disease
        - Mitral valve prolapse with regurgitation or thickening, isolated mitral stenosis, tricuspid valve disease, pulmonary stenosis, hypertrophic cardiomyopathy
        - Secundum atrial septal defect, ischemic heart disease, previous coronary bypass surgery, mitral valve prolapse without thickening or regurgitation
        - Fever > 38°C

- ○ Vascular phenomena: arterial emboli, septic pulmonary infarct, mycotic aneurysm, intracranial hemorrhage, conjunctival hemorrhage, Janeway lesions
  - Not petechiae and splinter hemorrhages
- ○ Immunologic phenomena: glomerulonephritis, Osler's nodes, Roth spots, rheumatoid factor
- ○ Microbiologic findings not meeting major criteria:
  - Positive blood cultures not meeting major criteria, or
  - Serologic evidence of active infection with organisms consistent with endocarditis
    - But not single cultures of coagulase-negative Staph or organisms unlikely to cause endocarditis
- Definite diagnosis
  - 2 major criteria
  - 1 major criterion and 3 minor criteria
  - 5 minor criteria
- Possible diagnosis
  - 1 major criterion and 1 minor criterion
  - 3 minor criteria

THERAPY

Therapy for endocarditis is focused on elimination of bacteremia and sterilization of vegetations to prevent recrudescence. Four to six weeks of therapy is often required.

- Antibiotic choice is based on cultured organism and sensitivity.
- Emerging antibiotic resistance is an ongoing problem, frequently requiring double or triple antibiotic therapy.
- Empiric therapy may be necessary until the infectious organism is known.
  - Acute endocarditis therapy should cover *S. aureus*, streptococci, and some Gram-negative bacilli
    - ○ Nafcillin, ampicillin, and gentamicin. Vancomycin is substituted for nafcillin if it appears likely that methicillin-resistant *S. aureus* (MRSA) is present.
  - Subacute endocarditis therapy should cover strptrococci, including *E. faecalis*.
    - ○ Ampicillin and gentamicin
- Surgery should preferably precede hemodynamic deterioration or perivalvular extension, which worsen prognosis.
  - Major indications:
    - ○ Moderate to severe CHF
    - ○ Periannular/myocardial abscess
    - ○ Prosthetic valve dehiscence
    - ○ Persistent bacteremia despite appropriate antibiotics
    - ○ Fungal infection

- ○ Pacemaker or ICD leads endocarditis generally requires removal of the leads
  - ▪ The device pocket is also assumed infected and, after antibiotic therapy, contralateral device implantation is preferred.
- Relative indications
  - ○ Recurrent embolism
  - ○ Staphylococcal and Gram-negative bacillus infections, especially with prosthetic valve
  - ○ Enlarging vegetation despite antibiotics
  - ○ Endocarditis due to *Pseudomonas, Brucella, Coxiella burnetti,* and drug-resistant enterococci
  - ○ Prosthetic valve endocarditis

PROPHYLACTIC THERAPY

Traditionally prophylactic antibiotic therapy was used to prevent endocarditis in high-risk patients undergoing invasive procedures that might induce bacteremia leading to endocarditis. There is a dearth of evidence that prophylactically administered anitbiotics are effective at preventing endocarditis. Use of preventive antibiotics is not free of risk for the individual patient; unnecessary use contributes to the growing problem of antibiotic resistance. Therefore the American Heart Association (AHA) guidelines now recommend restriction of prophylactic therapy to patients with the *highest risk of adverse outcome from infectious endocarditis.* Many fewer people are recommended for IE prophylaxis than in the past.

- Prosthetic cardiac valve, or prosthetic material used for valve repair
- Previous infectious endocarditis
- Some forms of congenital heart disease (CHD; no longer recommended for other CHD)
  - Unrepaired cyanotic CHD, including the presence of palliative shunts/conduits
  - Completely repairied CHD with prosthetic material for the first 6 months after the procedure
  - Repaired CHD with residual defects at site or adjacent to a prosthetic valve or other prostetic device.
- Cardiac transplant patients who develop cardiac valvulopathy.

Therapy is also only recommended in the settings of:

- All dental procedures that involve manipulation of gingival tissue of the periapical region of teeth or penetration of the mucosa
- Invasive respiratory tract procedures involving incision or biopsy of respiratory tract mucosa (such as tonsillectomy/andenoidectomy)
  - For high-risk patients undergoing respiratory tract procedures to treat an established infection, such as drainage of an abscess (not prophylaxis), an antiobiotic active against the known/suspected organism should be used.

ANTIBIOTIC PROPHYLACTIC REGIMENS

Administered 30–60 minutes prior to the procedure
- Standard: amoxicillin 2 g PO
- Unable to take oral medications:
  - Ampicillin 2 g IV/IM, or
  - Cefazolin 1 g IV/IM, or
  - Ceftriaxone 1 g IV/IM
- Allergic to penicillin:
  - Clindamycin 600 mg PO, or
  - Cephalexin 2 g PO, or
  - Azithromycin 500 mg PO or clarithromycin 500 mg PO
- Allergic to penicillin and unable to take oral medications:
  - Clindamycin 600 mg IM/IV, OR
  - Cefazolin 1 g IV/IM (note some cross-reactivity between cephalosporins and penicillin), OR
  - Ceftriaxone 1 g IV/IM (note some cross-reactivity between cephalosporins and penicillin)

17 ■ BRADYARRHYTHMIAS

INTRODUCTION

Bradycardia is a ventricular rate (at rest) less than 50 bpm (cycle length 1200 ms). Some references use 60 bpm (cycle length 1000 ms) as the lower limit of normal. Bradycardia is not a disease in and of itself in the absence of symptoms. Trained athletes, especially endurance athletes, usually have resting bradycardia.

Symptoms of bradycardia are many and are nonspecific (meaning the symptom is not necessarily directly correlated to the bradycardia). The symptoms include: fatigue, generalized weakness, lack of energy, dyspnea, dyspnea on exertion, lightheadedness, presyncope, syncope.

Since all rhythm disturbances are either: *disorders of impulse formation*, or *disorders of impulse propagation*, the bradycardias can be readily classified by mechanism.

SINUS NODE DYSFUNCTION (BRADYCARDIC DISORDERS OF IMPULSE FORMATION)

Sinus node dysfunction, also called sick sinus syndrome (SSS), is defined as inadequate heart rate for the body's demands. There are several typical variants.

- Symptomatic sinus bradycardia at rest.
  - There may be an escape rhythm, most commonly a "junctional" rhythm, with a normal narrow QRS complex.
  - If the QRS of the escape is wider, it may arise more distally in the conduction system or it may still be junctional with *aberrant* conduction (such as a bundle branch block or fascicular block). The more distal the origin of the escape, the less reliable it is.
- *Chronotropic incompetence:* The resting sinus rate may be abnormally slow, with or without symptoms. The inability to accelerate in response to physiologic demand (especially exercise) is a variant of SSS.
- *Tachy-brady syndrome:* The patient experiences both tachycardia (e.g., atrial fibrillation with rapid ventricular rate), and bradycardia when in sinus rhythm (often limiting rate control therapy for the tachycardia). Classic variant: a long pause and/or profound bradycardia (possibly with syncope) when the tachycardia terminates.

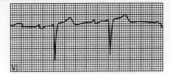

FIGURE 17-1 AV Block, 1°

AV CONDUCTION DISORDERS (BRADYCARDIC DISORDERS OF IMPULSE PROPAGATION)

Abnormal conduction from the atria to the ventricles. The defect is in the "AV junction," which is comprised of the compact AV node, the His bundle, and the proximal left and right bundles.

- AV Block is classified by the pattern of AV conduction seen on ECG:
  - First-degree AV block (NOT truly AV block) (**Figure 17-1**): prolongation of the PR interval beyond the upper limit of normal (200 ms).
  - Second-degree AV block: intermittent failure of A-V conduction:
    - Mobitz type 1 or Wenckebach block (**Figure 17-2**): a non-conducted P-wave after a series of conducted P-waves with varying PR intervals (almost always progressively lengthening). The lengthening may be subtle. The best way to assess it is to measure the PR immediately prior to a blocked beat and the PR immediately after a blocked beat. The latter should be shorter.
    - Mobitz type 2 block (**Figure 17-3**): Intermittent failure of AV conduction without variability in the PR of the conducted beats.
      - High-degree AV block: intermittent success of conduction rather than intermittent failure. If there are no consecutive conducted beats, there can be no variability of the PR.
        - High-degree block may be thought of as more advanced block than typical Mobitz type 2 block

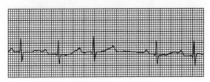

FIGURE 17-2 AV Block, 2°—Mobitz Type I (Wenckebach)

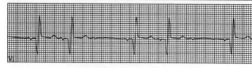

FIGURE 17-3 AV Block, 2°—Mobitz Type II

- ○ 2:1 AV block (**Figure 17-4**): Every other P-wave is conducted. 2:1 block is neither Mobitz 1 nor Mobitz 2 block (because consecutive PR intervals cannot be assessed).
- • Third-degree AV block (complete heart block) (**Figure 17-5**): There is no conduction from the atrial to the ventricles. Diagnosis of complete heart block essentially requires that the atrial rate is faster than the ventricular rate to ensure that normal physiologic refractoriness is not the reason for failure to conduct (e.g., failure of conduction from the atria to the ventricles during VT is not complete heart block).
- • Usually, first-degree AV block and Mobitz type 1 AV block are associated with parasympathetic activity, not irreversible structural disease. Mobitz type 2, high-degree, and complete heart block are typically associated with structural disease of the His-Purkinje system.
- • **2:1 AV block** may proceed from parasympathetic activity on the AV node or from progression of infranodal structural heart disease.
  - • **Assessing 2:1 AV block**
    - ○ Change the autonomic afferent:
      - ▪ Exercise or atropine: Speeds the sinus rate and increases AV nodal conduction (and shortens the AV node's refractory period).
        - ▪ If AV block improves (e.g., from 2:1 to 1:1), the block was probably intranodal.
        - ▪ If AV block worsens (e.g., from 2:1 to 3:1), the block is probably infranodal.

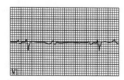

FIGURE 17-4 AV Block, 2:1

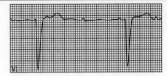

FIGURE 17-5 AV Block, 3°

- Carotid sinus massage or Valsalva: Slows the sinus rate and slows AV nodal conduction (and prolongs the AV node's refractory period).
  - If the AV block improves, the block was probably infranodal.
  - If the AV block worsens, the block was probably intranodal.

THERAPY

- **Urgent short-term therapy.** Persisting profound bradycardia/asystole must be treated urgently.
  - Temporary transcutaneous pacing: very painful to the awake patient
  - Parasympathetic withdrawal (anticholinergic agents; block muscarinic acetylcholine (ACh) receptor):
    - Glycopyrrolate (more commonly used by surgeons and anesthesiologists)
    - Atropine: 1 mg IV; may repeat after 5 min (x 2)
      - Avoid smaller doses, which may have a "partial agonist" effect on the receptor and worsen the bradycardia.
      - May not improve rate in AV block.
  - Beta-agonist therapy: Isoproterenol: 1–10 µg/min IV infusion
  - Temporary transvenous pacing
- **Long-term therapy**
  - Permanent pacemaker implantation is the only reliable therapy
    - Highly effective at controlling slow heart rates
    - Indicated in all patients with symptomatic bradycardia not due to a reversible cause
      - Sick sinus syndrome
      - Any second- or third-degree AV block
    - Indicated even in asymptomatic patients if at high risk for profound bradycardia and syncope with injury.
      - Mobitz type 2 AV block, 2:1 infranodal block; complete AV block
  - Theophylline has been used, mostly unsuccessfully, in sick sinus syndrome in hopes of avoiding pacemaker implantation.

18 ■ TACHYARRHYTHMIAS

INTRODUCTION

Tachycardia is the heart rate exceeding 100 beats per minute. Sinus tachycardia is a normal response to physiologic demand, exercise, emotional or physical stress, fever, and volume depletion. Tachycardias arising from other sources are tachyarrhythmias.

MECHANISMS OF TACHYARRHYTHMIAS

Tachycardias, like all arrhythmias, are either disorders of impulse formation or disorders of impulse propagation.

- Disorders of impulse formation: focal tachycardias. A single ectopic (not the sinus node) site generates propagating impulses that overdrive the sinus node. The two mechanisms are difficult to distinguish clinically.
  - **Abnormal automaticity**: Automaticity is gradual depolarization of the "resting" (Phase 4) membrane potential to the point of the action potential threshold. Automaticity is abnormal when an ectopic site's rate of automatic discharge is accelerated to overdrive the natural heart rate. Potential contributors to abnormal automaticity include relative depolarization of the resting (Phase 4) membrane potential (as in ischemia); changes in transmembrane Na^+, Ca^{2+}, and K^+ balance; and abnormalities in the sarcolemmal ion channels.
  - **Triggered activity**: The occurrence of *afterdepolarizations*, sarcolemmal depolarizations that occur after the initial phases of the action potential. Triggered activity may lead to polymorphic VT, *torsades de pointes*, or VF. There are two types of afterdepolarizations:
    - ○ *Early afterdepolarizations (EADs)*: Occur during the plateau (phase 2) or repolarization (phase 3) of the action potential. Appear to be associated with Ca^{2+} overload. Clinically associated with prolonged QT and torsades de pointes.
    - ○ *Delayed afterdepolarizations (AEDs)*: Occur after repolarization (phase 3) is complete. Associated clinically with digoxin toxicity.
- Disorders of impulse propagation: *Reentry* occurs when there is a functional circuit allowing the electrical impulse to circulate repeatedly. Reentry requires:
  - A functional circuit (which may be defined by an anatomic obstacle, such as an MI scar or the tricuspid valve; or it may be physiological, such as created by an area of refractoriness)
  - Unidirectional block in one limb of the circuit (typically created by refractoriness to a premature impulse)

If the refractory limb recovers excitability as the impulse returns in the retrograde direction, the impulse will circulate as long as the wavefront meets excitable muscle. The portion of the circuit that is excitable is the *excitable gap*.

- Fibrillation is the chaotic, disorganized activation of the muscle. It may involve both abnormal impulse formation and impulse propagation.

CLASSIFICATION OF TACHYARRHYTHMIAS

- Supraventricular
  - Mechanism confined to the atrium (atrial arrhythmias)
  - Mechanism *requiring* supraventricular structures (atrial, AV node) (paroxysmal supraventricular arrhythmias—PSVTs)
- Ventricular: The rhythm originates in ventricular structures (usually myocardium, but may also originate in the His-Purkinje system).

SUPRAVENTRICULAR TACHYCARDIAS (SVTS)

- **Atrial arrhythmias:** The mechanism is confined to the atria. May be reentrant, focal, or fibrillatory.
  - Atrial fibrillation (AF) **(Figure 18-1)**: Fibrillatory activity in the atria. An active area of investigation, atrial fibrillation appears to have different mechanisms in different patients. There may be multiple reentrant wavelets, or one or more focal "drivers" of the chaotic rhythm. These two mechanisms may coexist. Ultimately the mechanisms at work in the individual patient may be used to tailor therapy.
    Clinically it is useful to classify AF base on its persistence:
    - Paroxysmal: AF terminates spontaneously (though its duration may be minutes to weeks). Initiation may occur with an easily identified trigger (caffeine, stimulants, exertion, stress) or with no clear trigger.
    - Persistent: AF does not terminate spontaneously, though sinus rhythm may be maintained for some period of time after cardioversion.

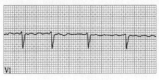

FIGURE 18-1. Atrial fibrillation in lead V1. Note the low amplitude, disorganized atrial activity and irregular ventricular response.

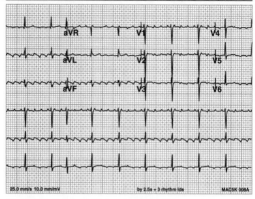

FIGURE 18-2. Typical atrial flutter with variable AV block. In leads II, III, and aVF the flutter waves are negative and relatively narrow, yielding the typical "sawtooth" pattern.

- ○ Permanent: AF is constant and attempts at cardioversion appear futile either due to failure or immediate recurrence of AF. Hope for success with catheter or surgical procedures has led many to replace the term *permanent* with *long-standing persistent*.
- Atrial flutter: Rapid, but with a "monomorphic" repetitive atrial activity, usually mediated by reentry within the atrium:
  - ○ "Typical" atrial flutter (**Figure 18-2**): The most common reentrant circuit is in the right atrium, circulating around the atrial side of the tricuspid annulus. Viewed from the right ventricular apex, the electrical wavefront travels counterclockwise (up the septum, across the roof from medial to lateral, down the lateral wall and then medially across the isthmus of muscle delineated by the tricuspid valve annulus and the inferior vena cava. Generates the classic "sawtooth" pattern of narrow, negative flutter waves in the inferior leads of the 12-lead ECG. Usually occurs at about 300 cycles per minute (200 ms cycle length or 1 large box on the ECG grid). Very commonly, there is consistent 2:1, 3:1, or 4:1 AV block, yielding a ventricular rate of 150, 100, or 75 beats per minute. Variable AV block is also possible, yielding a more irregular ventricular pattern (and pulse).

- - "Atypical" atrial flutter: any other flutter
    - A special case is "clockwise" isthmus-dependent flutter; it is identical to typical "counterclockwise" flutter described above, except the wave circulates in the opposite direction.
  - Focal atrial tachycardia. Atrial tachycardia originating from single site (usually presumed due to abnormal automaticity). Maybe difficult to distinguish from flutter, but reentry in the atria (flutter) usually generates very fast rates (> 180 bpm) compared to a focal atrial tachycardia.
  - Multifocal atrial tachycardia (MAT). Diagnosis requires at least 3 consecutive *differing* P-waves, at a tachycardic rate. May look like coarse atrial fibrillation, but the P-waves should be more distinct. Highly associated with pulmonary disease, and often the best treatment is treatment of underlying cause.
  - Junctional ectopic tachycardia (JET), arising from the AV node or AV junction. Rare in adults, though may occur in postoperative patients. More common in the pediatric population.
- **"Paroxysmal" supraventricular tachycardia (PSVTs).** Reentrant arrhythmias whose mechanism requires some part of the supraventricular structures of the heart (the atria, the AV node, the His bundle).
  - AV nodal reentrant tachycardia (AVNRT) (**Figure 18-3**): the substrate is "dual AV nodal physiology," which may be thought of as 2 pathways. Anatomically, these pathways appear to be inputs into the compact AV node. The compact AV node lies at the apex of the triangle of Koch. At the base of the triangle of Koch is the ostium of the coronary sinus. One leg of the triangle is the border of the tricuspid annulus and the other is the tendon of Todaro, which proceeds from the CS os in the inferior atrial septum toward the compact AV node, which is in the superior AV septum.
    - A fast pathway, which conducts quickly, but has a relatively long refractory period. The fast pathway is the superior input into the compact AV node from high septal right atrium. Sinus rhythm conduction usually utilizes the fast pathway, generating a normal PR interval.
    - A slow pathway with a shorter refractory period. Anatomically, the slow pathway is the inferior input into the compact AV node, coursing between the CS os and the tricuspid annulus. Ablation therapy is usually directed at the slow pathway.
    - AVNRT may be of the *typical* (*slow-fast*) or *atypical* (*fast-slow*) variants.
      - In typical (slow-fast) AVNRT, antegrade conduction is in the slow pathway, and the PR interval is long. Retrograde conduction is via the fast pathway; the RP interval is therefore short and can be so short as to be unseen.
      - In atypical (fast-slow) AVNRT, antegrade conduction is via the fast pathway, and the PR interval is relatively short. Retrograde conduction is via the slow pathway; the RP is longer than the PR.

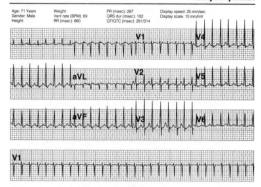

Age: 71 Years	Weight:	PR (msec): 267	Display speed: 25 mm/sec
Gender: Male	Vent rate (BPM): 69	QRS dur (msec): 102	Display scale: 10 mm/mV
Height:	RR (msec): 860	QT/QTC (msec): 291/314	

FIGURE 18-3. 12 lead ECG of typical AVNRT. In this example, the retrograde p-waves are prominent at the end of the QRS. The classic appearance is as a "pseudo-S" wave in lead II and/or a "pseudo-R'" wave in V1. Since the P-wave is retrograde and propagates from the septum to the left and right atria simultaneously, it's negative and brief (narrow). Since the reentry occurs in the AV node, activation of the atria can occur virtually simultaneously with the ventricle. In this case the QRS may completely obscure the P-wave.

AVNRG is a typical reentrant rhythm. It is usually triggered by a PAC that meets refractoriness in the fast pathway. The impulse may conduct slowly through the slow pathway, which is less likely to be refractory. If the fast pathway recovers from refractoriness to allow retrograde conduction, reentry can occur.

- AV reentrant tachycardia (utilizing an accessory pathway) (AVRT); also called circus movement tachycardia (CMT) and AV reciprocating tachycardia (AVRT)
  ○ Orthodromic AVRT (**Figure 18-4**): Activation wave travels anterograde (or *antegrade*) through the normal conduction system and retrograde (from the ventricle to the atrium) through the accessory pathway. Orthodromic AVRT (sometimes "ORT") is the most common of the accessory pathway-mediated SVTs; it can occur with any accessory pathway that conducts retrograde (regardless of whether it can conduct antegrade). Orthodromic tachycardia produces a narrow QRS complex or one that is consistent with supraventricular origin (e.g., there may a typical conduction defect, such as LBBB or RBBB).

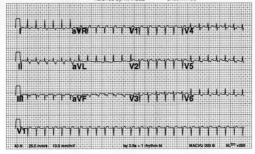

Referred by: MARBLE   Unconfirmed

FIGURE 18-4. 12 lead ECG of orthodromic AVRT. In this case, prominent retrograde P-waves are seen, occuring after the QRS. Unlike typical AVNRT, the atrial are activated (via the accessory pathway) after the ventricles. Orthodromic AVRT is a "short RP" SVT, but the RP is longer than in typical AVNRT.

- ○ Antidromic AVRT: The activation wave travels retrogradely through the AV node from the ventricle to the atrium, then antegrade through the accessory pathway. *Antidromic AVRT occurs only with manifest/latent accessory pathways.* Antidromic tachycardia always has a wide QRS complex, as the His-Purkinje system is not utilized to activate the LV. (Antidromic tachycardia is, therefore *not* part of the differential diagnosis for narrow complex tachycardia.)
- Manifest accessory pathways and Wolff-Parkinson-White syndrome. Manifest accessory pathways conduct antegradely, and therefore conduct to the ventricle during sinus rhythm, resulting in *pre-excitation* of the ventricular myocardium, signified by a *delta wave* (a slow, slurred initial part of the QRS) **(Figure 18-5)**. Wolff-Parkinson-White syndrome requires a delta wave on ECG in sinus rhythm and rapid palpitations.
  - ○ Orthodromic AVRT
  - ○ Antidromic AVRT
- "Latent" accessory pathways. An accessory pathway that produces little ventricular pre-excitation on the resting sinus rhythm ECG; usually these are left lateral. Latency occurs because rapid conduction through the normal conduction system completes most of ventricular activation before the accessory pathway route can excite much of the ventricle. Latency can be diminished or removed by slowing the

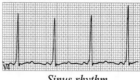

Sinus rhythm

FIGURE 18-5. Sinus rhythm with ventricular preexcitation. The PR interval is short and there is a delta wave.

normal conduction system: carotid sinus massage, adenosine, beta-blockers, calcium channel blockers. Physiologically, latent pathways are no different from manifest pathways. They are part of Wolff-Parkinson-White syndrome and may contribute to:
  ○ Orthodromic AVRT
  ○ Antidromic AVRT
- Concealed accessory pathways. An accessory pathway that conducts solely in the retrograde direction (from ventricle to atrium). Concealed accessory pathways mediate only:
  ○ Orthodromic AVRT

VENTRICULAR TACHYCARDIAS (VTS)

- Monomorphic VTs are those with a single QRS morphology, suggesting a stable site of origin (**Figure 18-6**).
  - *Idiopathic VTs* are those occurring in the absence of structural heart disease. They are typically well tolerated and the prognosis is good. They may be highly symptomatic, including palpitations, presyncope, and syncope. Typically thought to arise from a focus of abnormal automaticity. There are some exceptions, including an LV VT that appears to arise from "micro-reentry" involving the His-Purkinje system.

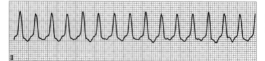

FIGURE 18-6. Monomorphic VT in lead II. Careful examination reveals P-waves dissociated and slower than the rapid ventricular rhythm.

- ○ A large majority of them arise from the right ventricular outflow tract, typically generating a QRS complex with a left bundle branch block pattern and an inferior axis.
  - ▪ The RVOT is also the most common site of origin of PVCs. The same QRS morphology as a VT or nonsustained VT is seen.
  - ▪ Idiopathic VTs may arise from many other sites, including the LV outflow tract, the sinuses of Valsalva (just above the aortic valve), the His-Purkinje system, and the epicardial LV.
- VT associated with structural heart disease
  - ○ Reentrant VT associated with old MI scar
  - ○ VT associated with acute MI or ischemia
    - ▪ May be due to focal mechanism (abnormal automaticity or triggered mechanism), particularly in the setting of ongoing ischemia.
    - ▪ Reentrant rhythms are also possible, particularly if there is preexisting scar from previous MI.
  - ○ VT due to other cardiomyopathy
    - ▪ Idiopathic dilated cardiomyopathy
      - ▪ Often reentrant, associated with scar or areas of infiltrative lesion.
      - ▪ May conceivably be due to abnormal automaticity or possibly triggered activity.
- Bundle branch reentry (BBR) is a special case where a rapid reentry utilizing the right bundle and left bundle generates a monomorphic VT. BBR usually occurs in the setting of dilated, non-ischemic cardiomyopathy. One of the bundles must be the retrograde limb of the VT and one must be the antegrade limb. The QRS morphology should have a typical right or left bundle branch block appearance.
- Polymorphic VT and ventricular fibrillation: less organized electrical activity in the ventricles. The ECG may show low-amplitude chaotic activation or it may show distinct multiple QRS complexes (polymorphic VT).
  - May often arise from active ischemia (as in sudden cardiac arrest during an acute MI), inflammation
  - May be triggered by PVCs
  - A special case is the polymorphic VT in which the VT is associated with a prolonged QT interval (torsades de pointes)

READING THE ECG IN TACHYCARDIA

- *Treat the patient, not the ECG!*
- **Narrow complex tachycardias** are narrow because the ventricles are activated normally, via the rapidly conducting His-Purkinje system. In general, narrow complex tachycardias are supraventricular rhythms (including those whose mechanism is confined to the atrium [sinus tach, atrial tach, atrial fibrillation, atrial flutter, etc.], and

including the "paroxysmal" SVTs [AVNRT, orthodromic—but not antidromic—AVRT]).

- **Wide complex tachycardias** are wide because of failure (or nonparticipation) of the rapid His-Purkinje system. Myocardial conduction is slower than His-Purkinje system conduction. Slower conduction prolongs the time for the ventricles to be fully depolarized, widening the QRS complex. The differential diagnosis of wide complex tachycardia is **(Figure 18-7)**:
  - VT
  - SVT with aberrancy (e.g., any SVT with right or left bundle branch block)
  - Pre-excitation (e.g., antidromic SVT in WPW syndrome, atrial fibrillation, or flutter in WPW)
    - Antegrade conduction through an accessory pathway is required.

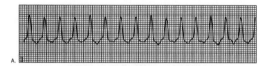

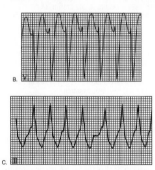

FIGURE 18-7. Three wide complex tachycardias with different mechanisms. A. Ventricular Tachycardia. B. Supraventricular tachycardia with aberrancy (Left Bundle Branch Block) in lead V1. C. Atrial fibrillation with ventricular preexcitation. Note the irregularity of the rate and QRS width.

- Orthodromic AVRT (the more common sort in WPW) is *not* pre-excited. Antegrade conduction proceeds via the normal conduction system and is narrow.

THERAPIES FOR SVT

- Direct current (DC) cardioversion—application of a high voltage field across the heart, depolarizing the entire heart, allowing normal sinus rhythm to return. Cardioversion does not influence the rhythm after the acute event; recurrence of arrhythmia is not a failure of cardioversion, it is failure to maintain sinus rhythm.
- Medical therapy: Can be used to attempt cardioversion and/or to maintain sinus rhythm.
  - AV nodal blocking agents (calcium channel blockers such as diltiazem and verapamil [not dihydropyridines]; beta-blockers; digoxin)
    - May slow the ventricular rate in rhythms whose mechanism is confined to the atria (atrial fibrillation, atrial flutter, atrial tachycardia).
      - May have suppressive effect on focal atrial tachycardia
    - May terminate or prevent the paroxysmal SVTs by blocking/slowing AV nodal conduction
  - Antiarrhythmic agents (Vaughan-Williams Class I and Class III drugs)
    - May terminate focal or reentrant tachyarrhythmias and atrial fibrillation
    - May maintain sinus rhythm in patients prone to paroxysmal (reentrant) SVTs, focal atrial tachycardias, atrial flutter, and atrial fibrillation
- Ablation therapy
  - Ablation therapy is heating (or, for cryoablation, freezing) myocardial tissue to denature the proteins and create a (small) scar that is electrically inactive. Mapping during electrophysiology study can reveal the origin of an arrhythmia or an isthmus of muscle that sustains reentry, or an abnormal pathway, such as an accessory pathway. If the site can be destroyed, it can no longer mediate the arrhythmia.

THERAPIES FOR VT/VF

- Direct current cardioversion/defibrillation. Especially for urgent therapy in the setting of sudden death or hemodynamically ill-tolerated ventricular arrhythmia. The shock should be *synchronized* to the QRS if there is an identifiable complex. Asynchronous defibrillation is reserved for VF.
- Implantable cardioverter defibrillator (ICD). Indicated for patients at high risk for malignant ventricular arrhythmia and sudden cardiac death (either for primary or secondary prevention). The ICD monitors the patient's rhythm continuously and delivers therapy (either

antitachycardia pacing or a high-energy shock) in the event of a rapid rate.

- Medical therapy. Antiarrhythmic agents (usually Vaughan-William Class III drugs) may be used as urgent therapy as an adjunct to defibrillation shocks. Their main role is maintaining sinus rhythm in patients at high risk for ventricular arrhythmia and ICD shocks. Their use alone, in the absence of an ICD, for prevention of sudden death has been disappointing.
- Ablation therapy may also be used for ventricular arrhythmias. Usually a focal source, or a critical isthmus for a reentrant arrhythmia is sought. If a VT cannot be induced and mapped, empiric ablation can be performed with by mapping suspected substrates (e.g., scar) for VT.

ANTIARRHYTHMIC DRUGS

The Vaughan-Williams system is an imperfect but widely used scheme for classifying the antiarrhythmic agents by mechanism: The classification is summarized in **Table 18-1**.

SOME IMPORTANT ANTIARRHYTHMIC AGENTS

Adenosine (Adenocard)
- Indications: Termination of supraventricular tachycardias utilizing the AV node. Diagnostic use: creates AV block in order to assess atrial activity for fibrillation of flutter.
- Dose: IV only
  - 6 mg IV push with rapid flush. May give second dose of 12 mg IV, and 12 mg IV may be repeated.
  - Use central line if possible.
- Potent slowing/block of AV node conduction. Usually causes transient heart block.
- Metabolized very quickly by red blood cells. Elimination half-life is < 10 seconds.
- Avoid in wide complex tachycardia, unless mechanism is known to be reentry involving the AV node.
  - Contraindicated with atrial fibrillation or flutter with ventricular pre-excitation.
- May cause bronchospasm

Amiodarone (Cordarone, Pacerone)
- Indications: ventricular arrhythmias; atrial arrhythmias (unapproved)
- Dose:
  - For life-threatening ventricular arrhythmias:
    - 150 mg IV over 10 min.; then 1 mg/min IV for 6 h; then 0.5 mg/min over 18 h
  - Oral loading: 800–1600 mg daily for 1–3 weeks, then 400–800 mg for 1 month
  - Oral maintenance: lowest effective dose, usually 200 mg/day

TABLE 18-1: The Vaughan-Williams Classification of Antiarrhythmic Agents

Class	Mechanism	Action	Examples
IA	Na^+ channel blockade K^+ channel blockade	—Slows depolarization; slow conduction/propagation; decreases excitability. —Prolongs action potential and refractoriness.	**Quinidine** **Procainamide** **Disopyramide**
IB	Na^+ channel blockade (with rapid association/dissocation)	—Slows depolarization; slow conduction/propagation; decreases excitability. —May shorten action potential and refractoriness. —No significant action on atrial cells.	**Lidocaine** **Mexiletine**
IC	Na^+ channel blockade (with slow association/dissociation)	—Slows depolarization; slow conduction/propagation; decreases excitability. —*Use dependence:* increased pharmacologic activity with high heart rates.	**Propafenone** **Flecainide**
II	Beta-adrenergic blockade (with varying levels of alpha-adrenergic blockade)	—Slows sinus rate, slows AV node conduction —Negative inotropy —arteriolar vasodilation	**Metoprolol** **Atenolol** **Propranolol** **Carvedilol**
III	K^+ channel blockade	—Prolongs action potential and refractoriness.	**Amiodarone** (has effects of multiple classes) **Sotalol** **Dofetilide** **Dronedarone** **Vernakalent** **Ibutilide** (may have a different mechanism)
IV	Some Ca^{2+} channel blockers	—Slows sinus rate and AV node conduction. —May decrease excitability in the setting of celluar Ca overload.	**Verapamil** (a phenylalkylamine) **Diltiazem** (a benzothiazepine)

- Large volume of distribution and delayed pharmacokinetics
  - Elimination half-life is at least 25 days.
- Initiation usually done with ECG monitoring for bradycardia, QT prolongation/torsades de pointes.
- Multiple end-organ toxicities, including thyroid, lungs, liver, eye, skin, but not the kidneys
  - Monitor TFTs, LFTs
  - PFTs and ophthalmologic exams as indicated
- Multiple drug interactions
  - Plasma protein binding increases level drugs, including:
    - Warfarin
    - Digoxin
    - Phenytoin
  - May increase levels of substrates of CYP450 system
  - May increase QT prolongation effect of QT-prolonging drugs
    - Avoid with Class IA and Class III agents.
- Beware toxicity and drug interactions after discontinuations, since elimination half-life is long
- Vaughan-Williams Class III primarily, but has effects of Class I, II, and IV agents as well
- Metabolized in the liver by the CYP3A4 system

Disopyramide (Norpace)
- Indications: VT, VF, atrial fibrillation; now rarely used to due to alternatives and adverse risk/benefit ratio
- Sometimes used to improve ventricular filling and decrease obstruction in hypertrophic obstructive cardiomyopathy (HOCM)
- Dose: 400–800 mg daily in divided doses
  - For immediate release formulation: divided every 6 hours
  - For extended release formulation: divided every 12 hours
- Prolongs QT interval; risk of torsade de pointes; should be initiated with ECG monitoring
- Potent negative inotrope and positive lusitrope (facilitates myocardial relaxation)
- Anticholinergic side effects common: urinary retention, constipation, dry mouth
- Vaughan-Williams Class IA: Na^+ channel blocker and K^+ channel blocker
- Metabolism/clearance: kidney, liver; avoid with hepatic or renal impairment

Dofetilide (Tikosyn)
- Indications: atrial fibrillation and atrial flutter
  - Prescribing limited to those who have completed education concerning dosing, toxicity, and proarrhythmia
  - Initiation limited to hospitals with ECG monitoring, ability to monitor ECG, QT, and creatinine clearance and to provide cardiac resuscitation
    - Minimum 3-day hospital stay with telemetry for initiation
    - 12-lead ECG after each dose

- Dose is closely indexed to QTc and creatinine clearance (see Tikosyn website for detailed instructions: www.tikosyn.com):
  - Not used if baseline QTc > 440 ms (500 ms in presence of ventricular conduction abnormalities, e.g., bundle branch block)
    - Use QT without correction if heart rate < 60 bpm
  - Creatinine clearance:
    - \> 60 mL/min: 500 mcg every 12 hours
    - 40–60 mL/min: 250 mcg every 12 hours
    - 20–40 mL/min: 125 mcg every 12 hours
    - < 20 mL/min: not used
  - QT changes: If QTc increases by >15% or beyond 500 ms (550 in presence of ventricular conduction abnormalities), the dose should be stepped down.
    - Further increase after second dose should prompt discontinuation.
- Cleared by the kidney and metabolized in the liver by the CYP3A4 system.
  - Coadministration with inhibitors of the CYP3A4 system is contraindicated due to the risk of elevated levels of dofetilide and proarrhythmia.
    - Macrolide antibiotics, azole antifungals, protease inhibitors, serotonin reuptake inhibitors, amiodarone, cannabinoids, diltiazem, grapefruit juice, nefazodone, norfloxacin, quinine, zafirlukast.
  - Other drugs contraindicated for coadministration:
    - Cimetidine, verapamil, trimethoprim (with or without sulfamethoxazole), ketoconazole, hydrochlorothiazide (with or with triamterene).
  - Cosubstrates of the renal cation transporter should be with care
    - For example, triamterene, amiloride, metformin.
- Vaughan-Williams Class III: blockade of the rapid component of the delayed rectifier K$^+$ current (I$_{Kr}$).

Dronedarone (Multaq)
- Indications: atrial fibrillation/flutter; reduces risk of cardiovascular hospital admissions
- Dose: 400 mg PO twice daily
- Not to be used with current or recent CHF decompensation
- May contribute to bradycardia, AV block
- Metabolized in liver CYP3A4 system
- May increase serum creatinine without affecting renal function
- Vaughan-Williams Class III (primarily): K$^+$ channel blockade
- Developed as analog of amiodarone without iodine moieties in hopes of eliminating amiodarone's toxicities
- Efficacy is not necessarily equivalent to amiodarone.

Flecainide (Tambocor)
- Indications: Atrial fibrillation and atrial flutter; reentrant PSVT, particularly utilizing an accessory pathway.
- Dose: Start 50–100 mg PO every 12 hours. Max dose: 200 mg every 12 hours.

- Unapproved: 200–300 mg PO single dose for conversion of atrial fibrillation ("pill in the pocket" dosing).
- Not to be used in the setting of structural heart disease, particularly previous MI.
- Proarrhythmic, particularly in setting of previous MI scar.
- May also convert atrial fibrillation to flutter with 1:1 AV conduction with wide QRS due to flecainide's conduction-slowing properties. Flecainide flutter may resemble VT and be just as malignant.
  - Usually used with an AV node–slowing agent.
- Vaughan-Williams Class IC: Na⁺ channel blockade
- Excreted by the kidney primarily. Also metabolized in the liver by the CYP2D6 system.

Ibutilide (Corvert)
- Indications: Cardioversion of atrial fibrillation and atrial flutter)
- Dose (IV only): 1 mg IV over 10 min. (If patient weight < 60 kg, 0.01 mg/kg over 10 min).
  - May repeat once if no cardioversion after 10 minutes.
  - Stop infusion if the rhythm converts to sinus.
  - ECG monitoring for 4 hours after the dose is recommended.
- Proarrhythmic: prolongs the QT and may induce torsade de pointes. Should only be given with careful ECG monitoring and resuscitation available.
- Avoid with severe LV dysfunction
- Atypical Vaughan-Williams Class III: appears to promote opening of a slow Na⁺ channel (rather than K⁺ channel blockade), prolonging the action potential, the refractory period, and the QT.
- Metabolized by the liver, and metabolites (one of which has mild antiarrhythmic effect) are cleared by the kidney. Elimination half-life is about 6 hours.

Lidocaine
- Indications: ventricular arrhythmias, particularly in ischemia or myocardial infarction
- Dose:
  - Initiation: 1–1.5 mg IV over 1–2 minutes; then 0.5–0.75 mg/kg every 10 min to maximum dose 3 mg/kg
  - Maintenance: 1–4 mg/min
- Not effective for atrial arrhythmias
- Not for routine prophylaxis in myocardial infarction
- Therapeutic level: 1.5–5 mcg/mL
- Central nervous system side effects (sleepiness, slurred speech, confusion, hallucinations)
- In overdose may cause asystole or myocardial depression with hypotension/shock
- Vaughan-Williams Class IB: Na⁺ channel blockade without prolongation of the action potential
- Metabolized by the liver. Accumulation of metabolites (particularly in renal failure) may contribute to CNS side effect.

Mexiletine (Mexitil)
- Indications: recurrent VT and VF
- Dose: Start 150–200 every 8 hours; max: 400 every 8 hours
- Take with food to minimize nausea, GI distress.
- More effective in presence of baseline depolarization:
  - Ischemia
  - In combination with a K^+ channel blocker (amiodarone, sotalol, procainamide, quinidine)
- CNS side effects (headache, gait unsteadiness) may limit dosing.
- Vaughan-Williams Class IB: Na^+ channel blockade without prolongation of the action potential
- Effects similar to lidocaine
- Not effective for atrial arrhythmias.
- Metabolized in the liver

Procainamide (Procan, Pronestyl)
- Indications: atrial fibrillation and flutter; ventricular tachyarrhythmias. Alternatives and adverse risk/benefit ratio have decreased use.
- Dose:
  - IV: 20 mg/min IV until arrhythmia terminated or 17 mg/kg (1 g max) has been infused (may be given at 50 mg/min in emergency)
    - Stop infusion for 50% widening of QRS, hypotension.
  - In cardiac arrest, has been given 100 mg IV push every 5 min
  - Oral: start 50 mg/kg/day; total dose 2–6 g/day
    - Immediate release formulation: dose divided q 3–4 hours
    - Sustained release: dose divided every 6 hours or every 12 hours (Procanbid)
- Prolongs the QT interval: risk of torsade de pointes. Initiate with ECG monitoring.
- Risk of bone marrow suppression, agranulocytosis, lupus-like syndrome
  - Monitor blood cell counts.
- Vaughan-Williams Class IA: Na^+ and K^+ channel blockade
- Metabolism: Acetylated in the liver to n-acetyl-procainamide (NAPA), an active metabolite with an elimination half-life of about 6 hours
  - About half of the population are rapid acetylators and NAPA levels may exceed procainamide levels.
    - Lupus-like syndrome associated with procainamide rather than NAPA and is less common in rapid acetylators
  - Avoid with renal impairment, risk of toxic procainamide and NAPA levels.
  - Therapeutic levels:
    - Procainamide: 3–10 mcg/mL
    - NAPA: 10–30 mcg/mL

Propafenone (Rythmol)
- Indications: atrial fibrillation and atrial flutter; reentrant PSVT, particularly utilizing an accessory pathway
- Dose: Start 150 mg PO every 8 hours. Max dose 300 mg every 8 hours.

- Unapproved: 600 mg PO single dose for conversion of atrial fibrillation ("pill in the pocket" dosing).
- Not to be used in the setting of structural heart disease, particularly previous MI
- Proarrhythmic, particularly in setting of previous MI scar
- May also convert atrial fibrillation to flutter with 1:1 AV conduction with wide QRS due to propafenone's conduction-slowing properties. Flutter may resemble VT and be just as malignant.
  - Less common with propafenone than flecainide due to its intrinsic AV node–slowing beta-blockade. Use of a separate AV node–slowing drug is still advisable.
- Vaughan-Williams Class IC: Na^+ channel blockade
- Metabolized in the liver in part by the CYP2D6 system
  - 5-hydroxypropafenone is an active metabolite, though with less beta-blockade effect.
  - About 10% of patients are slow metabolizers and are at higher risk for adverse effects.

Quinidine
- Indications: VT, VF, atrial fibrillation. Now rarely used due to alternatives and adverse risk/benefit ratio, particularly in atrial arrhythmias.
- Dose:
  - Quinidine gluconate (extended release): 324–628 mg every 8–12 hours
  - Quinidine sulfate (immediate release): 200–400 mg every 6–8 hours
  - Quinidine sulfate (extended release): 300–600 mg every 8–12 hours
- Prolongs QT interval; risk of torsade de pointes; should be initiated with ECG monitoring.
- Vaughan-Williams Class IA: Na^+ channel blockade and K^+ channel blockade.
- Metabolized in the liver; cleared by the kidney. Risk of toxicity, proarrhythmia increase with liver or kidney impairment.

Sotalol (Betapace)
- Indications: atrial fibrillation and flutter; ventricular arrhythmias
- Dose: Start 80 mg PO twice daily. Usual maintenance dose: 80–200 twice daily. Max dose: 320 mg PO twice daily.
- Has significant beta-blockade properties
  - May contribute to asthma or reactive airways disease
  - Contributes to bradycardia
  - May contribute to myocardial depression
    - Avoid in decompensated heart failure.
- Prolongs the QT interval; risk of torsade de pointes, especially with low serum K^+. Should be initiated with ECG monitoring.
- Sotalol is a racemate of:
  - d-sotalol, a Vaughan-Williams Class III antiarrhythmic drug: K^+ channel blockade, prolonging the action potential, refractory period, and the QT interval

- l-sotalol, a beta-blocking agent
  - The presence of the beta-blocking function is thought to reduce the risk of proarrhythmia.
- Cleared, unchanged by the kidney
  - Avoid with renal dysfunction.

19 ■ SYNCOPE

DEFINITION AND INCIDENCE

Syncope is transient loss of consciousness and postural tone due to hypoperfusion of the brain. Syncope is very common. One estimate suggests that > 40% of the population is likely to experience syncope sometime in their lifetime.

THE PROBLEM OF DIAGNOSING SYNCOPE

There are several potential etiologies, but evaluation is limited by the transient nature of the problem. Medical assessment almost always occurs in retrospect, with no physiologic data from the episode. Therefore, an accurate diagnosis cannot be known.

Texts and guidelines frequently overlook this point. Even those that acknowledge the difficulty may quote sensitivity and specificity—impossible when there is no gold standard for the diagnosis.

Syncope can be anxiety-inducing in those who know it may be a warning sign of serious events. Yet the prognostic value of syncope is poor in the absence of other abnormalities, particularly cardiovascular ones. In the absence of underlying heart disease, syncope is not a risk factor for mortality.

Therefore, the best initial approach to syncope is *risk stratification*—assimilating the fact of the patient's syncope with other factors. The physician's goal is to seek or exclude conditions in which syncope, as an additional risk factor, indicates a specific treatment.

In some cases, prospective observation (such as with an ECG monitor) can allow a diagnosis. But a clear arrhythmia (for example) with syncope/near syncope in one instance still does not prove that the index syncopal spell was arrhythmic at all. Similarly, a clearly neurocardiogenic episode seen during evaluation does not exclude a malignant arrhythmia as the cause of a previous syncopal spell in a patient with severe cardiomyopathy. Nor does it eliminate the possibility of a future episode of malignant arrhythmia and sudden death in such a patient.

POSSIBLE CAUSES OF SYNCOPE

Understanding cardiovascular and neurologic physiology can help predict causes of syncope, and observation of actual events has provided some information about relative incidence. These causes need not be mutually exclusive. Hypovolemia, for example, may be a contributor to syncope from any of the other causes.

- Neurocardiogenic syncope: Hyperactivity of the parasympathetic nervous system results in vasodilation (*vasodepressor*) or bradycardia (*cardioinhibitory*) response, or both. It is probably the most common cause (to the extent that it can be determined). There are multiple potential triggers:
  - The Bezold-Jarisch reflex is the proposed response to poor venous return, provoking tachycardia, and in turn, LV wall stress, LV mechanoreceptor stimulation, and parasympathetic surge. Poor venous return may result from:
    - Hemorrhage
    - Venous pooling with prolonged standing
  - Other triggers:
    - Carotid sinus hypersensitivity (syncope may be associated with head turning, tight neckware)
    - Pain
    - Acute emotional stress (e.g., seeing blood)
    - Bladder pain/fullness
    - Defecation
    - Cough
    - Micturition
    - Swallowing
    - Laughing
- Orthostatic hypotension
  - Hypovolemia
  - Hemorrhage
  - Poor oral intake
  - Diuretics
  - Diarrhea
  - Dysautonomia
- Cardiac. Any mechanism that reduces the efficiency of the heart may, in some cases reduce cardiac output enough to contribute to syncope or presyncope.
  - Tachyarrhythmias
    - Supraventricular: Not considered life threatening, but could contribute to syncope
    - Ventricular: can lead to sudden cardiac death. The idiopathic VTs are an exception.
      - Idiopathic VTs (those that occur in the structurally normal heart)
        - Prognosis is similar to SVTs .
        - Most commonly from the RV outflow tract. The LV outflow tract, the left His-Purkinje fascicles, and the aortic root (the sinuses of Valsalva) are other sites of origin.
      - VT/VF associated with coronary artery disease
        - Ongoing ischemia (frequently polymorphic VT or VF)
        - Chronic MI scar (more likely to be monomorphic VT)

- - - Other VT/VF
    - Nonischemic dilated cardiomyopathy
    - Long QT syndrome (polymorphic VT known as torsades de pointes)
    - Hypertrophic cardiomyopathy (also a potential nonarrhythmic cause if there is outflow tract obstruction)
    - Brugada syndrome, which predisposes to polymorphic VT
    - Catecholaminergic polymorphic VT
  - Bradyarrhythmias
    - o Sinus node dysfunction
      - Tachy-brady syndrome: classically, a prolonged pause or profound sinus bradycardia after termination of a tachyarrhythmia (such as AF)
      - Other sinus node disease
    - o AV node dysfunction may lead to syncope.
      - 2nd-degree type 1 block may occur with high vagal activity. It may be symptomatic (syncope/near syncope) even though progression to complete heart block is uncommon.
      - 2nd-degree type 2 block, higher degree AV block
        - Usually represent structural infranodal disease
        - May progress to complete heart block
      - Complete heart block
        - Junctional, fascicular, and ventricular escape rhythms are unreliable, and failure typically leads to syncope.
    - o Other conduction system disease that may progress to complete heart block:
      - The ill-named *trifascicular block* suggests risk of progression to heart block, sometimes with intermittent episodes of block and conduction.
        - Right bundle branch block, left anterior or posterior fascicular block, PR prolongation
        - Left bundle branch block and PR prolongation
      - Bifascicular block may also progress to heart block.
        - Right bundle branch block with left anterior or posterior fascicular block
  - Mechanical
    - o Valvular stenosis
    - o Prosthetic valve failure or thrombus
    - o Myxoma
    - o Hypertrophic obstructive cardiomyopathy with severe outflow tract obstruction
    - o Pericardial tamponade
    - o Pump failure, due to acute MI or worsening chronic dysfunction
- Vascular
  - Aortic dissection
  - Pulmonary embolism
  - Pulmonary hypertension

- Subclavian steal
- Vertebrobasilar insufficiency
- Carotid stenosis/dissection
- Neurologic (may rarely produce a syndrome similar to syncope, but does not meet the formal definition of syncope)
  - Seizure
  - CVA/TIA
  - Migraine
- Other nonsyncopal loss of consciousness
  - Hypoglycemia
  - Hypoxia
  - Anemia
  - Psychogenic

EVALUATION OF SYNCOPE

As detailed earlier, since the episode of syncope has usually already occurred at the time of medical evaluation, the focus can be on risk stratification for future events, including syncope, mortality, and/or the progression of other underlying disease.

- The history
  - Both the patient's own history and the history of any witnesses can be helpful. Though some patterns of history have been linked to specific syndromes, the history alone is rarely diagnostic. Even these textbook descriptions cannot rule out other causes, especially since the memory of events may be very poor.
    - Sudden loss of consciousness without prodrome with sudden regaining of consciousness and feeling normal soon after awakening has been described as typical for arrhythmic syncope.
    - A prodrome of nausea, lightheadedness, and visual changes, possibly associated with a full bladder has been associated with neurocardiogenic syncope. On regaining consciousness, reorientation may be slow and patients often feel unwell for minutes to hours.
  - The past medical history is critical, since patients with known heart disease face a more negative prognosis. Examples:
    - A syncopal spell with known aortic stenosis may be an indication to change course to surgical therapy.
    - Syncope with known cardiomyopathy increases the risk for malignant ventricular arrhythmias; an ICD may be indicated.
- The physical examination may help reveal conditions that predispose to or cause syncope. In some cases it can lead to directed diagnostic testing for a condition which places the patient at risk for recurrent syncope or sudden death.
  - Orthostatic vital signs have been called "high yield" for a diagnosis (but this is misguided in the absence of a gold standard diagnosis, as discussed earlier).

- Take the vitals supine. Have the patient stand and wait for 1 minute. Take the vital signs again.
  - ≥ 20 mmHg decrease in SBP or
  - ≥ 10 bpm increase in HR
- Orthostatic hypotension is a sign of volume depletion that may certainly contribute to syncope in many of the conditions described (e.g., vasovagal syncope, aortic stenosis, cardiomyopathy, bradyarrhythmias, tachyarrhythmias). But since it is not mutually exclusive to these conditions, a finding of orthostatic hypotension does not rule out other conditions for which we are risk stratifying.

- The cardiovascular examination is particularly important since many of the important conditions are cardiovascular.
  - Jugular venous pressure
  - Tachy-brady arrhythmias (if ongoing)
    - Note that if an arrhythmia is ongoing in an alert patient, it is difficult to attribute a previously occurring episode of syncope to an arrhythmia that is being well-tolerated at present. However, changes in autonomic activity *may* cause dramatic changes in vascular tone during the course of an arrhythmia. So the arrhythmia may be the primary culprit and certainly must be treated. But, as discussed, this does not rule out another condition that would change the risk stratification. (For example, a pacemaker would obviously be indicated for a syncopal patient in complete heart block. That doesn't mean the patient doesn't have a cardiomyopathy and congestive heart failure with high risk of malignant tachyarrhythmia and sudden death. In such a case, a pacemaker/defibrillator is indicated.)
  - Murmurs may indicate a significant valvular disease or septal defect or other congenital heart disease.
- Assess medication use, including noncompliance, overdosage, and of course, use of illicit drugs.
- Electrocardiogram is an essential tool that may be diagnostic of many conditions closely associated with syncope (e.g., heart block, acute MI, prolonged QT, Brugada syndrome, ventricular pre-excitation).
- **Other diagnostic tests**. There is a host of diagnostic tests that can be brought to bear in syncope.
  - **Echocardiogram** is probably the single most useful additional test for risk stratification. *In the absence of structural heart disease, a syncopal episode does not increase mortality.* Therefore, if echocardiogram and the basic evaluation reveal no heart disease and no significant suspicion of noncardiac disease, prospective evaluation (such as ambulatory ECG monitoring) can be undertaken.
  - **Ambulatory monitoring** is for the detection of transient ECG events (primarily rhythm events) that can cause syncope or other symptoms. In the patient without structural heart disease and recurrent

syncope, it is an important tool for *prospective* monitoring to diagnose the *next* episode of the syndrome

- Holter monitoring, usually 24 or 48 hours of continuous monitoring
  - Records much that is not of interest during asymptomatic periods, and short-term recording lowers the likelihood of capturing an event
- Loop/event monitors are typically worn for 30 days, increasing the likelihood of capturing an event. They record when activated by the patient (or a bystander) or when they detect an abnormally fast or slow rhythm.
- Continuous ambulatory monitoring is similar to telemetry worn in the hospital, continuously transmitting the ECG to a central location where it is analyzed by technicians and automatic alarm algorithms. The patient can transmit symptom information to correlate with ECG findings. Like a Holter monitor, continuous monitoring often records large amounts of data not related to any symptoms/problems. *Not* a substitute for in-hospital or ICU monitoring in patient at high risk for severe arrhythmias.
- Implantable loop recorders. Implanted subcutaneously with battery usually lasing longer than a year. Can be activated by patient/bystander or automatically by bradycardia or tachycardia. Implantable loop recorder monitoring is more likely to yield a diagnosis than tilt table testing and electrophysiology study.[41]
- Further additional tests should be driven by clinical index of suspicion.
  - Ischemia evaluation: stress testing or coronary angiography when there is suspicion of ischemic heart disease. Isolated syncope (without chest pain, ECG changes, enzyme [troponin, creatine kinase] abnormalities) is a very poor "anginal equivalent."
  - Neurologic testing (EEG, CT, MRI) are of little use in absence of additional neurologic risks and should probably be done under direction of a neurologist.
  - Vascular studies (carotid Doppler, angiogram, MR angiogram) should be used only if the index of suspicion is raised by other evaluation.
  - The utility of electrophysiology (EP) study is very limited. It can assess the inducibility of arrhythmia, sinus node function, and conduction system function.
    - Risk for bradyarrhythmia is usually assessed by ECG and by ambulatory monitoring.
    - For risk of tachyarrhythmias, inducibility of VT at EP study has limited predictive value in presence of coronary artery disease and much less value in the setting of other heart disease.
      - In presence of significant LV dysfunction, syncope places the patient at high risk for malignant arrhythmia and ICD may be indicated. EP study adds little to risk stratification.

○ Cardiac MRI can used to assess for structural heart disease. Its value over echocardiography is limited. It is often used to assess for arrhythmogenic RV dysplasia (ARVD), but should only be used in the presence of other indicators of the disease.

○ Tilt table testing is a test for vasovagal syncope, which is essentially a diagnosis of exclusion, made on clinical grounds. With no gold standard other than clinical suspicion, it is impossible to quantify sensitivity and/or specificity, though such figures are frequently quoted.

■ The patient is placed on a table with a footrest. The table is tilted near upright. Vital signs are monitored. A positive response is loss of consciousness (preferably with reproduction of the clinical syndrome) with a decrease in heart rate (cardioinhibitory) and/or blood pressure (vasodepressor) (though a cuff blood pressure may not be able to record a low value quickly enough). The table is returned to a supine position for the patient to recover.

■ The reproducibility is poor, probably due to "training effect," making it less likely for the patient to suffer a vasovagal spell on repeated trials. This has led to the concept of "tilt training" in which repeated exposure to the upright tilt apparently conditions the patient to decrease the predisposition to activation of the Bezold-Jarisch reflex.

ALGORITHM FOR EVALUATING AND TREATING SYNCOPE

- Evaluation
  - A complete history and physical examination (including orthostatic hypotension) is necessary.
  - In most cases, an echocardiogram is desirable to assess for structural heart disease.
  - Other testing is based on the index of suspicion for the disorder that can be tested.
- Any potential underlying cause uncovered by initial evaluation and follow-up testing should be treated.
- If the heart is structurally abnormal, the risk of malignant arrhythmia and sudden death must be considered.[42,43,44] Defibrillator implantation may be indicated if LV function is depressed.
- If no underlying disease is found, no ECG abnormalities are present, and there is no structural heart disease.
  - For a single syncopal spell, no further evaluation or treatment is necessary.
    ○ The most likely cause of any future event is vasovagal.
  - Recurrent events with no development of underlying disease are likely to be vasovagal.

- ○ Extended monitoring can assess for arrhythmia, including bradycardia.
  - Profound bradycardia causing symptoms is an indication for pacemaker.
  - Though permanent pacemaker implantation has not been helpful in vasovagal syncope overall, it may be useful in vasovagal syncope with a prominent bradycardic component. This is best seen by ECG monitoring.
- ○ Treatment of recurrent vasovagal syncope is difficult.
  - Encourage volume repletion.
  - Avoid triggers.
    - Gradual changes in position to avoid orthostatic triggers.
    - Lie down for blood draws or other similar triggers.
    - Compression stockings may improve venous return.
  - Medical therapy has mixed (at best) success.
    - Fludrocortisone
    - Midodrine
    - Selective serotonin reuptake inhibitors (e.g., Paroxetine)
    - Beta-blockers have been used, but more recent trials have shown no benefit.
    - Selective serotonin/norepinephrine reuptake inhibitors may be of some benefit (e.g., venlafaxine)
  - Attempt to abort or minimize an episode.
    - Immediate assumption of supine position in the event of the prodrome
    - Isometric exercises (e.g., pressing the palms together, squatting) to attempt to increase peripheral vascular resistance to improve blood flow to the brain.
      - ▫ Avoid breath-holding and Valsalva maneuver!
      - ▫ Avoid pressure on the carotid bodies!

20 ■ SUDDEN CARDIAC ARREST

INTRODUCTION

Sudden cardiac death (SCD), also called sudden cardiac arrest (SCA), is the sudden loss of cardiac output, which results in loss of end-organ perfusion (particularly to the brain). It is usually lethal unless treated immediately. For most cardiologists, the term implies a malignant ventricular arrhythmia (ventricular fibrillation [VF] or ventricular tachycardia [VT]). Conditions leading to pulseless electrical activity (PEA) without a primary arrhythmia (such as pericardial tamponade, massive pulmonary embolism, severe acidosis) are also causes.

Since the diagnosis must often be made after the fact and without witnesses, epidemiologic and research definitions cannot require documentation of an arrhythmia. Definitions are based on the unexpected nature and the brief time period between onset of any syndrome and death.

EPIDEMIOLOGY

- Estimates range from 200,000 to 450,000 sudden deaths per year in the United States.[45]
- Assuming a population of approximately 300 million, the incidence is about 1 per 1000 per year.
- More men are affected than women (primarily reflecting the comparative prevalence of coronary artery disease).
- African Americans suffer more SCA than other ethnic groups, possibly related to the prevalence of hypertension, left ventricular hypertrophy, and diabetes, as well as access to health care.

MECHANISM AND SUBSTRATE

Ventricular fibrillation is thought to be the rhythm underlying most SCD, although it is difficult to know how often another rhythm (such as monomorphic VT) occurs initially and then deteriorates to VF.

- Bradycardia leading to asystole seems to be relatively rare.
- Bradycardia-induced tachyarrhythmias (such as polymorphic VT and VF) may be more common causes of SCD than bradycardia itself.
- SCD associated with profound progressive heart failure is more likely to be ultimately caused by electromechanical dissociation (EMD), bradycardia/asystole, or both.

In general, it appears that the occurrence of SCA (particularly due to tachyarrhythmias) requires an interaction between a proarrhythmic *substrate* and an inciting *trigger*.

- **Substrate** is an underlying heart disease that predisposes to electro-physiologic instability, introducing vulnerability to arrhythmia.
  - Scarring in the ventricular myocardium disrupts normal patterns of myocardial arrangement, allowing arrhythmogenic inhomogeneities of conduction, depolarization, and repolarization.
    - The most common substrate is myocardial scarring due to previous myocardial infarction.
    - Scarring my also be detected in dilated idiopathic cardiomyopathies.
    - Infiltrative and inflammatory diseases produce similar substrates to scar:
      - Sarcoidosis
      - Amyloidosis
      - Hemochromatosis
      - Myocarditis
      - Lymphoma
    - Arrhythmogenic RV dysplasia (ARVD) is characterized by fatty infiltration into the RV myocardium, which may be arrhythmogenic similar to scarring. In addition, intercellular conduction is deranged by abnormalities of connexons and gap junctions.
    - Chronic cocaine use may induce a cardiomyopathy with myocardial scarring.
  - Electrical substrate implies an abnormality in the cellular physiology that makes the myocardium vulnerable to arrhythmia.
    - Congenital diseases
      - Long QT syndromes
      - Brugada syndrome
      - Catecholaminergic polymorphic VT appear to be due to a mutation that affects the Ryanodine receptor (the sarcoplasmic reticulum Ca^{2+} release channel, which mediates Ca^{2+}-induced Ca^{2+} release). The abnormality disrupts intracellular Ca^{2+} management.
      - Short QT syndrome
      - Idiopathic VF
    - Acquired
      - Drug-induced proarrhythmia
        - QT prolonging drugs, including class IA and class III antiarrhythmic drugs
        - Class IC antiarrhythmic (such as flecainide and propafenone) drugs slow conduction. In combination with other substrates (such as myocardial scar), slow conduction may allow reentry to occur where it was previously unsustainable.
    - Electrolyte abnormalities
      - Hypokalemia
      - Hyperkalemia
      - Magnesium deficiency
      - Calcium deficiency

- A **trigger** event is usually required to induce a lethal arrhythmia. In most cases, a normal rhythm exists in the context of a lethal substrate, until a trigger sets off the arrhythmia. Presumably most of the triggers either caused by fortuitously timed ectopy that may set off torsades de pointes, polymorphic VT, or VF in the vulnerable substrate. Some triggers may intensify a proarrhythmic substrate such that a previously minimal stimulus becomes effective. For example, catecholamines shorten refractoriness and increase membrane excitability. Minimal ectopy may then initiate VF or polymorphic VT in the setting of myocardial scar or other myocardial abnormality.
  - Acute ischemia depolarizes the resting membrane potential and increases automaticity. Since coronary disease is common and produces both substrate (myocardial infarction scar) and trigger, it is certainly one of the most common causes of SCA. In addition to atherosclerotic coronary disease, acute ischemia may also occur with:
    - Coronary spasm
    - Congenital coronary anomalies
    - Coronary embolism
    - Aortic dissection
  - Other triggers:
    - Exertion
    - Autonomic changes
      - Increased sympathetic activity
      - Decreased parasympathetic activity
    - Mental stress
    - Stimulants, including caffeine, cocaine, beta-adrenergic agonists

THERAPY

- Urgent therapy for sudden death
  - Restore cardiac output and perfusion immediately
    - Chest compressions
  - Restore normal-rhythm cardiac function (to the extent possible).
    - ACLS protocols are tailored to the presenting rhythm/problem.
      - Early defibrillation of ventricular tachyarrhythmias is a focus.
      - Pharmacologic support and pacing for profound bradycardia.
      - Reversal of other causes, such as draining pericardial effusion in tamponade.
  - Treatment or removal or acute triggers if possible
    - Ischemia
    - Electrolyte abnormalities
    - Proarrhythmic drugs
    - Beta-adrenergic stimulation

PREVENTION

- **General prevention.** Survival rates of SCA are very poor; thus preventive therapy is important. However, most SCA occurs, not in identifiable high-risk groups, but in the general population of people without known heart disease. Specific therapies (anti-arrhythmic drugs and implantable cardioverter-defibrillators (ICDs)) are expensive and potentially noxious, and are therefore not suited for widespread use.
  - Since structural heart disease plays such a large role in the substrate for SCA, and LV dysfunction is the single most important predictor of SCD, prevention and treatment of these problems is the most effective strategy for prevention of SCA in the general population.
    - Coronary artery disease is the most common of structural heart diseases, but nonischemic cardiomyopathies, congenital heart disease, and other structural heart diseases all bear consideration.
  - Treatment to prevent death from malignant arrhythmias focuses on immediate defibrillation to terminate the arrhythmia (not on preventing the occurrence of the arrhythmia in the first place).
    - The emergency medical service was instituted in part to allow rapid defibrillation and trained early response to SCA.
    - The proliferation of automatic external defibrillators in public places may prevent death by providing earlier defibrillation than even the emergency medical services can provide.
- **Secondary prevention.** Survivors without an immediately reversible cause of SCA are at very high risk of recurrent SCA.
  - Antiarrhythmic drugs have had some success in preventing SCA, but they are suboptimal due to proarrhythmia, side effects, and toxicity.
  - Implantable cardioverter defibrillators (ICDs) have been shown to be successful in preventing death in secondary prevention populations. As with the emergency medical services and bystander defibrillation, the strategy is not to prevent the occurrence of arrhythmias, but to terminate them immediately when they occur.
- **Primary prevention in high-risk populations.** Patients with significant left ventricular dysfunction and some other conditions (severe hypertrophic cardiomyopathy, ARVD, long QT syndrome) have been found to be at relatively high risk for SCA.
  - ICDs are indicated for primary prevention in high-risk groups. See Chapter 30: Implantable Defibrillator Therapy, pp. 2-19.
  - Antiarrhythmic drugs have a high incidence of toxicity, side effects, and proarrhythmia. They are therefore not routinely used for primary prevention.
    - The growth of defibrillator implantation has essentially provided a new indication for antiarrhythmic agents. In patients who have suffered painful ICD shocks for arrhythmias, antiarrhythmic

agents may have a favorable risk:benefit ratio. The intention
is less to prevent death, but to reduce the need for painful ICD
therapy.
- Indications for ablation of ventricular arrhythmias have grown
  in the same way.

21 ■ ADULT CONGENITAL HEART DISEASE

INTRODUCTION

Advances in the management and surgical treatment of children born with cardiac anomalies have dramatically improved survival of these patients well into adulthood. This has created a burgeoning population of adults that require expert care by physicians familiar with the unique challenges of managing the long-term sequelae of not only the lesions themselves but the repairs performed to "correct" them.

Adult congenital heart disease (ACHD) care requires careful attention to the following general principles:

- Know the history! Detailed knowledge of the original anomaly and the timing and approach of surgeries/procedures performed is essential.
- In general, there are no "cures" in surgical repair of congenital heart disease (CHD). Even simple lesions have long-term consequences.
- Know the natural history of the specific condition and the anticipated durability and consequences of the repair.
- You cannot always wait for symptoms. Imaging surveillance and close follow-up is particularly important in complex disease.
- Common maladies (HTN, CAD/ischemia, arrhythmias) may impose undue stress on these patients with less predictable tolerability of both disease and treatment.

ACYANOTIC LESIONS

Sometimes referred to as "simple," these anomalies do not involve right-to-left shunting if discovered and treated early.

ATRIAL SEPTAL DEFECTS

- Definitions (see **Figure 21-1**)
    - *Ostium secundum:* the most common ASD (75%) localized to the fossa ovalis region
    - *Ostium primum:* less common (15%), localized to the inferior aspect of the atrial septum; also called partial AV septal defect
    - *SVC sinus venosus:* less common (10%), located near the septal aspect of the SVC-RA junction
    - *IVC sinus venosus:* rare (<1%), located at the septal aspect of the IVC-RA junction
    - *"Unroofed" coronary sinus:* rarest form, with absence of wall separating coronary sinus from atria allowing interatrial communication

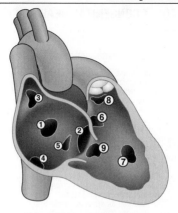

FIGURE 21-1. Atrial Septal Defects (ASDs) and Ventricular Septal Defects (VSDs). 1. Ostium secundum ASD. 2. Ostium primum ASD. 3. Superior Sinus venosus ASD. 4. Inferior Sinus Venosus VSD. 5. "Unroofed" Coronary Sinus (ASD). 6. Perimembranous VSD. 7. Muscular VSD. 8. Supracristal VSD. 9. Inlet VSD.
Adapted from Aboulosn JA, Child JS. Chapter 84: Congenital Heart Disease in Adults in *Hurst's The Heart, 13th ed.* Fuster V, Walsh RA, Harrington RA, eds. New York: McGraw Hill Medical. pp. 1884-1913.

- Clinical presentation
  - Most patients are asymptomatic. When present, symptoms are non-specific and include fatigue or dyspnea on exertion, usually indicating that chronic left-to-right shunting has led to chamber dilatation and volume overload. Atrial arrhythmias are common.
  - Physical exam: signs of right-sided volume or pressure overload (fixed, split S2(loud P2); systolic flow murmur; RV heave and/or PA tap)
  - ECG findings: incomplete RBBB, right axis deviation (secundum), left axis deviation (primum), atrial enlargement, RVH, prolonged PR, atrial arrhythmias
  - Echocardiography is essential for diagnosis and assessment of shunting consequences (e.g., chamber enlargement, RV dysfunction, shunt magnitude, elevated pulmonary pressures). Transesophageal echo is required for diagnosis of sinus venosus variants and for careful assessment of pulmonary vein drainage. It is also helpful in confirming site and size of the more common defects.
  - Additional lesions are common. These include: partial anomalous pulmonary venous return, cleft mitral valve, mitral valve prolapse, pulmonic stenosis, coarctation, PDA, VSD.
- Management
  - All "significant" (RV volume overload and/or large shunt Qp:Qs > 1.5:1.0) ASDs should be closed, regardless of age.
  - Contraindications to closure: significant LV dysfunction, irreversible pulmonary arterial hypertension, small ASDs without evidence of right chamber enlargement.
  - Catheter-based device closure is performed at most experienced centers for isolated secundum ASDs.
  - Surgical closure is required for all others and secundum ASDs that are too large (> 4 cm) or lack sufficient rims of tissue for device seating or those associated with valvular or pulmonary vein drainage abnormalities.
  - If repaired early (before age 25), survival is not reduced. Without repair, late complications also include heart failure, pulmonary hypertension (pHTN), paradoxical embolism/stroke.

VENTRICULAR SEPTAL DEFECTS

- Definitions (see **Figure 21-1**):
  - *Muscular VSD:* Defect is surrounded entirely by ventricular myocardium and can be seen anywhere in the muscular septum (apical, anterior, mid-muscular, inlet, outlet).
  - *Perimembranous VSD:* Most common (70%), located at the base of the ventricle involving the fibrous portion of the septum, often with extension into the trabecular, inlet, or outlet portions of the muscular septum.

- *Supracristal/infundibular VSD:* Rare defect in the outlet septum above the *crista supraventricularis.*
- *Inlet VSD:* extending from the annulus of the tricuspid valve to the muscular septum. May be isolated or associated with an *ostium primum* ASD as part of the AV canal complex.

- Restrictive versus nonrestrictive VSDs:
  - *Restrictive:* Small defect associated with large interventricular pressure gradient with minimal shunting ($< 1.5:1.0$) and, therefore, no significant hemodynamic consequences.
  - *Nonrestrictive:* Large shunt ($> 2.5:1.0$), associated with LV volume overload leading to chamber enlargement, pulmonary hypertension, and eventually shunt reversal (Eisenmenger physiology) if not repaired early.

- Clinical presentation:
  - Symptoms depend on the size and hemodynamic consequences of the defect. They include dyspnea, fatigue, decreased exertional capacity, and other symptoms of heart failure.
  - Restrictive defects generate a loud, harsh holosystolic murmur that may produce a thrill. Other exam findings that should warrant concern for larger shunts or chamber enlargement include S3, displaced PMI, loud P2, or diminishing murmurs on subsequent visits.
  - ECG findings: If small, ECG is normal. Large VSDs may produce ECG evidence of left atrial enlargement, ventricular hypertrophy, and right axis deviation.
  - CXR: Signs of LV enlargement and prominent pulmonary vascularity. With severe pulmonary hypertension (pHTN), pruning of the visible distal pulmonary vasculature occurs.
  - Echo: Location, size, and consequences of the defect. Aortic valve dysfunction (aortic insufficiency) can be seen in supracristal VSDs.
  - Cardiac MRI: Detailed imaging and functional flow assessment across the defect.
  - Cardiac catheterization: Direct measurements of right heart hemodynamics and shunt ratio.

- Management:
  - In general, small, restrictive VSDs do not require repair and can be followed with yearly imaging if asymptomatic. Moderately sized and large VSDs should be surgically repaired as early as possible before chamber enlargement ensues or irreversible pHTN develops.
  - If repair is delayed and pulmonary hypertension is already present at diagnosis, then surgical closure should still be pursued if the net left-to right shunt is $> 1.5:1.0$ or if pHTN is "reversible" based on response to pulmonary vasodilators.
  - Catheter-based device closure is reasonable in defects that are not in close proximity to the valves.

ATRIOVENTRICULAR SEPTAL DEFECTS (ENDOCARDIAL CUSHION DEFECT)

- Definitions:
  - *Partial AVSD:* ostium primum ASD with cleft mitral valve and intact ventricular septum
  - *Transitional or intermediate AVSD:* primum ASD with small, restrictive VSD and distinct, but malformed, AV valves
  - *Complete AVSD (also called complete AV canal):* primum ASD with contiguous large VSD separated by common AV valve
- Clinical presentation:
  - Most patients are asymptomatic with partial or intermediate AVSD. Dyspnea may indicate a more significant shunt or mitral regurgitation.
  - Complete AVSD is most often associated with Down syndrome and presents early in childhood with heart failure.
  - Physical exam should reflect the presence or absence of findings consistent with heart failure (S3, displaced PMI, elevated JVD) and/or pHTN (RV heave, PA tap, loud S2) in addition to holosystolic murmurs generated by VSDs, enhanced flow, and/or AV valvular regurgitation.
  - ECG: PR prolongation, left axis deviation, RBBB or incomplete RBBB
  - As described in the previous septal defects, echo, cardiac MRI, and cardiac catheterization aid in defining type, size, hemodynamic effects of the defect, with additional emphasis on defining competency of AV valves.
- Management:
  - In the absence of irreversible pHTN, surgical repair focusing on defect closure (typically via pericardial or Dacron patch) plus repair/reconstruction of the AV valve malformation should be performed at an experienced center.
  - These patients should be followed at least annually after repair. Late complications include recurrent mitral regurgitation, atrial arrhythmias, manifest residual defects, and AV or aortic valvular stenosis.

COARCTATION OF THE AORTA

- Definition:
  - Ridge-like luminal narrowing of the aorta typically at the site of the ligamentum arteriosum just beyond the left subclavian artery. Many variants exist including narrowing proximal to the subclavian, a long tubular stenosis of the distal arch, and, rarely, descending/abdominal aorta coarctation.
- Clinical presentation:
  - Male predominance
  - Associated lesions: bicuspid aortic valve (20–50%), cerebral aneurysms (5–10%), Turner's syndrome
  - Most patients are repaired in childhood. Unrepaired or undiagnosed patients develop hypertension and extensive thoracic collaterals and

have poor survival (average age 35 years). Most common causes of death include CHF (25%; 3rd–5th decade of life), aortic rupture (21%; 2nd–3rd decade), endocarditis complications (18%; 2nd–3rd decade), and intracranial hemorrhage (12%; 1st–5th decade)

- Symptoms: Most neonates present with heart failure. Adults may be asymptomatic and present only because of hypertension or exam findings. Other complaints may include epistaxis, headache, dizziness, or claudication. Symptoms of heart failure or aortic dissection are particularly concerning.
- Physical exam: Hypertension, discrepant upper and lower extremity pulses and blood pressure, murmurs (from coarctation, thoracic vessel collaterals, or aortic regurgitation), opening click (if bicuspid aortic valve)
- ECG: LVH
- CXR: "Figure 3" sign (formed by the dilated aortic knob, the coarct itself, and post-stenotic dilation of the aorta), rib notching (from large intercostal collaterals)
- Echo: Careful evaluation of aortic valve structure and competency. Doppler assessment of aortic outflow, including suprasternal notch "views" to assess gradient. Gradients > 30 mmHg are considered significant and warrant repair.
- Cardiac MRI, CT, aortography: Helpful in delineating extent and nuances of coarctation (including extent of collateral circulation) before repair and useful in follow-up when concerned for recurrence.
- Cerebral MRI: Controversial. May obtain to evaluate for presence of aneurysms.
- Management:
  - Surgical repair in childhood is typical. Techniques have evolved over the years and include resection with end-to-end anastomosis with or without an interposition graft (most common; adults often require graft), subclavian flap aortoplasty (weak pulse in LUE; ischemia is rare), patch aortoplasty (abandoned due to frequency of aneurysm formation), and bypass with long prosthetic tube grafts (reserved for complex or complete stenosis)
  - Catheter-based stenting of lesions have shown promise and are frequently utilized in adults with discrete lesions and in recurrent lesions.
  - Follow-up imaging is important to survey for recurrence, aneurysm formation, or aortic valve stenosis or regurgitation.

CYANOTIC LESIONS

These patients are defined by the presence of arterial oxygen desaturation due to shunting of deoxygenated venous blood into the systemic arterial circulation. Survival beyond childhood is dependent on the degree of shunting and timely repair of these "complex" lesions.

TETRALOGY OF FALLOT

- Definitions:
  - *Tetralogy of Fallot (ToF):* cyanotic CHD caused by right ventricular outflow tract obstruction, nonrestrictive VSD, overriding aorta, and RVH; occasionally (~5%), an ASD is also present ("pentology")
  - *Acyanotic Fallot or "pink Tet:"* the same constellation of defects with minimal RVOT obstruction
  - *Blalock-Taussig (BT) shunt:* original palliative procedure to increase pulmonary blood flow by anastomosing the subclavian artery to the pulmonary artery (*classic:* end-to-side; *modified:* via interposed graft)
  - *Potts shunt:* descending aorta to left pulmonary artery
  - *Waterston shunt:* ascending aorta to right pulmonary artery.
- Clinical presentation:
  - Timing of presentation depends largely on degree of RV outflow obstruction. Usually, the outflow obstruction is substantial and the resultant murmur, right-to-left shunting, and cyanosis lead to diagnosis shortly after birth if the defect went undiscovered during prenatal evaluation.
  - Surgical repair typically occurs early in life. It is rare for adults to present with undiagnosed ToF. With mild RVOT obstruction, shunting and cyanosis are minimal and the lesions can be tolerated for some time. Dyspnea and diminished exertional capacity may be seen.
  - Common associated lesions: right-sided aortic arch, anomalous coronary arteries, atrial septal defect.
  - Physical Exam(pre-repair): Cyanosis and clubbing, holosystolic murmurs, RV lift.
  - Exam (post-repair): RV lift, systolic murmurs (from RVOT obstruction, residual VSD, VSD patch leak, or TR from RV enlargement), diastolic murmurs (PI, AR), soft/delayed or absent P2. Patients with history of Blalock-Taussig shunt will have a diminished or absent ipsilateral upper extremity pulse
  - ECG: RBBB (almost all), RVH
  - CXR: normal-sized, "boot-shaped" heart
  - Echocardiography: Reveals these defects. Careful assessment of shunting across septal defect and gradient across RVOT. Following repair, echo is vital in assessing success of repair, degree and progression of pulmonary insufficiency, and RV and LV size and systolic function.
  - Cardiac MRI and catheterization can provide further information on severity and location of shunting, degree/level of RVOT obstruction, coronary and aortic anomalies, ventricular size and systolic function, and post-repair issues (PI, AR, residual septal defect or outflow obstruction, RVOT-patch aneurysmal dilatation, progressive chamber dilation, and systolic dysfunction)

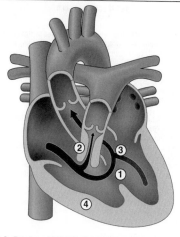

FIGURE 21-2. Tetrology of Fallot. The tetraology consists of: 1. Large VSD; 2. RV outflow tract (infundibular) stenosis; 3. Aorta "overriding" the VSD and receiving RV and LV blood; 4. RV hypertrophy.
Adapted from Brickner EM, Hillis LD, Lange RA. Congenital Heart Disease in Adults: Second of Two Parts. *N Engl J Med.* 2000; 342: 334-342.

- Management:
  - Palliative procedures to temporarily increase pulmonary flow (listed above) were previously common and, therefore, many surviving adults have a history of them preceding complete repair.
  - "Complete" repair involves patch closure of the VSD with transannular patch repair or surgical resection of the outflow obstruction with reconstruction of the RVOT.
  - Following repair, annual visits should always address the following:
    - "Red-flag" symptoms: worsening dyspnea, diminished exertional capacity, syncope, palpitations
    - Quantitative right ventricular size and systolic function
    - Degree of pulmonary regurgitation and/or residual outflow tract stenosis
    - Sudden cardiac arrest (SCA) risk stratification
  - Risk factors for SCA include: QRS duration > 180 ms, history of palliative shunts, prior ventriculostomy, elevated LVEDP (> 12 mmHg), nonsustained VT, inducible sustained VT.
  - ICD implantation should be considered in high-risk patients for primary prevention and offered to all patients with aborted sudden death, unexplained syncope, or sustained VT/VF (in the absence of contraindications to ICD).
  - Pulmonic regurgitation is well tolerated for years and, if one waits for symptoms to develop, irreversible RV dilation and dysfunction may occur. PI murmurs are unreliable indicators of severity as they are often subtle and short as RVOT and PA pressures equalize quickly in severe PI.
    - Timing of PV replacement (PVR) is trending earlier in experienced centers with low operative risk. Ideally, PVR will occur before irreversible RV dysfunction ensues but not too early, as many patients will require repeat surgery every 10 years.
  - New arrhythmias (atrial or ventricular) should trigger concern for adverse change in hemodynamics due to valvular regurgitation and/or ventricular enlargement and dysfunction.

TRANSPOSITION OF THE GREAT ARTERIES (TGA)

Transposition of the great arteries refers to anomalous origin of the aorta from the RV and pulmonary artery from the LV (see Figure 21-3). Distinction of the subtypes depends on the relative orientation of the ventricles and atrioventricular relationship caused by normal or abnormal looping of the heart tube during development.

- Definitions:
  - *Complete transposition of the great arteries (dextro-transposition; D-TGA):* Defect is marked by ventriculoarterial discordance with typical looping of the ventricles (flow: venous blood to RA to tricuspid valve to RV to aorta; oxygenated blood to LA to MV to LV to pulmonary artery) generating 2 separate, parallel circulations that would be

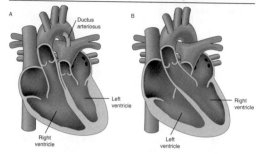

FIGURE 21-3. Transposition of the Great Arteries. In both d-transposition and l-transposition, the Aorta is anterior to the pulmonary artery. A. D-Transposition. The positions of the morphologic LV and RV are switched, as are the connections of the aorta and pulmonary artery. In the absence of shunts, the pulmonary and systemic circulations are separate. No oxygenated blood reaches the systemic circulation, and no deoxygenated blood reaches the pulmonary circulation. B. L-Transposition. The positions of the morphlic LV and RV are switched, but the aorta and pulmonary artery maintain their normal ventricular connections. The path of blood circulation is normal, but the systemic ventricle is relatively weak and subject to failure.

Adapted from Sommer RJ, Hijazi ZM, Rhodes JF. Pathophysiology of Congenital Heart Disease in the Adult: Part III: Complex Congenital Heart Disease. *Circulation*. 2008; 117:1340-1350.

incompatible with life if a shunt (PFO, ASD, PDA, VSD) is not present or created.

○ The RV (or pulmonic ventricle) actually has the morphology (thick muscular walls) normally seen in the LV. Meanwhile, the LV has the thin-walled morphology normally seen in the RV.

○ *Imagine switching the positions of the ventricles with their associated arteries (the pulmonary artery and the aorta)*

○ The separated systemic and pulmonary circulation circuits prevent appropriate flow of oxygenated blood to the systemic circulation and deoxygenated blood to the pulmonary circulation

  ▪ **Memory aid: "Ds Die"** (in the absence of shunt, as noted above).

- *Congenitally corrected TGA (levo-transposition; L-TGA):* Transposed great arteries (aorta anterior to PA) with fortuitous atrioventricular discordance. Abnormal looping during development places the systemic, morphologic RV posterior and to the left. Several terms have been used to describe this "two-wrongs-make-a-right" anomaly including "ventricular inversion" or "double switch." (Flow: RA to mitral valve to LV to pulmonary artery to lungs to pulmonary veins to LA to tricuspid valve to RV to aorta).

  ○ The morphology of the ventricles is again reversed from normal: The pulmonic (anteriorly located) ventricle is thick walled; the systemic (posteriorly located) ventricle is thin walled and subject to failure.

  ○ *Imagine switching only the ventricles (and AV valves), but leaving the arteries (the pulmonary artery and the aorta) in place.*

  ○ The course of oxygenated and deoxygenated blood flow is the same as in a person without the defect (except for the morphology of the ventricles).

    ▪ **Memory aid: "Ls Live"** (since the blood circulation is normal)

THERAPEUTIC PROCEDURES

- *Blalock-Hanlon septostomy:* Palliative surgery to create large atrial septal defect to allow for left-to-right shunting in D-TGA.
- *Rashkind procedure:* Minimally invasive, transcatheter balloon septostomy accomplishing the same palliative result as surgical septostomy without need for cardiopulmonary bypass and thoracotomy.
- *Atrial switch* **(Figure 21-4A)**: Blood is diverted at the atrial level via baffles created out of native atrial tissue (*Senning procedure*) or Dacron or pericardium (*Mustard procedure*), restoring the normal physiologic relationship of the systemic and pulmonic circulations, but leaving the RV as the systemic ventricle. Most adult D-TGA survivors had an atrial switch as it was the operation of choice until the 1980s.
- *Rastelli procedure:* Operation performed for D-TGA with associated VSD and pulmonary stenosis, involving an LV-to-aorta baffle via the VSD and a valved RV-to-PA conduit.
- *Jatene procedure* **(Figure 21-4B)**: The procedure of choice currently for D-TGA, consisting of an "arterial switch" restoring the RV and LV

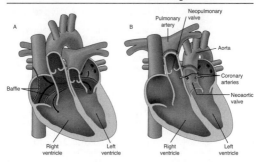

FIGURE 21-4. Surgical repair of d-Transposition of the Great Arteries. A. Atrial switch procedures (e.g., Senning, Mustard) create flow from the veins to the appropriate atrium and ventricle for normal circulation. The systemic ventricle remains thin-walled and subject to failure. B. Arterial switch procedure (Jatene) creates ventriculo-arterial concordance, and the thick-walled morphologic LV serves as the systemic ventricle, as is desirable. The coronary arteries must be relocated to the aorta.

Adapted from Brickner EM, Hillis LD, Lange RA. Congenital Heart Disease in Adults: Second of Two Parts. *N Engl J Med.* 2000; 342: 334-342.

as the pulmonic and systemic ventricles, respectively. The coronary arteries are removed from the root of the vessel coming off the RV and attached to the neo-aortic root leaving the LV.

- *"Double switch" operation:* Arterial and atrial switch to restore LV as systemic ventricle in L-TGA.
- Clinical presentation:
  - The D-TGA infant becomes progressively more cyanotic as the *ductus arteriosus* closes. Without a natural or created palliative shunt, the defect is lethal.
  - L-TGA patients can remain undiagnosed into adulthood. They often present with heart failure symptoms due to systemic ventricular dysfunction (morphologic RV) and/or systemic atrioventricular (TV) valvular regurgitation.
  - Associated lesions are common, especially with L-TGA (VSD ~ 70%; pulmonic stenosis ~ 40%; systemic AV valve abnormality ~ 90%; AV block ~ 2% per year).
- Physical exam:
  - L-TGA: Single S2 +/− systolic murmur from an associated lesion (VSD, AV valve regurgitation, pulmonic stenosis)
  - D-TGA: depends on repair
    ○ Atrial switch: RV heave, single S2, holosystolic murmur (systemic "TR")
    ○ Arterial switch: unremarkable
- ECG:
  - D-TGA: rightward axis, RVH, bradycardia, atrial arrhythmias
  - L-TGA: prolonged PR, heart block, inferior and/or right precordial Q waves
- CXR: "egg-on-its-side" shape with narrow vascular pedicle
- Echocardiography:
  - Left-sided, trabeculated ventricle (RV) with left AV valve displaced more apically
  - D-TGA: "parallel" great arteries
- Cardiac MRI and catheterization: Assess for baffle leaks, systemic ventricular dysfunction, residual VSDs, etc., that may not be fully appreciated on echocardiography.
- Management:
  - At a minimum, annual follow-up is required with imaging (TTE and/or MRI). Adult patients should be followed for evidence of late complications including:
    ○ Baffle leaks or stenosis
    ○ Significant shunts: surgical or catheter-based intervention
    ○ Arrhythmias
      ▪ Bradyarrhythmias: Symptomatic bradycardia and advanced heart block should be treated with permanent pacing.
      ▪ Atrial tachyarrhythmias: Common, especially after atrial switch procedures. If burden is significant, pharmacologic therapy or catheter ablation should be considered

- ○ Systemic AV valve regurgitation
  - Timing of valve replacement for severe regurgitation must weigh "too early" (e.g., need for future surgery) against "too late" (e.g., irreversible ventricular dysfunction).
- ○ Systemic ventricular dysfunction
  - Although not studied in ACHD, most patients are placed on ACE inhibitors and/or beta-blockers.
  - Severe dysfunction with significant HF symptoms should be evaluated for advanced HF therapies or heart transplant.
  - ICDs are appropriate for secondary prevention of sudden cardiac death. Their role in primary prevention is less well defined.
- ○ Additional late complications
  - Arterial switch: pulmonary artery stenosis, neo-aortic valve regurgitation, and ostial coronary artery stenosis
  - Rastelli: conduit and/or subaortic stenosis, residual VSD

SINGLE VENTRICLE PHYSIOLOGY AND THE FONTAN SURGERY

Single ventricle patients possess a defect or constellation of defects that functionally lead to a single ventricle driving both circulations with early intervention required for survival. "Correction," in general, ultimately leads to creation of a surgical diversion of venous blood into the pulmonary arteries while utilizing the ventricle as the systemic pump. Although rare, they arguably represent the most complex patients in the ACHD clinic.

- • Definitions:
  - • *Hypoplastic left heart syndrome (HLHS):* Most common form of univentricular physiology. Characterized by atretic or stenotic mitral and aortic valves with hypoplasia of the LV and ascending aorta, typically with associated coarctation and ASD or PFO.
  - • *Tricuspid atresia:* Second most common form that is characterized by atretic tricuspid valve with resultant RV hypoplasia. There is often a VSD and/or pulmonic stenosis.
  - • *Double inlet left ventricle (DILV) or right ventricle:* Both AV valves empty into a large, functionally "single" ventricle that gives rise to a great artery. This ventricle is attached via defect to a rudimentary ventricle that gives rise to the other great artery. Associated TGA and pulmonic stenosis is very common.
  - • *Glenn shunt:* Palliative surgery to increase pulmonic blood flow via direct anastomosis between SVC and PA (cavopulmonary shunt).
    - ○ *"Classic" Glenn:* SVC to divided right PA (divided from the main and left PA) with ligation of SVC inferior to anastomosis
    - ○ *Bidirectional Glenn:* Ligated SVC to undivided PA
  - • *Norwood procedure:* A staged procedure specific to palliating HLHS
    - ○ *Stage 1 (1st week of life):* Establish RV as systemic ventricle without obstruction, allow unimpeded intra-atrial flow, and establish pulmonic flow via shunt.

- Aortic reconstruction using PA, hypoplastic aorta, and prosthetic patch with PV as neoaortic valve
- Atrial septectomy
- Systemic to PA shunt: B-T Shunt or *Sano modification* (RV-to-PA conduit)
  - *Stage 2 (4–6 months):* Create cavopulmonary shunt.
    - Bidirectional Glenn or hemi-Fontan
    - B-T Shunt or Sano taken down
  - *Stage 3 (2–3 years):* Complete separation of circulations.
    - IVC flow redirected to PA to complete Fontan circuit (see below)
- *Fontan surgery:* Operation to palliate single ventricle physiology involving diversion of systemic venous blood to the pulmonary artery, thus bypassing the (nonexistent) pulmonary ventricle and eliminating cyanosis and volume overload.
  - *"Classic" Fontan:* RA connected to PA originally via valved conduit then subsequently via direct anastomosis with RA appendage with closure of ASD; conceived initially for tricuspid atresia
  - *Bjork Modification:* RA-to-RV (hypoplastic) conduit for correction of tricuspid atresia
  - *Lateral-tunnel Fontan or total cavopulmonary connection (TCPC):* Systemic venous return is baffled from IVC through surgically isolated lateral aspect of RA to inferior aspect of divided SVC (from previous Glenn Shunt) into PA. A small *fenestration* is occasionally placed in the baffle to provide a relief valve for pressure overload.
  - *Extracardiac Fontan or TCPC:* IVC flow is redirected to PA via an extracardiac graft. SVC flow is already redirected to PA via Glenn shunt.
  - *Hemi-Fontan:* Bidirectional Glenn shunt with a second anastomosis of the inferior aspect of the SVC to the PA that is oversewn, facilitating future conversion to full Fontan.
- Clinical presentation:
  - These patients present with cyanosis and heart failure requiring early intervention and multiple surgeries throughout their lives to allow survival into adulthood. Although there are subtleties unique to each condition, in general, these patients have a similar course including the following:
    - 1–2 weeks: palliative shunt created to increase pulmonic flow via systemic arterial-to-PA shunt (e.g., B-T shunt) or cavopulmonary shunt (Glenn)
    - 4–6 months: cavopulmonary shunt (e.g., bidirectional Glenn) if not previously performed
    - 18 months to 4 years: Fontan procedure
- Physical exam: cyanosis, signs of right heart failure, systolic and diastolic murmurs from AV valve, or outflow stenosis and/or regurgitation

- ECG: Variable depending on anatomy. Bradyarrhythmias, PR prolongation, higher degree AV block, atypical patterns of hypertrophy, and atrial tachyarrhythmias are common.
- CXR: Pulmonary vasculature abnormalities are common and related to degree of pulmonary blood flow. Thus, depending on anatomy and obstruction to flow, enhancement, asymmetry, or oligemia can be seen.
- Echo: Characterize the AV connection as common, single, or double. Assess severity of AV valve stenosis and/or regurgitation. Assess for TGA and other associated lesions. Following repair, serial imaging vital for assessment of shunting, chamber enlargement, valvular abnormalities, and thrombosis or circuit obstruction.
- MRI/Catheterization: Useful supplement to echo to better define anatomy, function, and hemodynamics, particularly in those likely to need surgical intervention.
- Management:
  - Follow-up should be frequent (6–12 months at a minimum) and geared toward evaluation for inevitable long-term sequelae of the Fontan circuit.
  - Hypoxemia
    - Consider worsening of systemic ventricular function, shunting across fenestration or ASD, venous collaterals, or pulmonary AVMs/
  - Arrhythmia
    - Bradyarrhythmias and atrial tachyarrhythmias are very common and carry significant morbidity if poorly controlled. They are often indicative of compromised flow in the Fontan circuit.
    - Maintenance of SR and AV conduction (e.g., cardioversion, catheter ablation, antiarrhythmic drugs, pacing) should be aggressively pursued to avoid further hemodynamic deterioration.
    - In patients undergoing surgery, permanent epicardial pacing and right atrial MAZE procedure should be considered when appropriate.
  - Hepatic dysfunction
    - Chronic elevated right sided pressures can lead to hepatic congestion, hepatomegaly, and elevated liver function tests.
  - Protein-losing enteropathy (PLE)
    - Protein loss via GI tract due to chronically elevated venous pressures lead to refractory edema, ascites, pleural and pericardial effusions, and chronic diarrhea.
    - Low serum albumin and elevated fecal alpha-1-antitrypsin are diagnostic.
    - Reversible causes of Fontan obstruction should be sought and intervention (e.g., fenestration, stenting, surgical revision) should be considered early.
  - Ventricular dysfunction
    - Typical heart failure therapies are often prescribed empirically but careful titration is advised to avoid reduction in preload and deterioration of sinus node function or AV conduction.

- Thromboembolism
    - Sluggish flow in the setting of chamber enlargement, atrial arrhythmias, hepatic dysfunction, and/or protein losing enteropathy places the Fontan patient at significant risk for thrombus formation.
    - Anticoagulation is typical in patients with atrial arrhythmias and in those with known history of thromboembolism. Utility of anticoagulants or antiplatelet agents in other patients is unclear.
- In general, patients with earlier versions of the Fontan (atriopulmonary connections) are more susceptible to these complications. Surgical conversion to a TCPC (plus MAZE and/or epicardial pacemaker) has shown early promise in reducing this risk.

EISENMENGER SYNDROME

Eisenmenger syndrome represents the end-stage complication of a significant, unrepaired central shunt that causes chronic overloading and adverse remodeling of the pulmonary vasculature. Ultimately, severe pHTN develops with resultant shunt reversal (now right-to-left) and cyanosis.

- Clinical presentation:
    - Typically, dyspnea and diminished exercise tolerance develop in childhood or early adulthood. If undiscovered and/or unrepaired, shunting and hypoxemia worsen, causing progressive decline and development of right heart failure.
    - Most common etiologies: VSD, AVSD, PDA
    - Survival is abysmal with less than 50% alive at 25 years.
    - Physical exam: hypoxemia/cyanosis, digital clubbing, loud/palpable P2, RV heave, right sided S4, diastolic murmur of PI, holosystolic murmur of TR, defect- specific murmurs
    - ECG: RVH/LVH with repolarization abnormalities, right atrial enlargement, right axis deviation
    - CXR: enlarged RA/RV, prominent central vasculature with distal pruning
    - Echocardiography: reveals underlying defect with Doppler evidence of shunting and pulmonary hypertension; atrial and ventricular enlargement/hypertrophy
    - Cardiac catheterization: vasodilator challenge to determine degree and reversibility of pHTN
    - Laboratory results: erythrocytosis, thrombocytopenia, neutropenia, iron deficiency, hyperuricemia, hyperbilirubinemia, proteinuria
- Management:
    - Once irreversible Eisenmenger physiology develops, these patients are susceptible to a number of complications, and their tenuous hemodynamics make them difficult to manage.
    - In general, surgery to correct the underlying defect is not recommended as it does not improve and may worsen survival.

- Extreme caution should be taken with these patients. Any perturbation in blood pressure and volume status can have unpredictable, untoward results. Therefore, medication additions/changes, noncardiac surgery, infections, blood loss, pregnancy, heavy exercise, etc. should be avoided if possible.
- Hyperviscosity syndrome
  - Erythrocytosis from chronic hypoxemia may lead to hyperviscosity, particularly if there is iron deficiency and resultant RBC deformability.
  - Symptoms include changes in mental status, headaches, visual changes, myalgias, paresthesia, and generalized fatigue.
  - Iron deficiency and ample hydration should be emphasized. Phlebotomy is rarely required and should only be considered in situations were symptoms are severe.
- Bleeding/thrombosis
  - Paradoxically, these patients are at risk for bleeding (hemoptysis/pulmonary hemorrhage, mucocutaneous bleeding, ecchymosis) and thrombosis (embolic CVA, DVT/PE).
  - The benefit of warfarin is unclear and must be weighed against bleeding risk.
- Symptomatic gout from hyperuricemia is common. Treatment with steroids and colchicine for acute flares in addition to chronic suppression with allopurinol is typical. Aspirin and other NSAIDs should be avoided.
- Pulmonary vasodilators (CCBs, endothelin receptor blockers, prostacyclin) have shown early promise in improving symptoms and quality of life in these patients.
- Definitive therapy is heart-lung transplant or lung transplant with repair of the central shunt.

OTHER LESIONS

Ebstein's anomaly:
- A rare defect related to abnormal development of the tricuspid valve. Classically, there is apical displacement of the valve leaflets, particularly the septal leaflet, often with a "sail-like" anterior leaflet. This results in "atrialization" of a variable portion of the right ventricle (Figure 21-5).
- In approximately half the cases, there is an associated ASD or PFO.
- The degree of TR, right atrial enlargement, shunting, and RV dysfunction determine the clinical course.
- 25% of patients have accessory pathways, and atrial tachyarrhythmias are common.
- Surgical repair or valve replacement should be considered in patients with severe TR, worsening functional capacity, significant shunting, right-sided heart failure, paradoxical emboli, or refractory arrhythmias.

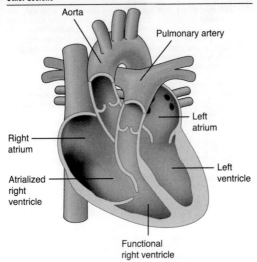

FIGURE 21-5. Ebstein's anomaly. The tricuspid valve is displaced apically, reducing the right ventricular chamber volume. A portion of ventricular muscle is on the atrial side of the valve ("atrialized" ventricle).

Adapted from Brickner EM, Hillis LD, Lange RA. Congenital Heart Disease in Adults: Second of Two Parts. *N Engl J Med.* 2000; 342: 334-342.

Coronary artery anomalies:
- **Left circumflex artery from right sinus of Valsalva (SOV):** Most common anomaly with circumflex passing posterior to aorta to reach territory. Typically, it has no clinical significance.

- **Left main artery from right SOV:** Less common but more malignant natural history. Multiple variants exist, including a course between the great vessels (aorta and pulmonary trunk) that can induce ischemia and sudden cardiac arrest (SCA). Often, the artery has a slit-like ostium.
- **Right coronary artery (RCA) from left SOV:** Traditionally thought to be of no clinical consequence, but its course between the great vessels and occasional slit-like orifice likely increase risk of ischemia and/or SCA.
- **Single coronary artery:** A single ostium from either the right or left SOV feeds the entire coronary circulation. In the absence of atherosclerosis, myocardial bridging, or a course between the great vessels, this anomaly is typically benign.
- **Left coronary artery from pulmonary artery (LCAPA):** Malignant anomaly, also known as Bland-White-Garland syndrome, leading to LV hypoxemia with resultant LV dysfunction/dilatation and severe MR. Significant collaterals form from the RCA leading to coronary steal toward the lower pressure system. Surgical intervention is typically required once diagnosed.
- **RCA from pulmonary artery (RCAPA):** Rare defect with similar pathophysiology and treatment to LCAPA.

OTHER ISSUES IN ACHD

Pregnancy:
- Contraception and preconception counseling are important tasks for those caring for ACHD patients with careful consideration of risks to patients and their babies.
- Many of the therapies prescribed to these ACHD patients can have adverse effects on the fetus.
- Contraception options are complicated by the fact that many of these conditions place the patient at increased risk for thrombosis and certain agents would increase that risk.
- Conditions that portend a particularly poor prognosis in pregnancy that should prompt repeated discussion at each office visit include:
  - pHTN
  - Cyanotic heart disease
  - Severe left-sided obstructive lesions (e.g., mitral stenosis, aortic stenosis)
  - Eisenmenger physiology
  - Aortic disease in Marfan syndrome

Spontaneous bacterial endocarditis (SBE) prophylaxis:
- In 2007, the guidelines for SBE prophylaxis were revised (see Chapter 16). The cardiac conditions that warranted prophylaxis were substantially reduced to only those at highest risk:
  - Prosthetic valve
  - Previous infective endocarditis

- Unrepaired cyanotic CHD
- Recent (< 6months) repair of CHD utilizing prosthetic material or device
- Repaired CHD with residual defect next to prosthetic material or device
- Specific procedures that warrant prophylaxis include all dental procedures, invasive respiratory tract procedures, and surgical procedures involving infected skin or musculoskeletal tissue.
  - GI/GU procedures do not warrant special prophylaxis, however, if antibiotics are utilized for procedure-related purposes then it is reasonable to include enterococcus coverage in the regimen.

22 ■ PERICARDIAL DISORDERS

ANATOMY OF THE PERICARDIUM

The normal pericardium is a double-layered sac; the visceral pericardium is a serous membrane that is separated by a small quantity (15–50 mL) of fluid.

- The pericardium exerts a restraining force that prevents sudden dilation of the cardiac chambers, especially of the right atrium and ventricle.
- Total absence of the pericardium, either congenital or following surgery, does not produce obvious clinical disease.

ACUTE PERICARDITIS

- Pericarditis is a frequent cause of chest pain. There are numerous causes for pericarditis **(Table 22-1)** Pericarditis accounts for 5% of the final diagnoses among patients consulting in the emergency department for chest pain.
- Pericardial tamponade and constriction as a complication of the disease are infrequent and most patients have a benign clinical course; however recurrences are frequent.

TABLE 22-1. Causes of Pericarditis

Malignant tumor
Idiopathic pericarditis
Uremia
Bacterial infection
Anticoagulant therapy
Dissecting aortic aneurysm
Procedures: perforation during electrophysiologic and cardiac catheterization
Connective tissue disease
Postpericardiotomy syndrome
Trauma
Tuberculosis
Radiation
Drugs that induce lupus-like syndromes (procainamide)
Chylopericardium
Post-myocardial infarction syndrome (Dressler's Syndrome)
Fungal infections
Acquired immunodeficiency syndrome-related pericarditis

TABLE 22-2. ECG in Acute Pericarditis vs. Acute (Q-Wave) MI

ST-Segment Elevation	ECG Lead Involvement	Evolution of ST and T Waves	PR-Segment Depression
PERICARDITIS			
Concave upward	All leads involved except aVR and V1	ST remains elevated for several days; after ST returns to baseline, T waves invert	Yes, in majority; PR elevation in aVR
ACUTE MI			
Convex upward	ST elevation over infarcted region only; reciprocal ST depression in opposite leads	T waves invert within hours, while ST still elevated; followed by Q wave development	No

Symptoms: Chest pain, which may be intense, mimicking acute MI, but characteristically sharp, pleuritic, and positional (relieved by leaning forward); fever and palpitations are common.

Physical Findings: Rapid or irregular pulse, coarse pericardial friction rub (the sound is described as two pieces of leather being rubbed together;, it may vary in intensity and is loudest with the patient sitting forward.

Electrocardiogram (Table 22-2)

- Diffuse ST elevation (concave upward) usually present in all leads except aVR and V_1.
- PR-segment depression may be present.
- PR-segment elevation occurs in aVR (very useful to differentiate from early repolarization and myocardial infarction).
- Days later, ST segments return to baseline before T-wave inversion develops.
- Serial ECGs may be of benefit to discriminate between pericarditis and acute infarction since the latter may have more dynamic changes (Table 22.2).
- ST-T ratio < 0.25 with early repolarization, but > 0.25 in pericarditis.
- ST elevation is more diffuse in pericarditis.
- ST elevation involves V_5 and V_6 infrequently.

Laboratory:

- Selected use of the following may suggest a causal diagnosis:
  - Tuberculin skin test
  - Serum albumin and urine protein measurement (nephrotic syndrome)
  - Serum creatinine and BUN (uremia)
  - Thyroid function tests (myxedema)
  - ANA (SLE and other collagen-vascular disease)
  - Age-appropriate screening for a primary tumor (especially lung and breast)

- Cardiac troponin concentrations are elevated in 35–50% of patients with pericarditis, a finding that is thought to be caused by epicardial inflammation rather than myocyte necrosis.
  - The magnitude of elevation in the serum troponin concentration appears to correlate with the magnitude of the ST-segment elevation, and the concentration usually returns to normal within 1 to 2 weeks after diagnosis.
- An elevated troponin concentration does not predict an adverse outcome, although a prolonged elevation (lasting longer than 2 weeks) suggests associated myocarditis, which has a worse prognosis.
- The serum creatine kinase and its MB fraction may also be elevated with pericarditis, but is less often observed than elevated serum troponin.

Chest x-ray:
- Increased size of cardiac silhouette if large (> 250 mL) pericardial effusion is present, with "water bottle" configuration.

Echocardiography:
- Most sensitive test for detection of pericardial effusion, which commonly accompanies acute pericarditis.
- If there is a drop in ejection fraction, there is myocardial involvement also present and the diagnosis of myopericarditis is made.

TREATMENT

- NSAIDs are first-line therapy for acute pericarditis.
- High-dose aspirin may be administered using 750 mg to 1 g/day PO three times per day, or ibuprofen 600 mg PO three times per day. Indomethacin may be used as a second-line agent (50 mg PO three times per day).
  - Co-administration with H2-antagonist or proton pump inhibitor may reduce risk of GI bleeding.
  - Colchicine co-administration may reduce the chances of recurrent pericarditis (1–2 mg for the first day followed by 0.6–1.2 mg/day for 3 months).
- For recurrent pericarditis, colchicine can be used with NSAIDs or as a replacement for NSAIDs (1–2 mg/day followed by 0.6–1.2 mg/day).
  - The lower dose may be selected for those who are intolerant due to GI symptoms.
  - Chronic kidney disease is a risk factor for side effects including bone marrow suppression.
- Steroids should be avoided as a treatment for pericarditis since recurrence rate is increased and the adverse side effect profile is poor.
  - Steroids can be considered for those who fail NSAID and colchicine therapy. Prednisone (0.2 to 0.5 mg/kg/day) for 4 weeks until symptoms and elevated C-reactive peptide have resolved.

- A very slow taper: 20% every 1–2 weeks until dose is 25 mg or less, then 15–20% every 2–4 weeks until dose is 15 mg or less, then 10–15% every 2–6 weeks as long as symptoms are controlled.
  - Colchicine and NSAIDs are introduced as the taper completes. If symptoms recur during steroid taper, an attempt at utilizing NSAIDs should be made before increasing the steroid dose.
  - Osteoporosis prevention should be utilized with steroids.
- Combination and immunosuppressive therapy (e.g., azathioprine, cyclophosphamide, methotrexate) have been utilized in some patients who fail steroid therapy.

CARDIAC TAMPONADE

A life-threatening emergency resulting from accumulation of pericardial fluid under pressure. The increased pressure around the heart leads to impaired diastolic filling of cardiac chambers despite increased filling pressures. Impaired filling can lead to decreased cardiac output, shock, and death.
Etiology:
- Similar to that of pericarditis
  - About 7–10% of those with pericardial effusion are at risk for developing tamponade.
  - Rapidly accumulating effusions are more prone to cause tamponade than effusions that accumulate slowly.
History:
As with pericarditis (see Table 22-1), any history of trauma, recent instrumentation (pacemaker, coronary intervention), anticoagulant use, chest radiation, cancer, or infection (pneumonia, HIV, tuberculosis, viral illness) should be elicited as potential causes. Subacute symptoms include dyspnea (occurs in 90% of patients with tamponade), edema, weakness, lethargy, and confusion.
Physical findings:
- Beck's triad
  - Hypotension (may develop abruptly)
  - Elevated jugular venous pressure with preserved x descent, but loss of y descent
  - Distant heart sounds
- Tachypnea
- Tachycardia
- *Pulsus paradoxus* (inspiratory fall in systolic blood pressure >10 mmHg)
  - To measure the pulsus paradoxus, inflate the blood pressure cuff to 20 mmHg higher than the systolic and very slowly release the pressure. The first intermittent Korotkoff sounds signify the upper value. Deflate the cuff until all the beats are audible. The pulsus paradoxus is the difference between the 2 pressures. An increased pulsus paradoxus may be seen in other disorders such as asthma.

- Egophony at the lower edge of the left scapula (Ewart's sign).
- Peripheral edema, hepatomegaly, and ascites are frequently present if tamponade develops subacutely.

Electrocardiogram:

- Low voltage (QRS amplitude < 10 mm in V_1–V_6 and < 5 mm in limb leads)
- Tachycardia
- Large effusions may cause electrical alternans (alternating size of QRS complex due to swinging of heart).

Chest x-ray:

- Enlarged cardiac silhouette if large (> 250 mL) effusion present.
- Cardiomegaly is present in 90% of patients with tamponade physiology with "water bottle–shaped heart."
- Pulmonary edema is rarely seen with cardiac tamponade.

Echocardiography:

- Note: Cardiac tamponade is a clinical and not an echocardiographic diagnosis.
- The pericardial pressure can exceed right atrial pressure leading to right atrial diastolic collapse. If the pressure increases further, there can be right ventricular or even left ventricular collapse.
- Other findings are a prominent decrease of transmitral inflow (25% of baseline) and increase of blood flow through the tricuspid valve (40% of baseline) during inspiration.
  - This is the echocardiographic corollary of the pulsus paradoxus and is due to exaggerated intraventricular dependence induced by a hyperdynamic intraventricular septum.

Cardiac catheterization:

- Right heart catheterization confirms tamponade physiology.
  - Elevation and equalization of diastolic pressures in all four chambers.
  - Preserved x and blunted y descent on right atrial pressure tracing.
  - The pericardial pressure waveform will track right atrial pressure.
  - Reduced cardiac output.

Management of cardiac tamponade:

- The first step is to determine whether pericardial tamponade is present by performing a targeted history and physical examination with measurement of the pulsus paradoxus.
  - An echocardiogram may be useful to determine the size of effusion and suitability for drainage. Urgency of this evaluation depends upon the clinical stability of the patient.
  - Surgical drainage is utilized for effusions that cannot be drained percutaneously
- Pericardiocentesis is usually done via the subxiphoidal approach or an apical approach utilizing pressure monitoring, echocardiographic, electrocardiographic and/or fluoroscopic guidance (see Chapter 39, Pericardiocentesis).
- Bedside pericardiocentesis is usually reserved for cardiac arrest.

CONSTRICTIVE PERICARDITIS

- The rigid pericardium in constriction leads to impaired cardiac filling, causing elevation of systemic and pulmonary venous pressures and decreased cardiac output.
- Constriction results from fibrosis in some patients with previous pericarditis.
  - Viral, tuberculosis, previous cardiac surgery, uremia, and neoplastic pericarditis are the most common causes.

History: Gradual onset of dyspnea, fatigue, pedal edema, abdominal swelling due to ascites, weight loss or gain, palpitations, symptoms of LV failure uncommon.

Physical findings:
- Tachycardia
- Jugular venous distention (prominent x and y descents)
  - May not become evident in patients who are volume depleted
- An increase in JVP upon inspiration is termed Kussmaul's sign
- "Pericardial knock" following S2 is a sharp diastolic sound that is sometimes present.
- Pleural effusion
- Hepatomegaly, ascites, and peripheral edema are common.
- Cachexia

Electrocardiogram:
- Low limb lead voltage
- Atrial arrhythmias are common.

Chest x-ray: A rim of pericardial calcification may be seen.

Echocardiography: Thickened pericardium, normal ventricular contraction; abrupt halt in ventricular filling in early diastole.

CT or MRI: More precise than echocardiogram in demonstrating thickened pericardium (> 2–5 mm thickness).

CARDIAC CATHETERIZATION

Right heart catheterization:
- Elevation and equalization of diastolic pressures in all chambers.
- Right ventricular pressure tracing may show "dip and plateau/square root."
- Greater fall in pulmonary capillary wedge pressure than left ventricular diastolic pressure during inspiration
- Some of these findings are also seen in cardiac tamponade. **Table 22-3** compares the findings of cardiac tamponade and constriction.
- By placing a pressure catheter into the left and right ventricle ventricular pressure, systolic discordance can be determined and is a very sensitive and specific sign of constriction.
  - Ventricular discordance stems from ventricular interdependence in constriction. Because venous return is augmented during inspiration, more blood enters the right ventricle.
  - The interventricular septum bulges toward the left since the pericardium constraints expand outward.

TABLE 22-3. Comparison of Cardiac Tamponade and Constrictive Pericarditis

	Cardiac Tamponade	Pericardial Constriction
Venous Return	Monophasic: Systole only, inspiratory increase intact	Biphasic: Systolic and diastolic. Inspiratory increase absent
Filling Pressures	Elevated and equalized	Elevated and equalized
JVP and RA	Prominent X and blunted y	Prominent X and Y
RV Pressure	No dip and plateau	Prominent dip and plateau
Pulsus Paradoxus	Nearly always present	Only found in 1/3
Kussmaul's	Unusual	Prominent

- Left ventricular filling is reduced and the left ventricular systolic pressure falls while the right systolic ventricular pressure rises, which is called ventricular discordance.
  - Ventricular discordance in constriction should be distinguished from restrictive cardiomyopathy where ventricular *concordance* is more typical because there is little interventricular dependence. **Table 22-4** compares the hemodynamic findings of constriction and restrictive cardiomyopathies.

TABLE 22-4. Discriminatory Criteria for Constriction vs. Restriction

	Constriction	Restriction
LVEDP-RVEDP, mm Hg	≤5	>5
RVSP, mm Hg	≤50	>50
RVEDP/RVSP	≥0.33	<0.3

TREATMENT

Surgical stripping of the pericardium is definitive treatment for constriction. Progressive improvement ensues over several months.

23 ■ PERIPHERAL ARTERIAL AND RENAL ARTERY DISEASE

- Occurs in approximately one-third of patients:
  - Over age 70
  - Over age 50 who smoke or have DM
- Strong association with CAD
  - Obvious associated risk of stroke, MI, cardiovascular death
  - 5-year nonfatal MI risk approximately 20%
  - Mortality 15–30% (three-fourths due to cardiovascular causes)
- Progressive disease in 25% with progressive intermittent claudication/limb-threatening ischemia
- Outcomes
  - Impaired quality of life (QoL)
  - Limb loss
  - Premature mortality

Spectrum of lower extremity disease:
- No symptoms, but evidence of PAD on noninvasive testing
- Claudication
  - Classically, symptoms start with walking and are relieved by rest within minutes. The pain is described as a cramping or aching sensation.
  - Localization of pain is helpful (may occur singly or in combination)
    - Buttock/hip
      - Aortoiliac occlusive disease (Leriche's syndrome) manifests with thigh claudication in some cases.
      - Bilateral disease is often associated with erectile dysfunction.
    - Thigh
      - Atherosclerotic occlusion of the common femoral artery may induce claudication in the thigh, calf, or both.
    - Calf
      - Cramping in the upper two-thirds of the calf is usually due to SFA.
      - Cramping in the lower one-thirds of the calf is due to popliteal disease.
  - Atherogenic claudication can be distinguished from pseudoclaudication (e.g., spinal stenosis):
    - Pseudoclaudication may occur either at rest or with activity. The pain is described as a paresthesia-like sensation, which may be relieved by rest (usually takes > 10 min) or by sitting, or leaning forward ("shopping cart sign") and walking,

TABLE 23-1. ABI (Ankle Brachial Index) Chart

Grade	Resting ABI	Post exercise ABI
Normal	>0.90	No change, or increase
Mild	0.66–0.90	>0.45
Moderate	0.5–0.7	>0.25–0.44
Severe	<0.5	<0.25

Adapted from: Feringa HH, Bax JJ, van Waning VH, et al. *Arch Intern Med.* 2006;166:529–535.

Diagnosis:
- ABI (ankle brachial index—either resting or resting plus exercise) determines presence or absence of PAD. Exercise portion can give hemodynamic information. **Table 23-1** categorizes severity of PAD based on ABI.
- SDP/PVRs (segmental Doppler pressures/pulse volume recordings) help localize disease by segment.

Anatomic imaging is utilized if intervention is to be planned.
- CT angiography: Assesses entire vascular tree. Requires contrast. Calcium artifact may limit ability to assess lesions.
- MR angiography: Assesses entire vascular tree. May overestimate stenosis.

Medical treatment:
- Risk factor modification
- Exercise training
  - Supervised walking program of 45–60 min 4 days per week for 6 months may improve symptomatic walking distance by 180%
- Medications
  - Aspirin 81–325mg daily
  - Clopidogrel bisulfate (Plavix) 75 mg daily
  - Cilostazol
  - Statin therapy
  - ACE inhibition
- Revascularization
  - Consider in patients who are disabled by claudication symptoms on medical therapy.
  - Consider in any patient with symptoms or signs of critical limb ischemia.
  - Endovascular approach: Consider in lesions that are stenotic but not totally occlusive and that are discrete (< 5 cm in length in the iliac region, and < 10 cm in the SFA region). Should not be considered for common femoral or SFA origin, or disease extending into the popliteal fossa or below
  - Stent placement should be considered if initial angiographic result is not sufficient, or dissection is noted.

- Surgical approach should be considered if multiple levels affected. Consider especially with involvement of common femoral and distal popliteal areas.

Acute occlusion due to thrombosis or embolism:
- Sudden onset of symptoms (< 5 hours)
- Symptoms include the 5 Ps (pain, pallor, pulselessness, paresthesia/paralysis, poikilothermy/polar).
- Initial approach should include urgent angiography and consideration of thrombolytic therapy with adjunctive endovascular or surgical therapies.

Aneurysmal disease:
- May see in any part of the lower extremity, but classically iliac (in concert with AAA), and popliteal areas
- May initially be asymptomatic; can cause compression of structures, thrombosis or embolism, infection, and rupture
- Consider a surgical approach

Less common causes of occlusive disease:
- Thromboangiitis obliterans
- Arteritis due to connective tissue disease or vasculitis (e.g., giant cell arteritis)
- Trauma
- Entrapment (e.g., popliteal entrapment syndrome)

SUBCLAVIAN/UPPER EXTREMITY DISEASE

Subclavian stenosis or occlusion (left side most commonly):
- May be asymptomatic (left arm may develop sufficient collaterals)
- Discovered by difference in arm BP

Subclavian steal phenomenon:
- Classically described with left subclavian stenosis/occlusion. It refers to the retrograde flow down the vertebral into the distal subclavian (past the subclavian lesion) in the setting of left upper extremity use. The blood is "stolen" away from the posterior circulation and can manifest with symptoms of vertebrobasilar insufficiency.

Coronary-subclavian steal phenomenon:
- Described in the setting of left subclavian stenosis/occlusion in a patient with a LIMA (left internal mammary artery) to LAD (left anterior descending coronary artery). When the left arm is used this can cause "stealing" of blood from the LIMA to the distal subclavian causing symptoms of coronary ischemia.

OTHER LESS COMMON PAD

Thromboangitis obliterans (Buerger's disease):
- This is a disorder of the small vessels with involvement of the upper extremity vessels in the arms and hands.

- It is most often seen in smokers under the age of 40 years.
- Patients may present with Raynaud's phenomenon, claudication, or ulceration (especially digital ulceration) depending on the severity of disease.
- These patients will have an abnormal Allen's test on physical examination.
- Smoking cessation is essential to slow the progression of this disease. Stopping smoking reduces the risk of amputation in this population.

Erythromelalgia:

- Hot, red, burning sensation of fingers or toes in response to warm temperatures or exercise.
- Can be a primary or secondary disorder.
- Most often secondary to myeloproliferative disorder.
- Treatment includes aspirin, betablockade, avoidance of warm temperature, and treatment of any underlying secondary disorder.

Pernio:

- A vasospastic disorder in which the patient experiences cold sensitivity.
- Results in bluish discoloration of fingers or toes, and may include blistering.
- Usually has onset in autumn and goes away in spring.
- Treatment includes alpha-blockade and avoidance of cold.

Raynaud's phenomenon and disease:

- A vasospastic disorder of the small arteries and arterioles of the extremities.
- Raynaud's phenomenon is classically seen in men older than 40 years old. Ischemic changes, ulceration, and gangrene can be seen in this condition. Treatment focuses on treating the underlying disorder as well as treatment to reduce ischemia. Raynaud's phenomenon is secondary to another disorder. Causes may be divided into 3 groups:
  - Systemic disease: Collagen vascular disease, cryoglobulinemia, cold agglutinin, myxedema, ergotism
  - Compression syndromes: carpal tunnel, thoracic outlet syndrome
  - Occupational trauma: hypothenar hammer syndrome, chainsaw operation
  - Arterial occlusion
- Raynaud's disease refers to the primary syndrome that is idiopathic in nature, and had to have been persistent for at least 2 years. It is seen in women younger than 40 years of age, and manifests as the classic "white, blue, and red" digits, brought on by cold exposure and emotional stressors.
  - The primary disease is not typically associated with ulceration or gangrene.
  - The mainstay of therapy is reduction of cold exposure (wearing gloves).
  - Low dose beta-blocker or nifedipine to prevent symptoms can be used.

Livedo reticularis:

- Mottling of skin in a lacy reticular pattern that is due to spasm or occlusion of arterioles of the skin. May be primary or secondary.

- Secondary causes are most commonly due to aneurismal disease and the showering of embolic debris.

Popliteal artery entrapment syndrome:

- Symptomatic calf or foot claudication seen mostly in young men.
- Its cause is due to entrapment of the popliteal artery by the medial head of the gastrocnemius muscle.
- The popliteal artery may potentially be occluded. Physical exam may demonstrate a diminished popliteal pulse with foot plantar flexion.
- MRA or contrast angiography may help to diagnose this condition.
- Popliteal duplex with maneuvers (e.g., plantar flexion) may also suggest the diagnosis.
- Surgery is warranted in symptomatic patients.

Thoracic outlet syndrome:

- Subclavian artery, vein, or nerve is compressed within the "thoracic outlet" which commonly consists of the space between the cervical or first rib and the clavicle.
- Symptoms may include thrombosis, pain, Raynaud's phenomenon, digital ulceration and cyanosis, arm claudication.
- Patients may have an abnormal Allen's test on physical examination.
- Diagnosis may be made with physical maneuvers or duplex ultrasound noting flow in both the normal and hyperabducted positions.
- MRA and contrast angiography may also be helpful.
- Therapy consists of resection of the first rib and revascularization if thrombosis of a vessel is present.

PERIPHERAL ARTERIAL AND RENAL ARTERY DISEASE

- Renal artery stenosis remains the most common cause of secondary hypertension, accounting for approximately 5% of cases
- Main causes include atherosclerotic renal artery disease and fibromuscular dysplasia
- Rate of progression: Numerous studies suggest those with lesions > 60% have progression of narrowing, and may progress to complete occlusion. Also, those with > 60% lesions may experience decrease in renal mass over time.
- Physical examination: bruits (systolic and diastolic) auscultated over the flank area are highly specific findings.
- Clinical presentations: progressive azotemia in patients with known PAD or CAD, progressive hypertension with worsening renal function.
- Progressive renal failure or acute renal failure with initiation of ACE inhibition or ARB (an increase in serum creatinine of > 15%)
- Acute congestive heart failure in the setting of hypertension and renal failure (flash pulmonary edema).
- Risk factors: Hypertension, age, diabetes, smoking, prior renal failure, atherosclerosis.

- Workup: serum creatinine, creatinine clearance, urinalysis, serology for SLE or vasculitis (ANA, C3, C4, ANCA), urinalysis, 24-hour urine collection (protein levels).
- Renal ultrasound: good screening tool, however, technically challenging, limiting sensitivity, and may fail to identify accessory renal arteries.
  - Helpful ultrasound criteria include the following:
    - Asymmetry of kidney size: > 1.5 cm
    - Velocity criteria: Olin criteria: PSV > 200 cm/s, EDV > 150cm/s, aortic to renal ratio > 3.5 predicts RAS of ≥ 60%
    - Renal resistive index: 1-(EDV/Max systolic velocity)
      - Renal resistive index > 0.8 is suggestive of small vessel renal disease (not likely to improve with renal artery revascularization).
      - Normal RRI = 0.6–0.7: suggests parenchyma is working and intrinsic renal function is preserved.
- MR angiography: provides accurate images of the renal arteries and entire aorta.
  - May be good for FMD.
  - Difficulties with use of gadolinium in the renal failure population due to nephrogenic systemic fibrosis; limit use.
  - May overestimate degree of stenosis.
  - May be limited if assessing a renal stent (artifact).
- CTA: requires contrast dye load which may be prohibitive in patients with known renal failure. Good for anatomic detail in patients with known normal renal function (e.g., congenital abnormalities, renal artery aneurysms).
- Angiography: should be used sparingly; only when possible renal intervention is planned or when there is discordance between other noninvasive imaging tests.
- Indications for percutaneous renal revascularization:
  - Accelerated (sudden or persistent worsening), resistant (to full doses of a 3-drug regimen that includes a diuretic)
  - Malignant (associated with end-organ damage) hypertension
  - Pulmonary edema associated with renal artery stenosis
  - Hypertension with unilateral small kidney
  - Hypertension with intolerance to medication
  - Other considerations: preservation of renal function, in those patients with solitary functioning kidney, or those with bilateral severe renal artery stenosis
  - Percutaneous intervention is particularly successful in younger patients with FMD and focal lesions.
  - Percutaneous approach to FMD is balloon-only angioplasty to break up the septae.
  - Bilateral renal artery lesions respond better than unilateral.
  - Less success in those patients with chronic parenchymal damage due to longstanding hypertension or diabetes.
  - If approached percutaneously, atherosclerotic disease usually requires stenting to cover the ostium.

The utility of renal artery stenting has been called into question. The ASTRAL trial[46] randomized patients with renal artery stenosis (lesions > 60%) to medical therapy versus renal stenting. There was no difference between the 2 groups with respect to blood pressure control, renal events, major cardiovascular events, and mortality.

Indications for surgical revascularization:

- FMD when it extends into segmental arteries
- Atherosclerotic renal artery stenosis when it involves multiple small renal arteries or early branching primary renal artery
- Renal artery stenosis undergoing pararenal aortic reconstruction for aortic aneurysms or aortoiliac occlusive disease
- Concurrent abdominal aortic aneurysm
- Renal artery aneurysm
- Renal artery rupture
- Acute renal artery occlusion after unsuccessful thrombolysis

Medical therapy: ACE inhibitor or ARB if tolerated, calcium channel blocker for hypertension, statin therapy.

24 ■ AORTIC DISEASE AND MESENTERIC ISCHEMIA

Arises from 2 main causes:

- Traumatic: tear in aortic intima leading to separation of intima and media, creating false lumen or flap
- Non traumatic: substrate degeneration of media, cystic medial necrosis leading to rupture, hemorrhage, dissection

Complications:

- Involvement of branch vessels leads to organ ischemia: coronary (RCA more commonly), cerebral, extremity, spinal, renal/adrenal, mesenteric vessels.
- Dissection can cause aortic regurgitation or cardiac tamponade.

Epidemiology:

- At least 2000 cases occur each year in the United States.
- If dissection flap involves ascending aorta, mortality is 1% per hour.
- "Acute" is defined as < 2 weeks from symptom onset.

Predisposing factors:

- Age
- HTN
- Aortic aneurysm
- Vasculitis: Takayasu's, giant cell, rheumatoid arthritis, syphilitic aortitis
- Collagen Disorders: Marfan's, Ehlers-Danlos
- Bicuspid aortic valve
- Coarctation of the aorta
- Prior cardiac surgery (especially aortic valve surgery)
- Cardiac catheterization
- Trauma
- Cocaine
- Family history of aneurismal disease
- Pregnancy

Classification systems:

Stanford (Daily system) more commonly used

- Type A: dissection involving ascending aorta
- Type B: dissection involving descending aorta

Debakey

- Type 1: ascending and descending thoracic aorta
- Type 2: ascending aorta
- Type 3: descending aorta

Ascending aortic dissection is 2 times more common than descending.

Clinical presentation:
- Chest pain
- Back pain
- Sharp or "tearing" (classic description)
- Stroke symptoms
- CHF
- Syncope

Physical examination:
- Blood pressure differential, pulse deficits
- Aortic insufficiency murmur: diastolic decrescendo (may be short in acute aortic dissection since aortic diastolic pressure may be similar to left ventricular end diastolic pressure)
- Jugular venous distention
- Cardiac tamponade (pulsus paradoxus)
- Hemothorax
- Complete Heart block (if involves the RCA)
- Neurologic deficits due to spinal cord involvement or cerebral ischemia
- Horner's syndrome
- Vocal cord paralysis

Key diagnostic features (prediction model)[48]:
- Sudden onset thoracic or abdominal pain with tearing or ripping or sharp character
- Mediastinal and/or aortic widening on CXR
- A variation in pulse or blood pressure

Incidence of dissection:
- No features: 7%
- Pain: 31%
- CXR features: 39%
- Variation in pulse or BP differential: ≥ 83%
- All three features: ≥ 83%

Differential diagnosis:
- Myocardial infarction
- Pulmonary embolism
- Aortic valvular disease (AS/AI)
- Pericarditis
- Esophageal disorders

ECG:
- Normal, nonspecific changes, LVH pattern, myocardial ischemia or infarction, heart block
- Note: from IRAD[49] database—coronary involvement is not necessarily reflected on ECG

Imaging:
- Computed tomography: ESC guidelines class II for acute dissection, IIa for chronic dissection
  - Differentiates dissection from intramural hematoma or penetrating ulcer
  - Allows for evaluation of aortic branch vessel involvement

- Echocardiography: ESC guidelines class I for acute dissection, IIa for chronic dissection (TTE followed by TEE)
  - Preferred modality for less stable patients
  - Renal dysfunction
  - Evaluates hemodynamics and flow within true and false lumens, and valvular involvement (AI)
  - Can localize flap origin but difficulty imaging near left subclavian artery
- Aortography: IIb for unstable patients, IIa for chronic dissection
- MRI: contraindicated in unstable patients, preferred modality for chronic dissection

Treatment:

- Type A dissections: surgery (surgical emergency), though contraindication with evolving CVA (increased risk of hemorrhagic transformation)
- Type B dissections: medical, unless evidence of progression or extension into pleural or retroperitoneal spaces, endovascular treatment may be considered in more stable patients

Adjunctive medical treatment:

- Goal is to lower shear stress, or dP/dt (rate of rise of LV pressure); this involves a combination of SBP and HR lowering
- Maintain arterial line and 2 large bore IVs
- If hypertensive, goal to lower SBP to 100–120, or MAP 60–65 and HR to < 60 in critical care setting
- Medications:
  - Labetalol: boluses (20 mg IV initially, with range between 20–80 mg) or IV infusion (0.5–2 mg/min)
  - Metoprolol: 5–10 mg IV push every 5 min
  - Esmolol: 80 mg IV load over 30 seconds, then 150mcg/kg/min IV, may increase by 50 mcg/kg/min IV to max of 300 mcg/kg/min IV
  - If beta-blocker intolerant, consider diltiazem or verapamil (bolus or infusion)
- Once HR is controlled, if still require SBP lowering, add nitroprusside (IV infusion 0.25–0.5 mcg/kg/min), however there is a risk of cyanide toxicity with prolonged use or at high infusion rates. Discontinue the drug if the blood pressure is not controlled after 10 minutes of use.
- Alternatives include IV ACE inhibition, nicardipine, diltiazem, and verapamil. Avoid hydralazine without adequate heart rate control (direct vasodilator reflex, tachycardia, increased shear stress).
- Ideally avoid inotropes (which increase shear stress), however, choose norepinephrine or phenylephrine (little effect on shear stress). Avoid epinephrine or dopamine.

Note: Although hemopericardium with tamponade are common mechanisms of death, exercise caution with pericardiocentesis: Removal of fluid may increase shear stress and accelerate dissection. In the absence of pulmonary edema, aggressive fluid resuscitation while preparations for surgical repair are made is preferred.

Management for observation and discharge:
- If patients are treated medically, the goal is to have patient free of pain and with adequate blood pressure control.
- Options: oral metoprolol or labetalol, diltiazem or verapamil if cannot tolerate BB.
- Consider adding amlodipine or ACE inhibitor once HR is stable.

Prognosis:
- Patients with Stanford A dissections have a higher mortality rate within the first 48 hours than those with type B dissections. However the operative mortality for type B dissections that fail initial medical therapy is 30–50%, compared with 10–15% for those with type A

AORTIC INTRAMURAL HEMATOMA

Pathology: Hematoma in aortic medial layer due to hemorrhage within vasovasorum or plaque.

According to 2010 guidelines[50] should be treated similarly to aortic dissection at the corresponding level.

PENETRATING AORTIC ULCER

Pathology: Ulceration in wall extending beyond intimal layer (penetration through internal elastic lamina)

Clinical consequences of this include formation of an intramural hematoma, formation of a saccular aneurysm, formation of a pseudoaneurysm, or transmural rupture.

Management: Intervention depends on whether or not the patient is having related symptoms.
- If asymptomatic, may undergo surveillance with noninvasive imaging, and control of hypertension.
- If the patient is symptomatic, referral is warranted for surgical or endovascular therapies.

ABDOMINAL AORTIC ANEURYSM (AAA)

Incidence has increased exponentially due to ultrasound detection programs.
- Typically becomes manifest in the 7th and 8th decades of life.
- 20% family history
- Expansion rate of aneurysm is 2–3 mm/year.
- Active smoking is an independent risk factor for accelerated expansion and rupture.

Rupture risk:[51]
- < 5 cm aneurysm: 1%/year
- 5–7 cm: 5–10%/year
- > 7 cm: 10–25%

Surveillance approach:
- United States Preventive Services Task Force recommends a screening ultrasound in men older than 65 years of age who have ever smoked.[103]

Elective approach:
- < 5 cm monitor with serial ultrasound
- 5–5.4 cm CT to define aneurysm and surrounding anatomy
- ≥ 5.5 cm consider for surgery or EVAR

Imaging modalities:
- Ultrasound
  - AP diameter is more accurate than transverse diameter.
  - Quality of study is related to technician skill and patient body habitus.
- Computed tomography
  - Allows for surgical or EVAR planning.
  - Can demonstrate the following anatomical considerations: aortic calcification, thrombus, "landing zone" in relation to major aortic branches, tortuosity, involvement of aneurysm with aortic bifurcation, renal arteries, thoracic aorta
- Aortography
  - Less reliable for determining diameter since plaque/thrombus may not allow for demonstration of outer margin

Urgent surgical indications:
- Known aneurysm with acute peripheral emboli
- Known aneurysm with acute tenderness at site or abdominal/back pain
- Rupture

Considerations prior to surgery:
- Cardiovascular risk assessment given that approximately 50% of patients also have CAD
- Assessment of carotid disease

Surgical mortality:
- Elective repair: 2–5%
- Emergent repair for rupture: 50–75%

Endovascular repair:
- Approximately 50% of U.S. repairs are now endovascular
  - 25% of EVAR patients will require graft-related intervention at 5 years compared to 2% for those who have undergone open repair.
- A randomized trial suggested that EVAR significantly decreases the risk of aneurysm-related death (but not all cause mortality) in patients who are ineligible for open repair.[52]
- A randomized trial comparing open repair versus EVAR showed that EVAR had a lower rate of operative mortality, but:
  - There was no difference in mortality from aneurysm related causes or overall mortality.
  - EVAR was associated with more graft complications and reinterventions and cost more than open repair.[53]

Endoleak is defined as incomplete sealing of the aneurysm sac after endograft placement. There are 4 categories:

- Type 1: Failure of primary graft to seal aneurysm (either at aortic neck or iliacs)
- Type 2: Bleeding into aneurismal sac from collateral supply (lumbars, inferior mesenteric)
- Type 3: Flow to aneurysm through junction points in graft
- Type 4: Flow into aneurysm through graft porosity

THORACIC AORTIC ANEURYSM

Causes:
- Atherosclerosis
- Hypertension
- Trauma
- Marfan syndrome
- Bicuspid aortic valve disease
- Giant cell arteritis
- Infection (syphilis)

Imaging:
- May be found incidentally on CXR
- Other imaging modalities to assess disease include:
  - CTA
  - MRA
  - TEE

Indications for surgery include:
- Symptoms which are attributed to the aneurysm
- Rapid expansion (> 0.5 cm/year in asymptomatic patient with thoracic aorta <5.5 cm)
- Post trauma
- Pseudoaneurysm
- Size > 4.5 cm in patient who also requires aortic valve surgery
- Size > 6 cm in patients without connective tissue disease
- Size > 4.0–5 cm in patients with Marfan syndrome, other genetic connective tissue diseases, bicuspid valve, familial thoracic aneurysm
- For women with Marfan syndrome contemplating pregnancy, surgery may be indicated prophylactically for size > 4.0 cm

Medical therapy includes:
- Smoking cessation
- Controlling lipid profile
- Minimizing other cardiovascular atherosclerotic risk (e.g., diabetes control)
- Hypertension control—beta-blockers reduce rate of expansion, also increase evidence for ACEI and ARB therapy

MESENTERIC ARTERIAL DISEASE

- Mesenteric arterial disease is common but clinical manifestation of mesenteric arterial disease is uncommon and is usually due to atherosclerosis.
  - Median arcuate ligament syndrome: compression of celiac axis with median arcuate ligament—controversial disease
- Less symptomatology due to numerous collaterals in setting of atherosclerotic or embolic disease
- Also, due to vague presentation and degree of stenosis/occlusion required before symptoms present, disease process may be very late in course, therefore therapies may be difficult.
- Additionally, these patients may suffer from multiple comorbidities and advanced panvascular disease, which may make any attempt at revascularization difficult, and overall prognosis poor.

Anatomic supply:
- Celiac axis—foregut, SMA—mid gut, IMA—hindgut
- Multiple collateral channels available
- Ischemic pain does not occur until two-thirds of mesenteric vessels have severe occlusive disease.

Clinical presentation:
- Chronic mesenteric ischemia: abdominal pain (usually beginning 30–60 min after eating) and weight loss—food fear, abdominal bloating, diarrhea
  - May have abdominal bruit on physical exam
- Acute mesenteric ischemia: due to thrombosis 40%, embolism 40%, intestinal hypoperfusion 20%
  - Classic presentation of abdominal pain out of proportion to physical exam
  - May progress to sepsis and shock
  - Early angiography is needed to salvage intestinal tissue.

Screening tools for chronic mesenteric ischemia:
- CT angiography
- MR angiography
- Duplex ultrasound
  - Criteria suggestive of > 70% stenosis on fasting exam: celiac PSV > 200 cm/s, EDV > 55 cm/s, reversed hepatic/splenic arterial flow; SMA PSV > 275 cm/s, EDV > 45 cm/s

TREATMENT

Acute mesenteric ischemia and chronic mesenteric ischemia are treated surgically and/or endovascularly.

CVA is a leading cause of disability in the United States and the third leading cause of mortality.

SYMPTOMATIC CAROTID DISEASE

TIA: Acute neurologic event lasting <24 hours and resolving spontaneously
- 30–50% risk of CVA once TIA has occurred
- 50% TIAs due to carotid disease (stenosis, thrombosis, ulcerated plaques)
- 50% TIAs due to atheroembolic event from heart, aortic arch, intracranial vessel, or hypercoagulable state, or unknown source

RIND: Acute neurologic event lasting >24 hours but then resolving spontaneously

CVA: Acute neurologic event lasting >24 hours with evidence of infarction
- Untreated CVA recurrence risk 10–20% per year
- Mortality with stroke recurrence is 35%

Symptoms of concern:
- Hemiparesis
- Hemiparesthesia
- Transient monocular blindness (amaurosis fugax)
- Aphasia

Major risk factors include:
- Hypertension
- Diabetes Mellitus
- Smoking
- Dyslipidemia

Causes of stroke include:
- Cardiac:
  - Intracardiac thrombus
  - Intracardiac mass lesions
  - Valvular disease
  - Infectious endocarditis
  - Paradoxical emboli through intracardiac shunt
- Vascular disease:
  - Carotid disease
    - Atherosclerotic
    - Fibromuscular dysplasia
    - Carotid body tumor

- ○ Carotid fibromuscular dysplasia
- ○ Carotid dissection
- ○ Carotid kinks and coils
- Large vessel: Aorta and major arch branch artery atheroma
- Small vessel disease due to diabetes and hypertension
- Vasculitis, arteritis
- Hematologic
  - ○ Polycythemia vera, leukemia, Anti-phospholipid antibody syndrome, thrombocytosis, thrombophilia, paraproteinemia

ASYMPTOMATIC CAROTID DISEASE

- 1% of U.S. population older than 65 years has carotid stenosis.
- Carotid bruits may be found in up to 5% of those older than 50 years.
- Bruit is not sensitive or specific for hemodynamically significant lesion.
  - Only 23% of bruits are associated with a hemodynamic lesion (>50%).
- Annual stroke risk is <1% for patients with carotid stenosis <60%, and 3–5% if carotid stenosis is greater than 80%.
- 10–15% of nonsignificant carotid lesions will progress to significant range.

Assessment of carotid disease:

- Carotid angiography remains gold standard; however, must be balanced against risk of invasive procedure: risk of neurologic event with angiography alone 4%, disabling stroke 1%, risk of death <0.1%.[54]
  - NASCET criteria: Measure from tightest stenosis in vessel and compare to normal internal carotid lumen distal to stenosis.
  - ECST criteria: Measure from tightest stenosis and compare to estimated probable origin diameter at site of maximal stenosis.
  - CC method: Measure tightest stenosis and compare to lumen diameter in proximal common carotid.
- Carotid ultrasound: Good for anatomic assessment, plaque characteristics, hemodynamic significance of lesions (**Table 25-1**).
  - Can miss subtotal occlusions
  - Can overestimate severity of stenosis
  - Cannot measure distal disease
- MR angiography
  - Can identify infarction immediately
  - May overestimate degree of stenosis
- CT Angiography
  - Identifies intracranial bleeding well.
  - Cannot identify immediate infarction well, which may take 24–48 hours to be visible on CT.
  - Calcification may limit ability to detect stenosis.

All imaging modalities can miss subtotal occlusions.

TABLE 25-1. Criteria for Classification of Internal Carotid Artery Disease by Duplex Scanning

Degree of stenosis, %	ICA/PSV, cm/s	Plaque estimate, %	ICA EDV, cm/s	ICA CCA PSV ratio
Normal	<125	0	<40	<2
<50	<125	<50	<40	<2
50–69	125–230	>50	40–100	2–4
>70	>230	>50	>100	>4
Subtotal occlusion	Variable	>50 Narrow lumen	>0	Variable
Total occlusion	0	>50	0	<1

CCA, Common carotid artery; *EDV*, end-diastolic velocity; *ICA*, internal carotid artery; *PSV*, peak systolic velocity.

Source: Reprinted from *JASE*, Volume 19, Issue 8, Gerhard-Herman M et al, Guidelines for noninvasive vascular laboratory testing: a report from the American Society of Echocardiography and the Society of Vascular Medicine and Biology, page 18, Copyright 2006, with permission from Elsevier.

MEDICAL THERAPY

Statins
- Antiplatelet agents
- Aspirin beneficial in secondary prevention
- Clopidogrel slightly more beneficial than aspirin in secondary prevention
- Aggrenox (Dipyridamole and Aspirin) slightly more beneficial than aspirin in secondary prevention
- Dual antiplatelet therapy with aspirin and clopidogrel contraindicated after stroke

Heparin or Coumadin: Can be used for TIAs of recent onset
Heparin: Not used in acute stroke due to risk of hemorrhagic conversion

CAROTID REVASCULARIZATION

Carotid Endarterectomy
    NASCET (North American Symptomatic Carotid Endarterectomy Trial)
- Those with >70% lesions had stroke risk of 26% at 2 years with medical therapy (antiplatelet) versus 9% with CEA (p < 0.001).
- Mortality was 12% medical therapy versus 5% (p < 0.01)
- Those with 50–69% stenosis had reduction in ipsilateral stroke (15.7% medical versus 22%, p = 0.045), and any stroke or death 33.3% vs. 43.3% p = 0.005) at 5 years

ACAS (Asymptomatic carotid atherosclerosis study) trial randomized patients with >60% carotid stenosis to carotid endarterectomy versus medical therapy.

- The event rate was 5% in the surgery group versus 11% in the medical therapy group.

Veterans Affairs Trial 309:[55] Examined patients with >50% asymptomatic carotid disease and found that randomizing patients to carotid endarterectomy plus medical therapy versus medical therapy alone resulted in:

- Reduction in ipsilateral neurologic events from 21% to 8%.

CAROTID ARTERY STENTING

Indications: Currently, carotid stenting is reserved for patients who are at high risk of a complication during carotid endarterectomy. High risk criteria include:

High-risk criteria for carotid stenting include the following:

- Age older than 80 years
- High carotid bifurcation or lesion which is not easily approached by surgery (intracranial, or approaching the thoracic region)
- Contralateral carotid occlusion
- Recurrent stenosis (post-CEA)
- Severe cardiovascular disease
- Severe pulmonary disease
- Contralateral recurrent laryngeal nerve palsy
- Prior neck radiation
- Radical neck surgery
- Stoma/tracheostomy

Several trials and registries have directly and indirectly compared carotid artery stenting versus carotid endarterectomy. The CREST trial[56] was a randomized trial that demonstrated that overall outcomes (stroke, MI, or death) for stenting versus surgery were similar (7.2% for stenting and 6.8% for surgery, $p = NS$).

- At 30 days the stroke rate was higher in the stenting group (4.1% versus 2.3%), however, the major stroke rate was similar in both groups and was <1%.
- Myocardial infarction was higher in CEA compared to stenting (2.3% versus 1.1%)
- The trial also suggested that those younger than 69 years did better with stenting, and those older than 69 years did better with CEA.

VERTEBROBASILAR INSUFFICIENCY

- Due to ischemia in midbrain and cerebellum
- Symptoms include ataxia, dysarthria, diplopia, dysphagia, vertigo, dizziness, and drop attacks.
- May be due to embolic phenomenon or hypoperfusion (more common)
- Posterior circulation CVA accounts for 25% of strokes
- Less evidence for surgery versus percutaneous approaches in this area

26 ■ PULMONARY HYPERTENSION

DEFINITION OF PULMONARY HYPERTENSION

Pulmonary hypertension (PH) is defined as sustained elevation of the mean pulmonary artery pressure (> 25 mmHg at rest or 30 mmHg during exertion) or of the systolic pulmonary artery pressure (> 40 mmHg). Pulmonary arterial hypertension (PAH) represents a heterogeneous group of disorders. The cause of death in patients with PH is usually right heart failure.

- Severe pulmonary hypertension: Mean PAH > 40 mmHg

PATHOPHYSIOLOGY AND CLASSIFICATION

- The lung parenchyma is normally a low-resistance circuit that can accommodate the entire cardiac output with a low-pressure gradient (5–10 mmHg normally) across the pulmonary vasculature
- Large increases in blood flow may occur with only small increases in the pressure gradient due to the recruitment of vascular beds
- World Health Organization (WHO) classification of PAH
  - WHO Class I: *Pulmonary arterial hypertension*—destruction/fibrosis of the pulmonary arteries or arterioles leads to a decreased cross-section for blood flow and elevation in pulmonary vascular resistance
  - IPAH (formerly primary pulmonary hypertension [PPH])/familial PAH
    - 10% of patients with IPAH may have familial disease
  - Collagen vascular disease (systemic sclerosis, HIV)
  - HIV infection
  - Drugs/toxins—fenfluramine, dexfenfluramine, cocaine, amphetamine
  - Congenital heart disease with pulmonary overcirculation (Eisenmenger's syndrome)
  - WHO Class II: *Cardiac dysfunction leading to elevated venous pressures*
    - LV systolic dysfunction
    - LV diastolic dysfunction
    - Valvular heart disease
  - WHO Class III: *Parenchymal lung disease and chronic hypoxia causing vasoconstriction*
    - COPD
    - Sleep-disordered breathing
    - Alveolar hypoventilation
    - Interstitial lung disease

- WHO Class IV: *Embolic disease to the pulmonary bed causing decrease in cross-sectional area* (chronic thromboembolic pulmonary hypertension)
- WHO Class V: *Diseases with unclear or multifactorial mechanisms*
  - Parenchymal lung disease with vascular involvement: sarcoidosis, lymphangioleiomyomatosis, neurofibromatosis, vasculitides
    - Metabolic disorders: thyroid disease, Gaucher disease
    - Renal failure, fibrosing mediastinitis

HISTORY

- Exertional dyspnea, fatigue, syncope, signs of right-sided failure (peripheral edema, abdominal distention), angina from RV ischemia

PHYSICAL FINDINGS

- Elevated jugular venous pressure
- Increased split S2
- Loud P2
- Tricuspid regurgitation
- Right-sided S3 and/or S4
- Right ventricular heave
- Lower extremity edema
- Ascites, pulsatile, enlarged liver, and jaundice (if liver failure develops)

ELECTROCARDIOGRAM

- Tall R waves in V_1 (> 7 mm)
- R:S>1 in V_1
- RBBB
- Right atrial enlargement (*P pulmonale*)
- Right axis deviation

CHEST X-RAY

- Enlarged PA
- Decreased peripheral vascular marking
- Right ventricular enlargement
- Signs of parenchymal lung disease as cause of PH

Echocardiography
- Enlarged RV and RA
- Tricuspid regurgitant jet can estimate pulmonary artery systolic pressure.
  - PA systolic pressure = RV systolic pressure = $4v_{regurgitant}^2$ + right atrial pressure where v is the velocity of the regurgitant jet.

- Signs of elevated right ventricular pressure (e.g., dilated or hypokinetic right ventricle, paradoxical septal motion, or a "D-shaped" right ventricle)
- May show signs of valvular heart disease or left ventricular dysfunction as causes of PH

DIAGNOSTIC EVALUATION

- A history of DVT/PE, obesity/hypoventilation, renal disease, COPD, cardiac disease, etc. should be elicited
- Signs of CHF, valvular heart disease, systemic illness on physical exam
- Chest x-ray—evaluation for intrinsic lung disease, PA enlargement, RV and RA enlargement
- Pulmonary function tests may diagnose obstructive or restrictive disease.
  - 50% of patients with IPAH have mildly abnormal PFTs. Avoid attributing PH to interstitial lung disease unless PFTs are severely abnormal.
  - A decreased DLCO is often the sole pulmonary function testing abnormality of patients with PH.
- Echocardiogram to evaluate for cardiac disease
- Perfusion scan/high-resolution CT to evaluate for thromboembolic disease and/or parenchymal lung disease
- 6-minute walk test
  - Determines WHO functional class
  - Prognostically important
- Laboratory evaluation
  - HIV, LFTs, RF, ANA, anti-Scl-70, ANCA
- Cardiac catheterization can diagnose *and* evaluate treatment for pulmonary hypertension. Right heart catheterization (Swan-Ganz catheter) can be used to measure:
  - Pulmonary pressures, right- and left-sided filling pressures, left-to-right intracardiac shunt, cardiac output, systemic and pulmonary vascular resistance
  - Elevated left-sided filling pressure is usually diagnostic of patients with WHO Class II pulmonary hypertension.
    - These patients should have diuresis so that the effect of intrinsic pulmonary disease can be measured.
    - Increased a-waves and flat x-descents on left atrial pressure tracing and/or a gradient between left atrium and left ventricle end diastolic pressure suggest mitral stenosis.
    - Large v-waves are consistent with mitral regurgitation or LV diastolic dysfunction.
  - Vasoreactivity test—especially useful in WHO Class I PH.
    - PA pressures measured while a vasodilator is given—either adenosine, nitric oxide, or epoprostenol.

- ○ Various definitions of "responsiveness" exist.
  - A decrease of more than 10 mmHg to a value < 40 mmHg with no change in cardiac output predicts a response to calcium channel blockers.
  - Another is a > 20% decrease in mean pulmonary artery pressure and more than a 20% decrease in pulmonary vascular resistance predicts a response to treatment with oral calcium channel blockers.

THERAPY

- "Primary therapy"—targeted to the underlying mechanism of PH
  - When primary therapy fails, "advanced therapy" with drugs that directly target the pulmonary vasculature are used.
- Treatment of patients in Class 2 is aimed at optimizing left-sided ventricular filling pressures and/or correction of valve pathology.
- For patients in Class 3, home oxygen administration has been shown to extend life.
  - In the NOTT trial, 19 hours per day of home O_2 was superior to nocturnal oxygen only. Three-year mortality was reduced from 42% to 22%.[57] Five-year survival increased from 46% to 67% among patients with COPD and RV dysfunction.[58]
- WHO Class IV pulmonary hypertension is caused by recurrent pulmonary emboli. All patients are started on anticoagulation. *There is no direct data that anticoagulation increases survival.*
  - Surgery (thromboendarterectomy) is possible in patients who:
    - ○ Remain incapacitated after 3 months of anticoagulation
    - ○ Have thrombi that are proximal enough to be accessible to surgical removal (usually main, lobar, or segmental arteries)
    - ○ Perioperative mortality < 5% in modern series. Four-year follow-up mortality 4% among patients who survive past 3 months post-op.[59]
- Drug therapy:
  - Vasodilator therapy has been demonstrated to improve pulmonary hemodynamics, right ventricular function, cardiac output, oxygen delivery, symptoms, functioning, and exercise.
    - ○ Abrupt discontinuation may lead to rebound PH and death.
  - Calcium channel blockers are utilized for those who are vasodilator responsive on provocative testing.
    - ○ Use cautiously given negative inotropic effect on RV.
    - ○ Nifedipine is commonly used but diltiazem may be preferred if there is resting tachycardia.
    - ○ Doses are increased cautiously given fear of circulatory collapse.
  - Prostaglandins
    - ○ Epoprostenol
      - Improves hemodynamics and survival in IPAH and scleroderma with NYHA Class III–IV symptoms
      - Given as continuous infusion

- ○ Treprostinil
  - Hemodynamic and symptomatic benefit shown in Class I PAH with NYHA Class II–IV symptoms
  - Given subcutaneously, IV or inhaled
- ○ Iloprost
  - Shown to have benefit in several PH classes
  - Inhaled 6–9 times per day
- Endothelin receptor antagonists
  - ○ Bosentan/Sitaxsentan
    - Hemodynamic and 6 minute walk improvement in Class I PAH
- PDE-5 antagonists
  - ○ Sildenafil, vardenafil, tadalafil
    - Both sildenafil and tadalafil shown to improve hemodynamics and 6-minute walk test in Class I PAH
- Some advanced-therapy drugs are *contraindicated* in certain types of pulmonary hypertension.
  - ○ Prostanoids may increase mortality in Class II PH for unclear reasons.
  - ○ In Class III, advanced therapy may worsen V/Q mismatch by increasing vasodilation, an effect that maybe restricted to epoprostenol, in patients with COPD.
- WHO Class IV and V—some benefit to drug therapy
  - ○ Data suggests hemodynamic improvement in patients who do not improve after anticoagulation or surgery.
- Diuretic therapy is indicated to control peripheral edema and ascites.
  - ○ Overdiuresis is common and can lead to decreased cardiac output and systemic hypotension.
- Increased intrathoracic pressure, decreased cardiac output, and syncope should be avoided through use of stool softeners for constipation or antitussives for chronic cough
- Atrial septostomy:
  - Palliative procedure to relieve obstruction to RV outflow, improve oxygen delivery despite desaturation.
  - Consider in patients with refractory pulmonary HTN and right heart failure, or patients with limited cardiac output and symptoms such as syncope.
  - Those with RAP > 20 mmHg, resting O_2 saturation < 80% may have an adverse outcome.
- Lung transplantation:
  - Three-year survival is ~50%
  - Refer for consideration of transplant when:
    - ○ NYHA functional class III/IV
    - ○ Mean RAP > 15 mmHg
    - ○ Mean PAP > 55 mmHg
    - ○ Cardiac index < 2.5 mL/min/m^2
    - ○ Failure to improve on maximal medical therapy

SECTION III

CARDIOVASCULAR THERAPEUTICS

INTRODUCTION

Coronary revascularization is the process of restoring blood flow (oxygen and nutrients) to the essential myocardium. The method of and indications for coronary revascularization are complex and often debated topics.

The basic goals of coronary revascularization include the following three items:

(1) Improve clinical symptoms
(2) Improve long-term survival
(3) Attempt to decrease the incidence of nonfatal outcomes such as myocardial infarction, congestive heart failure, and malignant arrhythmias

There are three common methods for approaching coronary revascularization:

- Percutaneous coronary intervention (PCI) is a generic term referring to any therapeutic procedure directed at treating the narrowed (stenotic) segments in coronary arteries using a combination of balloon angioplasty and stent implantation, coronary atherectomy, or thrombectomy.
- Coronary artery bypass surgery (CABG) is a surgical procedure directed at *bypassing* the stenotic coronary artery segments using vessels harvested from other places in the body (lower extremity veins or thoracic/abdominal arterial grafts).
- Fibrinolysis in the setting of ST-Elevation myocardial infarction (STEMI).

PERCUTANEOUS CORONARY INTERVENTION

- PCI involves repair of the artery by advancing equipment over a coronary guide wire that has been advanced past a blockage in the artery.
- PTCA (percutanous transluminal coronary intervention) angioplasty is when balloon inflation crushes the coronary plaque against the walls of the vessel, restoring blood flow to the downstream myocardium.
- Advanced adjunctive techniques are utilized for specific clinical scenarios and lesions subsets. Such devices include:
  - Rotational (diamond tipped drill) or laser atherectomy for calcified, noncompliant vessels
  - Manual or mechanical thrombectomy for large thrombus burden
  - Protection devices, utilized in saphenous vein grafts, to capture debris liberated during PCI, avoiding embolization downstream
    - No benefit demonstrated in native coronary arteries

- PTCA is now almost always accompanied by the implantation of a coronary stent.
  - Coronary stents are small (2.0–5.0 mm) metallic tubes that are mounted on balloons and advanced to the blockage over the coronary guidewire.
  - When the balloon is inflated, the stent is expanded and deployed against the wall of the vessel.
  - The stent creates a larger lumen, avoids abrupt closure related to vessel dissection and acts as a mechanical scaffold to prop open the vessel.
  - Compared with angioplasty alone, stents reduce restenosis, recurrent narrowing of the artery, abrupt closure, and early thrombosis of the vessel due to vessel dissection after angioplasty.
  - Restenosis still occurs with stents and is due to slow neointimal proliferation causing reblockage with scar tissue.
  - Stent thrombosis is an entity distinct from restenosis where there is abrupt clot formation within the stent. The latter most often presents as a recurrence of chest pain without infarction, while the stent thrombosis is generally an acute infarction with significant morbidity and associated mortality
- Uncoated bare-metal stents (BMS) were the first stents.
  - Restenosis rates were 10–30% or more with these.
- Stents coated with antiproliferative drugs (everolimus, sirolimus, paclitaxel, biolimus A9, and zotarolimus) were developed and reduced restenosis by approximately 60% or more.
  - Drug-eluting stents (DES) suppress restenosis by retarding neointimal proliferation by locally modulating healing, immune, and inflammatory responses to the stent.
  - Though DES have reduced restenosis and the need for repeat revascularization, one drawback has been the infrequent occurrence (≈1/400) of "late stent thrombosis" occurring 12 months or more after initial stent implantation.
- Plaque characterization and angiographically obscured or intermediate lesions can be characterized with intravascular ultrasound (IVUS) or optical coherence tomography (OCT).
- The hemodynamic significance of angiographically obscured or intermediate lesions can be assessed by measuring the fractional flow reserve (FFR).
  - FFR is assessed using a special wire with a pressure transducer on the end.
    - After the wire is advanced past the lesion of interest, induction of maximal hyperemia with adenosine administration is performed, and the pressure distal to the stenosis is compared to aortic pressure.
    - Hyperemia with adenosine induces coronary steal in hemodynamically significant lesions by redirecting blood flow away from arteries

where maximal vasodilation is present at baseline to areas where vasodilation is not maximal at baseline.
- FFR–guided revascularization compared with angiographically guided revascularization has been associated with improved outcomes.
- An FFR of < 0.75–0.80 is deemed hemodynamically significant.

RECOMMENDED GUIDELINES FOR REVASCULARIZATION

Unstable ischemic disease:
- PCI has been shown to improve clinical outcomes during STEMI (death, recurrent myocardial infarction) and moderate- and high-risk UA/NSTEMI (death, myocardial infarction, urgent revascularization)
- Controversy and outcomes are mixed for:
  - STEMI patients presenting > 12 hours post-symptom onset without ongoing symptoms of ischemic/clinical instability
  - Revascularization of non-culprit arteries before hospital discharge in patients who are clinically stable, without recurrent or provocable ischemia, and normal LVEF
  - After successful treatment of the culprit artery by PCI/fibrinolysis, if the risk of revascularization exceeds the estimated risk of the infarction or if significant comorbid conditions make survival unlikely despite revascularization

Stable ischemic disease in patients without prior CABG:
- See Chapter 11, Ischemic Heart Disease and Stable Angina, pp. 73
- For stable angina, revascularization is indicated to improve symptoms if there is failure of maximal anti-ischemic medical therapy.
  - Failure is defined as at least two classes of therapies to reduce anginal symptoms.
  - Patients with intermediate- or high-risk stress test findings (because a large amount of myocardium is in jeopardy and/or LM or 3-vessel coronary disease may be present) should be referred for angiography and/or revascularization (see Chapter 5, ECG Exercise Stress Testing, pp. 30):
    - Low-risk stress test findings: estimated cardiac mortality $<1\%$ per year
    - Intermediate-risk stress test findings: estimated cardiac mortality 1–3% per year
    - High-risk stress test findings: estimated cardiac mortality $>3\%$ per year
- Variable appropriateness guidelines (appropriate/uncertain or inappropriate) exist for numerous combinations of CAD vessel involvement, angina severity, and extent of medical therapy.
  - This section focuses on generally appropriate criteria as outlined in the guidelines for selected, common scenarios.

- Revascularization is appropriate in patients who have 1-, 2-, or, 3-vessel disease with or without involvement of the proximal left anterior descending (without left main stenosis), CCS III/IV angina, and low-risk stress test findings.
- Revascularization is appropriate in asymptomatic patients with 1- or 2-vessel disease with proximal LAD involvement (without left main stenosis) on appropriate medical therapy; patients with-3 vessel disease with no proximal LAD involvement and intermediate -or high-risk stress test findings are also candidates for revascularization.
- Revascularization is appropriate in patients with intermediate stress test findings who have CCS I–IV on maximal medical therapy with 1-, 2-, or 3-vessel disease, with or without proximal LAD involvement; patients with CCS III–IV symptoms with 1-, 2-, or 3-vessel disease with or without proximal LAD involvement and the intermediate-risk stress test findings are also candidates.
- Revascularization is appropriate in patients with high risk stress test findings and CCS I-IV symptoms on no/minimum/maximal medical therapy with 1/2/3 vessel with or without proximal LAD involvement

Among patients with advanced coronary artery disease, appropriateness for PCI and CABG are illustrated by the guidelines presented in Table 27-1:

- For patients where revascularization is necessary, CABG is appropriate in all of the advanced CAD clinical scenarios shown in Table 27-1.
- PCI is appropriate only in those patients with 2-vessel CAD and proximal LAD involvement and uncertain in patients with 3-vessel disease or those who are not candidates for CABG.
- CABG is clearly indicated in those patients with left main stenosis and/or LM stenosis with multi-vessel CAD.
- The revascularization guidelines in Table 27-1 are a topic of much debate and paradigms continue to evolve. For example, many patients with isolated left main coronary artery disease can be safely treated with PCI.

TABLE 27-1. Acute Coronary Syndromes.

	CABG			PCI		
	No DM, nl EF	DM	Low EF	No DM, nl EF	DM	Low EF
2 vessel CAD + prox LAD	A	A	A	A	A	A
3 vessel CAD	A	A	A	U	U	U
Isolated LM	A	A	A	I	I	I
LM stenosis + more CAD	A	A	A	I	I	I

A – appropriate, U – uncertain, I – Inappropriate

Source: Elsevier. Adapted from ACCF/AHA Coronary Revascularization guidelines. *J Am Coll Cardiol.* 2009;53(6):530-553.

- Randomized trials of PCI with DES vs. CABG suggest improved outcomes with CABG for patients with multi-vessel disease who have intermediate- or high-risk anatomy. PCI may be acceptable for those with low-risk anatomy (SYNTAX Trial[61]).
- Decisions are individualized based on individual patient circumstance (e.g., surgical risk and feasibility, anatomic risk for PCI, comorbid conditions, patient preference).

INTRODUCTION

The pacemaker is an artificial device that augments heart rate by electrical stimulation of the myocardium in response to bradycardia. Bradycardia requiring pacemaker therapy is usually symptomatic and due to sinus node dysfunction and/or advanced pathology of the conduction system, such as complete heart block. The pacemaker does *not* directly treat tachycardia—patients often have this misconception—and care must be taken to distinguish pacemakers from implanted cardioverter-defibrillators (ICDs), which primarily treat ventricular tachyarrhythmias. The fact that all ICDs possess pacemaker functionality in the event of bradycardia may be a source of such confusion. Also, in the inpatient setting, pacemakers are either temporary or permanent, whereas in the outpatient setting, all pacemakers are permanent. This chapter covers both types of pacemakers.

INDICATIONS FOR PERMANENT PACEMAKER (PPM)

Table 28-1 describes how the guidelines list indications for a therapy such as pacemakers.
- **Sinus node dysfunction (SND)** refers to abnormalities in atrial impulse generation from the sinus node. SND associated with symptoms, such as fatigue, lightheadedness, or syncope, constitutes a strong indication for PPM implantation. **Symptomatic SND** requiring a PPM should reflect one or more of the following characteristics:
  - Sinus rhythm with pauses ≥ 3 seconds
  - Awake heart rate < 40 bpm

TABLE 28-1. Classes of Indication Used by the ACC/AHA/HRS 2008 Guidelines for Device Based Therapy

ACC/AHA/HRS 2008 Guidelines for Device-Based Therapy (1) used most up to date clinical data to stratify a comprehensive set of indications for PPM implantation:
- Class I: PPM should be implanted, as benefit greatly outweighs risk
- Class IIa: PPM is reasonable, as benefit outweighs risk
- Class IIb: PPM may be considered, as benefit is at least greater than or perhaps equal to risk
- Class III: PPM should not be implanted, as benefit is less than or at best equal to risk

For the sake of brevity, this section will focus on the most common indications for PPM implantation based on these guidelines.

- Chronotropic incompetence—inability to intrinsically increase heart rate in response to physical stress or exertion
- Sinus bradycardia with the concomitant necessity for drugs which lower heart rate, such as beta-blockers in patients with paroxysmal tachycardias (e.g., rapid atrial fibrillation, atrial flutter)
- Postoperative or post-myocardial infarction SND which remains persistent and fails to show reasonable recovery

- **Acquired AV node or conduction system dysfunction**—3rd-degree or advanced 2nd-degree block regardless of anatomic level—also warrants a PPM in any one of the following circumstances:
  - Associated symptoms, such as fatigue, lightheadedness, or syncope
  - Sinus rhythm with pauses ≥ 3 seconds
  - Atrial fibrillation with pauses ≥ 5.0 seconds
  - 3rd-degree AV block or advanced 2nd-degree AV block at any anatomic level and arrhythmias requiring medications which themselves cause symptomatic bradycardia
  - Ventricular arrhythmias induced by AV node dysfunction
  - Advanced AV node or conduction system dysfunction with the concomitant need for drugs which may worsen conduction, such as beta-blockers in CAD
  - Postoperative or post-myocardial infarction 3rd-degree or advanced 2nd-degree AV block which remains persistent and fails to show reasonable recovery

- **Carotid sinus hypersensitivity syndrome** consists of recurrent syncope caused by stimulation of the carotid body, which lies in the carotid sinus at the bifurcation of the carotid artery. Such stimulation may occur with tight neckwear, head turning, or shaving. If carotid massage produces a pause of ≥ 3 seconds in the context of this syndrome, then a PPM is indicated.

- **Cardiac resynchronization therapy (CRT)** (see chapter 29) is pacing the free wall of the left ventricle in order to overcome delayed activation of a portion of the left ventricle (*dyssynchrony*). Dyssynchrony can be seen by imaging techniques such as echocardiography; however prolonged QRS duration (typically with left bundle branch block) is also indicative of ventricular conduction delay. Pacing from the septal side of the LV and free wall reduces dyssynchrony, increases ventricular efficiency, and reduces congestive heart failure.
  - CRT is indicated in patients with an LVEF ≤ 35% and QRS ≥ 120 ms and New York Heart Association Class III or IV congestive heart failure.

INDICATIONS FOR TEMPORARY PACING

- Profound bradycardia (or asystole) causing acute hemodynamic instability
  - Frequently used as a "bridge" to permanent pacemaker therapy (unless the cause of bradycardia is transient or reversible)
    - Awaiting resolution of issues preventing permanent pacemaker implantation, such as anticoagulation, infectious processes

PACEMAKER BASICS

- **Permanent implantable pacemakers.** Pacemakers consist of the pulse generator ("generator"), which contains circuitry, and a battery, and leads. The generator has sockets to receive the leads and set screws to secure the lead(s). The leads are insulated wires with exposed electrodes designed to contact the myocardium for sensing and pacing. Leads may be unipolar or bipolar for sensing and pacing. (Unipolar lead pacing requires that the case of the generator act as the second electrode.)
  - Transvenous permanent pacemaker
    - ○ Leads are implanted via an accessed vein (typically the subclavian, axillary, or cephalic vein).
    - ○ The generator is connected to the lead(s) and placed in a subcutaneous (or submuscular) pocket.
  - Epicardial permanent pacemaker
    - ○ Leads are secured to the epicardium and tunneled to the generator pocket.
    - ○ The generator is connected to the leads and placed in a pocket, which may be abdominal or pectoral.
- **Temporary pacing**
  - *Transcutaneous (external) pacing* utilizes large pad-electrodes (which can also be used for defibrillation).
    - ○ Noninvasive and can be initiated quickly
    - ○ Pacing impulses capture skeletal muscle as well as the heart; very painful
  - *Epicardial temporary pacing* leads are frequently placed during cardiac surgery. The leads can be connected to a temporary generator; programming is readily adjustable. Leads can be removed many days after surgery.
  - *Percutaneous, transvenous pacing* requires a lead to be positioned from a venous access site (femoral, subclavian, or internal jugular vein) and a temporary generator is used.
    - ○ For longer term temporary pacing, a lead designed to be permanent can be implanted percutaneously, connected to a generator remaining outside the body (which can be taped to the skin).
- **Pacing sites:** Endocardial leads are usually placed in venous (right-sided) chambers to minimize the risk of thromboembolism
  - Single-chamber pacing usually utilizes a lead placed in the right ventricle.
    - ○ Ventricular-only pacemakers are used in patients with permanent atrial fibrillation with no plans for return to sinus rhythm.
    - ○ Single chamber *atrial* pacing can be used for patients with sinus node dysfunction, but there is a risk of bradycardia/asystole if the patient subsequently develops heart block.

- Dual chamber: Leads are placed in the right atrium (RA) and right ventricle (RV).
  - Classically RV leads are placed in the RV apex, though active fixation (screw-type) leads may be implanted along the RV septum and in the RV outflow tract.
  - RA leads are conventionally placed in the RA appendage, though the appendage is usually amputated in cardiac surgery cases requiring cardiopulmonary bypass. Other RA sites can be effective and can be chosen by checking pacing parameters at other RA sites
  - Biventricular (resynchronization) pacing requires an additional lead to pace the left ventricle. Transvenous leads are guided to a left ventricular site via the coronary sinus and the left ventricular veins.

CLASSIFICATION OF MOST COMMON PPM MODES

The NASPE/BPEG (North American Society for Pacing and Electrophysiology/British Pacing and Electrophysiology Group) established a code in 1987 to describe pacing modes (Table 28-2):

- **First letter**: Pacing which chambers—that is, A = right atrium, V = R ventricle, D = both R atrium and R ventricle
- **Second letter**: Sensing from which chambers—that is, A, V, and D
- **Third letter**: Manner of responding to sensing—that is, 0 = none, T = triggered (a sensed event triggers a pacing stimulus), I = inhibited (a sensed event inhibits a pacing stimulus), and D = dual (an event in one chamber inhibits stimulus in that chamber but triggers a stimulus in the other chamber, after an appropriate delay, and if not inhibited)
- **Fourth letter** (optional): signifies additional features. For practical purposes, the only letter seen here is "R" for *rate responsiveness* (the lower rate limit rises when a device *sensor* perceives activity). If rate responsiveness is not used, the fourth position is usually blank.

TABLE 28-2. The NASPE/BPEG Pacing Code

Paced chamber	Sensed Chamber	Response to Sensed Events	Rate Responsiveness
A (Atrial)	A (Atrial)	I (Inhibited)	R (Rate responsiveness on; if no rate responsiveness, this position usually left blank)
V (Ventricular)	V (Ventricular)	T (Triggered)	
D (Dual)	D (Dual)	D (Inhibited and Triggered by event in the other chamber)	
0 (No pacing)	0 (No sensing)	0 (No response to sensed events)	

- **Most common PPM modes**
  - **DDD/DDDR**: Both atrium and ventricle are paced and sensed and AV synchrony is maintained. In this mode ventricular pacing *tracks* the atrium, and programmed *upper rate limit* is required to avoid very rapid pacing in atrial fibrillation and flutter. Commonly used mode, except in chronic atrial fibrillation.
  - **VVI/VVIR**: Only the ventricle is paced and sensed; sensing of intrinsic ventricular activity inhibits pacing. Can be used when bradycardic episodes are expected to be brief, thereby limiting AV dyssynchrony duration. Mode of choice in chronic atrial fibrillation, when the atrium cannot be paced and it is not desirable for ventricular pacing to *track* the rapid atrial rates.
  - **AAI/AAIR**: Only the atrium is paced and sensed; pacing is inhibited by sensed intrinsic atrial activity. Used when there is isolated sinus node dysfunction and no disease of the AV node/conduction system.
  - **DDI/DDIR**: Paces the atrium and ventricle and is inhibited by intrinsic events in both. Unlike DDD, ventricular pacing does not *track* the atrium, so if the intrinsic atrial rate is faster than the programmed lower rate limit (and there are no intrinsic ventricular events) the ventricle will be paced at the lower rate limit (and there will be AV dyssynchrony). When the intrinsic rate is below the lower rate limit, both the atrium and ventricle are paced.
    - Used to avoid rapid ventricular pacing with atrial tachyarrhythmias (atrial fibrillation, atrial flutter, ectopic atrial tachycardia).
- **Automatic mode switching**. Modern pacemakers are able to change modes automatically, depending on the circumstances. Two example are:
  - **Mode switch for atrial fibrillation**. If the device senses very rapid atrial rates, tracking of the atrial rhythm is not desirable and the device switches to VVI(R) or DDI(R). If the atrial tachyarrhythmia terminates, then mode switching reverses to DDD(R) to allow AV synchrony.
  - **Reducing ventricular pacing**. It has become apparent that unnecessary ventricular pacing (with its inherent ventricular dyssynchrony) is undesirable. Medtronic introduced an algorithm, *MVP (managed ventricular pacing)*, for dual chamber pacemakers to allow AAI(R) pacing, even if the PR interval is very long. If AV conduction block occurs, the mode will change to DDD(R).

INTERROGATION AND PROGRAMMING OF IMPLANTED PACEMAKERS

The most basic information about pacing performance comes from an ECG. *All pacemakers have a programmed response to placement of a magnet over the device and that response can be monitored by ECG.*

- Typically, the response to magnet application is *asynchronous* pacing (pacing without sensing—AOO, VOO, or DOO)
  - Most manufacturers build in a change in magnet rate with change in battery status, so the magnet rate indicates remaining battery life.

- Magnet application is the simplest programming maneuver and is used to ensure pacing in the setting of inhibition by *electromagnetic interference (EMI)*, which causes inhibition of pacing when sensed in most modes.
  - Surgical electrocautery is one common source of EMI. Magnet application (or reprogramming to VOO/DOO mode) during surgery protects against loss of pacing due to oversensing of EMI.

Noninvasive programming using a computer-based programmer was introduced in 1981. More modern pacemakers communicate wirelessly and without the need for a programmer probe to be placed on the patient at the site of the pacemaker. "Remote" (home) monitoring is now available via a telephone (usually a land line is required) and internet. No permanent reprogramming can be done remotely. Routine device checks as well as interrogation to assess the pacemaker in the event of symptoms can be done without requiring a trip to the hospital or clinic. There is now an abundance of information that can be derived from pacemaker interrogation, falling into a few general categories:

- Battery status: Not nearing end of life, elective replacement indicated (ERI), end of life (EOL)
  - The time between ERI and EOL is usually 3 months or more (making generator change elective)
  - When EOL is reached, pacing does not stop (at least for a while). The mode may switch to one that consumes less battery energy. Normal pacemaker behavior cannot be assured. Generator change is more urgent.
- Lead impedances
- Pacing thresholds
- Sensing thresholds (the amplitude of the sensed P- and R-waves, if any)
- Current programming (mode, AV delay, refractory periods)
- Stored data. Available data has increased dramatically over the years. It may include:
  - Heart rate and percentage-pacing data
  - Logs of events such as mode switches, high ventricular rate episodes, VPDs
  - Stored electrograms from high heart rate events
  - Logs from automatic measurements of impedances, sensing, and pacing thresholds

TROUBLESHOOTING IMPLANTED PACEMAKERS

Cardiologists are frequently called on to assess pacemaker function due to abnormal ECG findings or symptoms. Frank malfunction of the device is rare. Lead problems, unintended consequences of programming, electromagnetic interference, and changes in battery status are more common.

- First assess the apparent problem—examples are:
  - Failure to capture (though pacing spikes are present)

- Failure to pace ("failure to output"): There is an unexpected pause with no apparent attempt to pace.
  - Oversensing (inhibition of pacing due to sensing of events that are not actually P-waves or R-waves) is one common cause.
- Undersensing: Pacing spikes are seen despite the presence of intrinsic P-waves or QRS complexes.
  - It should be obvious that "undersensing" occurs with magnet application or in asynchronous modes (AOO, VOO, DOO).
- Interrogation of the pacemaker will then yield the programmed parameters, amplitude of sensed P- and R-waves, pacing thresholds, lead impedances, and battery status.
  - Rise in pacing threshold typically occurs in the 4–6 weeks after implantation and is attributed to local inflammation. It is rarely a problem since the introduction of steroid-eluting leads.
  - **Lead failure** such as lead fractures, insulation breaks, and dislodgements can often be discovered during device interrogation at the clinic or via home monitoring. May or may not be evident on chest x-ray.
    - **Lead fracture**: causes a significant rise in lead impedance from baseline. May also lead to inappropriate oversensing of atrial/ventricular activity due to electrical interference on the fractured lead.
    - **Insulation break** causes low-lead impedance. Current entry through insulation defect may lead to oversensing. Current leakage from the lead may lead to loss of capture.
    - **Lead dislodgement** may lead to loss of sensing and/or pacing. It is more likely to occur soon after lead implantation (before healing and scarring).
      - *Twiddler's syndrome* refers to the patient turning the generator through the skin (often unintentionally or unconsciously) and causing the leads to coil up and detach from the myocardium.
  - **Battery depletion** is also alerted via interrogation of the PPM or by audible warning beeps from the PPM itself.
    - **Elective replacement indication (ERI)**: Battery life is likely 3–6 months before system failure occurs due to low battery. Generator change should be scheduled soon.
    - **End of life (EOL)**: Depletion of battery is imminent; mode of PPM may change to conserve battery. Generator change becomes more urgent.

TRANSVENOUS PACEMAKER IMPLANTATION

- Local anesthesia with lidocaine during PPM pocket creation on L or R pectoral area.
- The pacemaker is usually placed on the patient's nondominant side, though exceptions occur due to structural constraints, such as upper venous occlusion due to prior instrumentation.

- Lead(s) inserted into subclavian vein via thoracic or extrathoracic (cephalic vein, extrathoracic subclavian as the vein crosses the first rib, axillary vein) approach.
- Sedation can range from minimal to deep, depending on patient preference and/or concerns for respiratory compromise.
- The patient is asked to limit ipsilateral arm movement and lifting for several weeks to avoid early dislodgement.

COMPLICATIONS POST-IMPLANTATION

- **Hematoma** at the pacemaker pocket is more likely to occur in anticoagulated patients and those with elevated venous pressure. Hematomas slow the return to full anticoagulation and increase the lengths of hospital stays.
  - Prevention
    - Antiplatelet agents (aspirin and clopidogrel) are not usually discontinued for pacemaker implantation.
    - Warfarin and dabigatran are traditionally discontinued, though many operators have to avoid bleeding complications with careful procedural attention to hemostasis.
    - Heparin and enoxaparin are avoided in the immediate postprocedure period.
      - In patients with urgent need for anticoagulation (mechanical mitral valves), the time without anticoagulation is usually limited to about 24 hours.
      - Heparin should be used as sparingly as possible after the waiting period, while warfarin is resumed.
    - Clotting activation agents (cellulose) or clotting factors (recombinant thrombin) can be placed in the pocket to minimize bleeding.
  - Treatment
    - Hold anticoagulation as much as possible considering other indications for anticoagulation
    - Evacuation of the pocket is only when unavoidable. Every opening of the pocket increases the risk of infection. Like pacemaker implantation, it should always be done in a sterile setting such as the electrophysiology laboratory of the operating room. Indications for pocket evacuation include:
      - Tension on the incision, risking dehiscence
      - Rapid expansion, suggesting arterial bleeding
- **Pneumothorax** is more likely using a needle puncture (modified Seldinger) approach for venous access, and it is more likely when access is difficult. Vigilance is required.
  - Chest x-ray should be checked after the procedure.
- **Cardiac perforation/pericardial tamponade** may be caused by an atrial or ventricular lead.
  - Hypotension should prompt evaluation for pericardial effusion and tamponade (usually with echo) after any instrumentation of the heart.

- Pericardiocentesis is the therapy. Lead revision is not desirable if lead function remains good and there is no significant lead tip migration.

- **Infection** is the most feared complication due to the difficulty of therapy. In general, infection of the pocket is also assumed to be infection of the leads, and infection of the leads (vegetations and bacteremia) must be assumed to involve the pocket and generator. Explantation is typically required.

  - Most common pathogen: *Staphylococcus epidermis. Staphylococcus aureus* (including methicillin resistant strains) is also common, particularly in hospitalized patients.

  - Presentation
    - Pocket: Swelling, erythema, warmth, tenderness, purulent drainage, fevers, rigors, chills
    - Lead infection: bacteremia, fever, rigors, chills

  - Prevention
    - In addition to meticulous sterile technique, IV antibiotics active against skin flora (cefazolin or vancomycin) infused immediately prior to the procedure have been shown to reduce infections.
    - Post-procedure antibiotics also appear to be effective, though the benefit is less certain.

  - Investigation
    - Examination of the pocket
    - Blood cultures
    - Consider echo and transesophageal echo to assess the presence of vegetations.
    - **Do not** *perform needle aspiration of a device pocket.*
      - High risk of introducing bacteria into the pocket.

  - Therapy. Infectious disease consultation is recommended to assess the nature of the infection and other patient factors.
    - Bacteremia with Gram-positive cocci typically warrants device explantation, long-term IV antibiotics, and reimplantation (in a different site) after a specified duration devoid of fevers and positive blood cultures.
    - Gram-negative bacteremia has been treated with long-term IV antibiotics only, with the device remaining in place. Failure to clear the infection requires explantation.
    - Lead explantation (of leads more than a few months old) is a highly specialized procedure with significant risk of urgent requirement for cardiac surgery and risk of death. It should only be performed by experienced personnel.

29 ■ CARDIAC RESYNCHRONIZATION FOR HEART FAILURE

DYSSYNCHRONY AND CONGESTIVE HEART FAILURE

The narrow width of the normal QRS complex reflects the rapidity of activation of the ventricles (< 100 ms). Conduction delay, particularly in the left ventricle in the form of left bundle branch block (LBBB), creates *dyssynchrony* of ventricular muscle contraction. Conventional right ventricular pacing also creates dyssynchrony.

- Dyssynchrony in the setting of congestive heart failure reduces the efficiency of contraction and contributes to systolic dysfunction and heart failure.
- Dyssynchrony is also associated with mitral regurgitation.
  - AV dyssynchrony is associated with functional (presystolic) mitral regurgitation.
  - Delayed papillary muscle contraction may exacerbate systolic mitral regurgitation.
- LBBB in congestive heart failure is associated with increased mortality and sudden cardiac death.[63]

EFFECTS OF RESYNCHRONIZATION

Cardiac resynchronization therapy (CRT) is achieved by pacing the free wall of the left ventricle (LV) to counteract the conduction delay. LV free wall and septal activation can thus be synchronized.

- Despite the term *biventricular pacing*, most of the benefit appears to proceed not from coordination of the left and right ventricles, but from LV *intraventricular* resynchronization.
  - LV pacing alone, correlated with intrinsic RV and septal activation could improve intraventricular synchrony.
    - However, simultaneous RV and LV pacing allows atrioventricular synchronization as well as intraventricular and interventricular synchronization.
  - AV synchrony with LV or biventricular pacing decreases late diastolic mitral regurgitation.[64]
- Importantly, the initial improvement in LV systolic function afforded by CRT can be attributed to the improvement in efficiency without requiring increased myocardial inotropy or metabolic cost.
- CRT reverses LV remodeling and improves systolic and diastolic function.[65]

Several trials have demonstrated positive clinical effect of CRT. In each, patients enrolled had:

- New York Heart Association (NYHA) Heart Failure Class III–IV symptoms
- LV ejection fractions ≤ 0.35
- Prolonged QRS duration (at least 120 ms)
- Stable, optimal medical therapy at the time of enrollment

The trials included:

- MUSTIC (Multisite Stimulation in Cardiomyopathies):[66] CRT improved 6-minute walk distance, peak oxygen consumption, NYHA Class, and reduced hospitalizations.
- Path CHF (Pacing Therapies in Congestive Heart Failure):[67] CRT (optimized based on hemodynamics at initial implant) resulted in improved exercise capacity, functional status, and quality of life.
- MIRACLE (Multicenter InSync Randomized Clinical Evaluation):[68] CRT improved 6-minute walk distance, NYHA Class, quality of life, and exercise time
- MIRACLE ICD (Multicenter InSync ICD Randomized Clinical Evaluation):[69] Implantation of a CRT defibrillator was associated with no change in 6-minute walk, but improvements in quality of life, functional status, and exercise capacity were seen. Use of CRT with a defibrillator appeared safe.
- COMPANION (Comparison of Medical Therapy, Pacing, and Defibrillation on Heart Failure Study):[70] CRT resulted in improvement in the combined endpoint of mortality and hospitalization. CRT with a defibrillator improved all-cause mortality. There was a trend toward improvement in mortality with CRT in the absence of a defibrillator, but it was not statistically significant ($p = 0.059$).
- CARE-HF (Cardiac Resynchronization-Heart Failure Study):[71] CRT therapy reduced occurrence of the primary endpoint, death, or cardiovascular hospitalization. There was also a reduction in overall mortality (a secondary endpoint) with CRT (in the absence of a defibrillator).
- A meta-analysis of 4 trials reporting the effect of CRT on mortality concluded that CRT reduces mortality from progressive heart failure and reduces heart failure hospitalizations. There was a trend toward reduction of all-cause mortality that was not statistically significant.[72]

After establishment of the benefit of resynchronization in advanced (NYHA Class III) heart failure, 2 studies have addressed prevention of progression or milder heart failure:

- MADIT-CRT:[73] in patients with:
  - LV ejection fraction ≤ 0.30
  - NYHA class I (if ischemic) or II (ischemic or nonischemic)
  - QRS duration ≥ 130 ms

CRT with ICD therapy (CRT-D) decreased the risk of the combined endpoint of death or heart failure event from 25.3% to 17.2% ($p = 0.001$). The reduction in the combined endpoint is attributable to the reduction in heart failure events; there was not reduction in all-cause mortality.

- Prespecified subgroup analysis showed more benefit in patients with:
  - NYHA Class II
  - QRS duration ≥ 150 ms
  - Age ≤ 65 years

Women also derived more benefit than men.

- RAFT (Resynchronization-Defibrillation for Ambulatory Heart Failure Trial):[74] In patients with NYHA Class II and III CHF and prolonged QRS undergoing ICD implantation, addition of CRT reduced mortality and hospitalization due to heart failure. There were more adverse events in patients undergoing CRT, which appear to be related to the additional challenges of implanting a left ventricular lead.

LEFT VENTRICULAR PACING LEAD IMPLANTATION

Lead implantation techniques:

- Initially, resynchronization was achieved by epicardial LV lead implantation. Since then, improvements in technique and technology have allowed transvenous placement of an LV lead in a lateral vein to become commonplace. In addition to improved delivery systems (introducer sheaths, guidewires), new LV leads are more versatile and most can be advanced over a guidewire. Typical steps in placing an LV lead include:
  - Venous access, similar to access used for other pacing/ICD leads
  - Use of a specially curved introducer sheath to cannulate the coronary sinus (CS), usually with a guidewire, a deflectable catheter, and/or contrast injections
  - A contrast venogram to evaluate the coronary venous system for lead implant targets
  - Use of a small caliber (0.014 inch) guidewire to cannulate the target vein.
  - Advancement of the lead over the guidewire to "wedge" it into place in the coronary vein.
    - In addition to typical pacing thresholds, care must be taken to test for capture of the phrenic nerve, which runs over the LV epicardium.
      - Phrenic nerve capture stimulates the diaphragm, with uncomfortable contraction with every heartbeat.
      - Choosing another tributary of the target vein or another target vein altogether may be required.
      - Sometimes, changing pacing electrode configurations can eliminate diaphragmatic stimulation.
  - Removal of the introducer sheath (without dislodging the lead!)

Target Sites for LV pacing:

- The proportion of nonresponders to CRT may be in part attributed to suboptimal LV lead position.

- Conventional wisdom is that the ideal LV pacing site is the site of latest activation before resynchronization. This may be difficult to determine without specialized imaging.
- Usually the mid-lateral or basal lateral wall is targeted.
  - Anterior sites are thought usually to be less effective.
  - The actual available pacing sites for transvenous leads are limited by coronary venous anatomy and by phrenic nerve pacing.

AV OPTIMIZATION

It is readily apparent that biventricular pacing must occur for CRT therapy to provide any benefit. For this reason, the CRT device must be programmed with an AV delay that is short enough to provide ventricular pacing. Yet, the AV delay cannot be so short as to disrupt ventricular filling. Several algorithms for "AF optimization" have been suggested.[75]

- It is possible to assess hemodynamic values invasively, though it may be hard to apply data from an invasive assessment to everyday conditions of variable exertion and heart rate.
- Echocardiography is noninvasive and readily available:
  - Some methods evaluate the mitral valve inflow pattern in order to maximize filling without truncating the A-wave (the "atrial kick").
  - Echocardiography can also be used to assess stroke volume, using the aortic or mitral velocity-time integral (VTI).
- There are now device-based algorithms for optimizing AV delay based on electrogram data that allows automatic optimization, which may be repeated often to maintain AV optimization with variable conditions.

However, a large clinical trial (980 patients) found that neither a device-based algorithm nor echo guidance was superior to a fixed empiric delay of 120 ms.[76] It is still likely that some individual patients, such as nonresponders to initial CRT, might benefit from AV optimization.

INDICATIONS FOR CARDIAC RESYNCHRONIZATION THERAPY

Guidelines published in 2008 by the American Heart Association (AHA), American College of Cardiology (ACC), and the Heart Rhythm Society (HRS) list indications for CRT:[77]

- Class I indication:
  - Patients with LVEF ≤ 0.35, QRS duration ≥ 120 ms, and NYHA Class III or ambulatory Class IV heart failure symptoms when already on optimal medical therapy for heart failure
- Class IIa indications:
  - Patients with LVEF ≤ 0.35, QRS duration ≥ 120 ms, atrial fibrillation, and NYHA Class III or ambulatory Class IV heart failure symptoms when already on optimal medical therapy for heart failure
  - For patients with LVEF ≤ 0.35, NYHA Class III or ambulatory Class IV heart failure symptoms when already on optimal medical therapy for

heart failure, and who have the requirement for frequent ventricular pacing

- Class IIb indication:
  - Patients with LVEF ≤ 0.35 with NYHA Class I or II heart failure symptoms, who are receiving optimal medical therapy for heart failure, and who are undergoing implantation of a pacemaker and/or ICD with anticipated frequent ventricular pacing.
- Class III indications (CRT not indicated):
  - Not indicated for asymptomatic patients with reduced LV function in the absence of other indications for pacing.
  - Not indicated for patients with limited functional status and life expectancy due to chronic noncardiac conditions.

After the publication of MADIT CRT, the U.S. Food and Drug Administration formulated additional acceptable indications for the prevention of progression of heart failure:[78]

- Patients with ischemic heart failure and:
  - EF ≤ 0.30
  - LBBB
  - QRS duration ≥ 130 ms
  - NYHA Class I or II heart failure symptoms
- Patients with nonischemic cardiomyopathy and:
  - EF ≤ 0.30
  - LBBB
  - QRS duration ≥ 130 ms
  - NYHA Class II heart failure symptoms

RIGHT BUNDLE BRANCH BLOCK

The initial clinical trials listed above did not exclude patients with right bundle branch block (RBBB). It is possible that those with RBBB have no significant LV dyssynchrony. On the other hand, the presence of RBBB does not exclude the possibility of poor conduction within the LV.

- The established indications reflect the fact that RBBB patients were enrolled in the initial clinical trials, though less commonly than LBBB.[77]
- The newer indications related to MADIT-CRT account for further subgroup analysis that suggests diminished benefit in RBBB.[78]

OTHER INDICATORS OF DYSSYNCHRONY

The QRS duration is the only manifestation of dyssynchrony utilized for patient selection for CRT. Yet CRT fails in up to about 30% of patients. Conversely, echocardiography and other imaging may detect dyssynchrony that is not reflected by the QRS duration. Two trials tested echocardiography as a predictor of response to CRT:

- PROSPECT (Predictors of Response to CRT) examined 12 echocardiographic parameters in patients with indication for CRT therapy.
  - The parameters were neither sensitive nor specific enough to be more useful than the QRS duration as a predictor of response.
- RETHINQ (Cardiac Resynchronization Therapy in Patients with Heart Failure and Narrow QRS) studied patients with EF $\leq$ 0.35, NYHA Class III heart failure symptoms, echocardiographic dyssynchrony, and QRS < 130 ms. Patients were randomized to CRT-D or ICD alone.
  - The CRT group had an improvement in NYHA Class.
  - CRT did not improve
    - Peak oxygen consumption
    - Quality of life
    - 6-minute walk

The results suggest that echocardiographically identified dyssynchrony (without QRS prolongation) is unlikely to respond to CRT.

Other imaging modes may ultimately be shown to be better suited to identify dyssynchrony that will respond to CRT.

30 ■ IMPLANTABLE DEFIBRILLATOR THERAPY

INTRODUCTION

- Implantable Cardioverter-Defibrillators (ICDs) have become the mainstay of therapy for malignant ventricular arrhythmias in patients at high risk for sudden cardiac death (SCD).
- ICDs monitor the heart rhythm via transvenous or epicardial leads which detect malignant ventricular arrhythmias and provide lifesaving therapies in the form of antitachycardia pacing, cardioversion, or defibrillation.
- The primary components of the ICD include the pacing circuitry, battery, charging circuit, and capacitor housed in a titanium shell.
- An ICD is essentially a pacemaker with additional capability of delivering a high-energy shock via a large capacitor.
  - When activated, the battery must charge the capacitor, which then discharges to deliver up to about 35 J of energy through the shocking electrodes.
- Defibrillation electrodes are required to deliver the shock energy.
  - Transvenous ICD leads have 1 or 2 exposed coils serving as defibrillation electrodes.
    - Additional coil electrodes may be added transvenously and placed in the subclavian vein or superior vena cava (if the RV lead does not have a proximal coil), in the azygos vein (posterior to the heart), or in the coronary sinus.
  - Subcutaneous electrode coils can be implanted in the left chest to allow the electrodes to more fully surround the heart.
  - Electrode patches may be surgically implanted:
    - Directly on the epicardium
    - Subcutaneously
  - In modern devices, the generator casing (which has a much greater surface area than a coil) usually also serves as an electrode.
  - Coil electrodes have also been implanted surgically in the pericardial space.
  - Entirely subcutaneous devices are in development. These consist of a generator subcutaneously positioned lead.
    - No need to implant intravascular hardware
    - No pacing capability
    - Sensing and detection or tachyarrhythmias must be achieved without a traditional endocardial (or epicardial) lead.

CLINICAL TRIALS OF ICDS FOR PRIMARY AND SECONDARY PREVENTION OF SCD AND INDICATIONS

- Landmark Trials for ICD therapy are shown in **Table 30-1**.

Indications for ICD therapy

Indications for ICD implantation have been established based on the data from clinical trials, including those listed in Table 30-1. Indications listed here are based on guidelines published jointly by the American College of Cardiology, the American Heart Association, and the Heart Rhythm society.[96] Since actual practice largely also depends on reimbursement, some the ACC/AHA/HRS guideline indications are modified by the policy of the U.S. Centers for Medicare and Medicaid Services (CMS).[97] Most health insurers/payers follow the policy of CMS. These indications are therefore an amalgam of the ACC/AHA/HRS guidelines and the CMS coverage policy.

- Class I Indications: ICD is indicated; potential benefits greatly outweigh the risks.
  - Survivors of cardiac arrest due to VF or hemodynamically unstable sustained VT in the absence of any reversible causes
  - Spontaneous sustained VT in association with structural heart disease
  - Syncope of undetermined origin with relevant, hemodynamically significant VT or VF induced at EPS
  - Ischemic heart disease and documented MI with EF ≤ 35%; ≥ 40 days post-MI and ≥ 3 months after revascularization; and NYHA class II or III congestive heart failure symptoms
  - Ischemic heart disease with EF ≤ 30%; ≥ 40 days post-MI and ≥ 3 months after revascularization, and NYHA class I
  - Ischemic heart disease with EF ≤ 40%; documented nonsustained VT; inducible sustained VT at electrophysiology study, which must be at least 4 weeks after any MI. ICD implantation should occur ≥ 40 days after the index MI.
  - Nonischemic cardiomyopathy with EF ≤ 35%. The cardiomyopathy must have persisted for more than 3 months after diagnosis; NYHA class II or III.
- Class IIa indications: ICD is reasonable; the benefits outweigh the risk.
  - Unexplained syncope, significant LV dysfunction, and dilated nonischemic cardiomyopathy
  - Sustained VT and normal or near-normal ventricular function in the absence of a reversible cause
  - Hypertrophic obstructive cardiomyopathy (HOCM) patients with one or more risk factors for SCD
  - Arrhythmogenic right ventricular dysplasia/cardiomyopathy (ARVD/C) with one or more risk factors for SCD
  - Long QT syndrome + syncope and/or VT/VF while on beta-blocker therapy
  - Nonhospitalized patients with heart failure awaiting cardiac transplantation

TABLE 30-1. Important Trials in the Development of ICD Therapy for Secondary and Primary Prevention of Sudden Death

Prevention Strategy	Trial Name	Patients Evaluated	Primary End-Point	Reduction in Primary Endpoint with ICD
Secondary	AVID[81]	-Resuscitated from VT -Syncope w/sustained VT -Sustained VT with EF ≤ 0.4 and -hemodynamic compromise	Mortality with ICD vs. antiarrhythmic agent	31% (p<0.02)
	CIDS[82]	-Sustained VT -Sustained VT with syncope -Sustained VT and EF ≤ 0.35 -Syncope with later spontaneous or inducible VT -Excluded MI within 72 hours prior to enrollment	Mortality with ICD vs. antiarrhythmic agent	20% (p = 0.1)
	CASH[83]	-Resuscitated from cardiac arrest w/documented sustained arrhythmia	Mortality with ICD vs. antiarrhythmic agent	23% (p = 0.2)
	Meta-analysis of AVID/CIDS/CASH[84]		Mortality with ICDs vs. antiarrhythmic agent	28% (p = 0.001)
Primary	MADIT[85]	Coronary disease, EF ≤ 0.35, NSVT, *and* inducible VT, not suppressed by procainamide	Mortality with ICD vs. antiarrhythmic agent	56% (p = 0.009)
	MUSTT[86]	*Coronary disease, EF ≤ 0.4, NSVT, *and* inducible sustained VT. Randomized to EP guided therapy, with ICD if inducible VT not suppressed by antiarrhythmic agent vs. best medical therapy without an antiarrhythmic agent).	Cardiac arrest or death with EP study-guided therapy vs. best medical therapy	27% (p = 0.04). All benefit attributable to ICD in EP-guided arm. No benefit to anti-arrhythmic agents

(Continued)

TABLE 30-1. Important Trials in the Development of ICD Therapy for Secondary and Primary Prevention of Sudden Death (Continued)

Prevention Strategy	Trial Name	Patients Evaluated	Primary End-Point	Reduction in Primary Endpoint with ICD
	MADIT II[87]	Previous MI, EF ≤ 0.3, NYHA Class I-III	Mortality with ICD vs. best medical therapy	31% (p = 0.02)
	CAT[88]	Non-ischemic cardiomyopathy, EF ≤ 0.3, and NYHA Class II-III, and CHF ≤ 9 months	Mortality with ICD vs. best medical therapy	No improvement (p = 0.6)
	AMIOVERT[89]	Non-ischemic cardiomyopathy, EF ≤ 0.35, NYHA Class I-IV	Mortality with ICD vs. best medical therapy	No improvement (p = 0.8)
	COMPANION[90]	Coronary disease, EF ≤ 0.35, QRS ≥ 120 msec, Chronic CHF, NYHA Class III-IV	Mortality or Hospitalization with resynchronization ICD vs. best medical therapy	20% reduction in primary endpoint (p = 0.01)
	DEFINITE[91]	Non-ischemic cardiomyopathy, EF ≤ 0.35, NSVT or frequent VPDs	Mortality with ICD vs. best medical therapy	35% but only nearing statistical significance (p = 0.08) (Significant decrease in sudden death as secondary endpoint).
	SCD-HeFT[92]	EF ≤ 0.35, NYHA Class II-III CHF > 3 months, no MI within 30 days	Mortality with ICD vs. best medical therapy	23% (p = 0.007)
	CABG-Patch[93]	Coronary disease undergoing CABG, EF ≤ 0.35, abnormal SAECG	Mortality with ICD vs. best medical therapy	No improvement p = 0.6
	DINAMIT[94]	Coronary disease w/recent MI, EF ≤ 0.35, NYHA Class I-III, depressed HR variability or elevated HR	Mortality with ICD vs. best medical therapy	No improvement (p = 0.7)
	Meta-analysis of Primary Prevention Trials[95]		Mortality with ICD vs. best medical therapy	25% (p = 0.003)

- Brugada syndrome with a history of syncope
- Brugada syndrome with documented VT in the absence of cardiac arrest
- Catecholaminergic polymorphic VT with syncope and/or documented sustained VT while on beta-blockers
- Cardiac Sarcoidosis, Giant cell myocarditis or Chagas disease
- Class IIb indications: ICD therapy may be considered; the benefits are equal to or greater than the risks.
  - NICM EF < 35% and NYHA class I
  - Long QT syndrome and risk factors for SCD
  - Syncope with advanced structural heart disease with invasive and noninvasive investigations having failed to define a cause
  - Familial cardiomyopathy associated with SCDs
  - Left ventricular noncompaction
- Class III indications: ICD is *not* indicated; the benefits are outweighed by the risks.
  - Expected survival < 1 year in a patient who otherwise would meet criteria based on the above recommendations
  - Incessant VT or VF
  - Psychiatric illnesses that may be aggravated by device implantation or may preclude systematic follow-up
  - NYHA Class IV patients with drug refractory CHF who are not candidates for cardiac transplantation or CRT
  - Syncope of undetermined cause in the absence of structural heart disease and negative EP study
  - VT or VF amenable to surgical catheter ablation (e.g., atrial arrhythmias associated with WPW, RV/LV outflow tract VT, idiopathic VT, or fascicular VT in the absence of structural heart disease)
  - Ventricular tachyarrhythmias due to a completely reversible disorder in the absence of structural heart disease (e.g., electrolyte imbalance, drugs, trauma)

IMPLANTATION TECHNIQUES/LEAD PLACEMENT/DFT TESTING

Transvenous ICD implantation is very similar to transvenous pacemaker implantation. A typical pre-pectoral implantation includes an infraclavicular incision, a subcutaneous pocket for the pulse generator, and venous access to advance and position the lead(s) in the right heart using fluoroscopy.

- Proper sterile technique is essential for the prevention of device infection with perioperative antibiotics directed toward Gram-positive skin flora (e.g., cefazolin, vancomycin) given to reduce infectious complications.
- For transvenous leads, venous access via the cephalic, subclavian, extrathoracic subclavian, or axillary veins may be used as described for pacemaker implantation.

- Most implanters favor an RV apical position for the RV lead.
  - Unlike a pacemaker, positioning the electrode for defibrillation efficacy is a consideration. A less apical position or a high RV septal position may be less efficacious for defibrillation.
  - R-wave sensing is of vital importance for ICDs, since VF waves are likely to be of much lower amplitude than normal intrinsic R-waves tested at the time of implant.
    - In rare cases, it is necessary to implant a separate ventricular pace/sense lead (a pacemaker lead) if poor sensing and/or pacing is found at the best site for defibrillation.
  - Ideally R-wave sensing should be > 5 mv with pacing thresholds preferably < 1.0. Impedance values that are too high (> 1000) or to low (< 100) suggest damage to the lead/improper placement and/or problems with the tissue-lead interface.
- A post-implantation CXR is desirable to evaluate for pneumothorax (if a needle puncture is used for venous access) and assess and document lead position.
- Defibrillation threshold testing (DFT) is often performed to reduce the risk of failed defibrillation and to help optimize the output settings of the device.
  - DFT testing involves induction of VF via burst pacing or a shock delivered on the T-wave during a ventricular pacing.
    - Sensing of VF, detection, and delivery of the high-energy therapy are all tested.
    - Traditionally, testing is performed with lower defibrillation energy than the maximum deliverable by the device to achieve at least a 10 J safety margin, though there is little data to support this.
  - There is emerging opinion that DFT testing is poorly predictive of performance in the field and that each defibrillation shock is deleterious to the heart. Therefore, in many cases DFT testing is omitted.
    - Omission of DFT testing also omits testing of sensing of VF wave amplitude and appropriate detection.
- Inadequate defibrillation safety margin (whether discovered by DFT testing or by failure of one or more defibrillation shocks in the field) should prompt consideration of action to improve defibrillation efficacy. Possible actions include:
  - Repositioning the RV lead
  - Use of a leads with proper spacing to keep the SVC coil in the innominate vein junction and testing with SVC coil on/off
  - Changing polarity
  - Adjustment of the pulse widths (depending on device manufacturer)
  - Addition of shock electrodes to lower impedance and/or improve the shock vector
    - Azygos vein coil
    - Additional subclavian or innominate vein coil
    - Coronary sinus coil

- Subcutaneous coil (or array or coils)
- Surgically positioned epicardial patch electrodes
- Surgically placed intrapericardial coil
- Addition of sotalol can lower the defibrillation threshold.
- Some antiarrhythmic drugs tend to raise the defibrillation threshold, sometimes negligibly. Consider DFT testing after initiation of:
  - Amiodarone
  - Lidocaine
  - Mexiletine

ICD FUNCTION

- Pacemaker function. All modern ICDs have pacemaker capabilities and can provide either single or dual chamber pacing.
  - In a dual-chambered system standard pace/sense atrial leads are used in addition to the RV defibrillation lead.
  - Some ICDs are capable of detecting and treating atrial fibrillation and other atrial tachyarrhythmias, though these features are not often used. This discussion will focus on ventricular tachyarrhythmias.
  - Most patients with indications for cardiac resynchronization pacing also have indication for an ICD, so resynchronization therapy (CRT) has been incorporated into ICDs. (CRT pacemakers are much less common).
- Sensing and detection
  - *Sensing* involves registering the intrinsic electrograms from the chamber in question.
    - Sensing utilizes amplifiers, filters, and adaptive thresholds and/or gain to avoid oversensing of cardiac (T-wave, far-field) and noncardiac activity while avoiding undersensing of low-amplitude cardiac activations during ventricular fibrillation.
    - Sensing algorithms are proprietary and vary with manufacturer.
  - *Detection* refers to the device's algorithms for comparing sensed events to programmed definitions of VT and VF.
    - Detection algorithms analyze the rate, timing, and (in some cases) the morphology of the sensed electrograms to determine the presence or absence VT or VF.
    - Discrimination algorithms for the discrimination of SVTs (atrial fibrillation, atrial flutter, sinus tachycardia, and others) with rapid ventricular rate from VTs that should be treated
      - Discrimination algorithms are also proprietary and vary with manufacturer. Some points of discrimination tachycardias include:
        - Onset: VT is more likely to have a sudden onset than sinus tachycardia.
        - Stability: VT is typically more regular than atrial fibrillation.
        - Morphology: Some devices evaluate electrogram morphology or width, since VT is more likely to produce a wide QRS and wide electrogram.

- A to V timing (in dual chamber ICDs): V-A dissociation is virtually diagnostic of VT. Some devices also utilize the relative timing between the atrial and ventricular electrograms even if there is no dissociation.
  - Detection zones (usually up to 3) can be programmed to allow *tiered therapy* (Figure 30-1):
    - Slower VT may be more hemodynamically stable, allowing for multiple attempts at pace-termination (antitachycardia pacing, ATP); see below.
    - ATP can be successful with faster arrhythmias. Usually fewer pacing trains are attempted before delivering a shock at rates that are likely to be hemodynamically unstable.
- Tachyarrhythmia therapy
  - ICD therapies include:
    - Antitachycardia pacing (ATP) for VT (low-energy therapies)
      - *ATP* is overdrive pacing to terminate reentrant VT. It is typically painless.
        - Burst pacing: A train of pacing impulse programmed at a percentage (e.g., 88%) of the tachycardia cycle length
        - Ramp pacing: A train in which each successive impulse occurs with shorter intervals
        - More "aggressive" ATP is more likely to transform a VT into VF or a faster VT.
          - Ramps and more rapid bursts are considered more aggressive.
    - High-energy therapies (shocks)
      - Painful if the patient is awake
      - Devices are programmed to deliver a maximum number of shocks (usually 6 to 8) for a single tachyarrhythmia episode.
      - Energies less than the maximum for the device may be programmed:
        - Allows faster charging
        - Is unlikely to make a significant difference in pain for the patient
      - Therapies
        - Synchronized cardioversion for VT
        - Unsynchronized defibrillation for VF if no R-wave can be synchronized
      - When the detection criteria are met, the capacitors are charged, which requires several seconds. After charging is complete, most detection algorithms confirm the continued presence of the VT/VF and then deliver the shock.
        - In some cases (e.g., subsequent shocks after the first in an episode), the shock is said to be *committed*. It is delivered without confirmation.
        - Once VT is detected, the ICD will charge and during this timeframe, the device will continue to sense. Once the device

has been fully charged, if the device continues to sense the tachyarrhythmia, then it will deliver therapy. If the device detects sinus rhythm during the charging process, then the shock will be aborted (for a noncommitted device).

- Charge times can be affected by the age of the device, battery status, and the condition of the capacitors
- Programming tachyarrhythmia therapies should aim for simplicity.
  - Unnecessary shocks are an important problem. Overprogramming can lead to painful therapy if the rhythm is life threatening.
    - For example, in a patient with no history of VT receiving a primary prevention ICD, complicated VT programming has a high risk of leading to unnecessary shocks.
    - Similarly, increasing the VF detect rate (compared to baseline settings) to about 200 bpm increases the specificity of detection.
      - Slower VTs are unlikely to cause death without accelerating to a faster rate or VF.

ICD INTERROGATION AND TROUBLESHOOTING

ICD interrogation is performed to:

- Assess any suspected malfunction
- Complete routine follow-up, particularly of battery life
- Assess any tachyarrhythmia event
- Interrogation of an ICD should involve a systematic approach that evaluates the following:
- How long has it been since the last interrogation?
- What is the battery life?
- What are the current atrial, ventricular, and shock coil lead impedances? What are the trends? Are they abnormally high or low?
  - Assists in assessing for fracture, dislodgement, insulation defect
- What are the atrial and ventricular pacing thresholds? Have they changed?
- What are the measured P- and R-waves, and is there an adequate safety margin? Is there inappropriate sensing secondary to noise/far-field sensing that results in inhibition of pacing or initiation of tachy therapies?
- Have any arrhythmias been detected?
  - If so, what therapy was provided and was it successful?
    - Modern ICDs store a great deal of information, including electrograms, plots of heart rate, and data about detected episodes.
  - Was detection and therapy appropriate or inappropriate?
    - Did inappropriate detection lead to an inappropriate shock?
    - If inappropriate, what was the cause?
      - SVT?
      - Electrical noise from lead fracture?

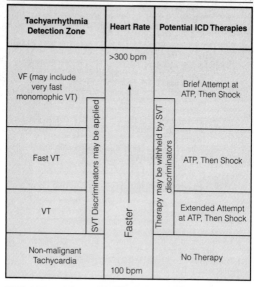

FIGURE 30-1 Tiered ICD Therapy. Detected tachyarrhythmias are distinguished by heart rate. A VF zone is always present; Fast VT and VT zones are optional. Rate for detection of each zone is programmable. Shock therapies are usually programmed; number and protocol of ATP attempts is programmable. SVT discriminators are algorithms designed to distinguish SVTs from VT: Lack of stability suggests atrial fibrillation; gradual onset suggests sinus tachycardia; 1:1 AV relationship may suggest SVT; normal electrogram morphology suggests SVT. SVT discriminators are programmable. ATP = antitachycardia pacing; bpm = beats per minute; SVT = supraventricular tachycardia.

- Ventricular oversensing?
  - T-wave oversensing
  - Far-field atrial electrogram
  - Skeletal muscle myopotentials
  - Electromagnetic interference (EMI)

- Based on the above, what changes should be considered?
  - Sensing and pacing parameters
  - Lead revisions and/or extractions
  - Change of VT/VF detection zones based on VT rate of detected rhythm(s)
  - Change of therapy
    - Addition or elimination of ATP cycle
  - Addition of an antiarrhythmic agent to suppress ventricular arrhythmias and spare the patient pain of therapies
  - Ablation of VT to minimize the need for painful therapies

PERIOPERATIVE/PERIPROCEDURE MANAGEMENT

- The surgeon and/or the anesthesiologist should:
  - Know indications for the device, model, and whether the patient is pacer dependent
  - Interrogate the device or have it interrogated to know the programming
  - Preoperative ECG
  - Determine likelihood of EMI from procedure, which causes oversensing and inhibition of pacing and delivery of unnecessary shocks.
    - Particularly from electrocautery, which should only be used in short bursts of cautery far from the patient's device site
    - Place magnet over ICD site
  - Suspend antitachycardia function of ICD by programming or continuous magnet application.
    - **Magnet application** (over an ICD) will temporarily turn off detection for tachy therapies but will not affect pacing parameters. That is, if a patient with an ICD is pacemaker dependent, the device needs to be programmed to asynchronous pacing.
      - Magnets usually make non-ICD pacemakers pace asynchronously.
  - If external defibrillation becomes necessary: Use anterior-posterior pad electrodes; use lowest energy possible.
- Lithotripsy: Focus beam away from generator.
- Radiation therapy:
  - Shield device; plan with radiation therapist.
    - Rarely, a device will exhibit bizarre, unpredictable behavior if the radiation beam is focused on the generator.
  - Consider changing device location only if it is clear that the device is interfering with radiation treatment.

31 ■ MANAGEMENT OF ATRIAL FIBRILLATION AND FLUTTER

INTRODUCTION

Owing to its "chronic, recurring" nature, its high prevalence, and the associated risk of thromboembolism, treatment of atrial fibrillation (AF) deserves attention apart from other arrhythmias.

Lately, much has been learned about the mechanisms of atrial fibrillation. For clinical purposes, it is acceptable to think of it as chaotic electrical activity in the atrium, generated by multiple small wavelets of action potentials. Some of the wavelets may behave like reentrant waves and others may arise from one or more focal sites. The sequelae of the electrical chaos are:

- **Very poor atrial contractility and blood transport.** Loss of the "atrial kick" in filling the left ventricles is of little consequence in most people. Those with heart failure may be affected hemodynamically.
- With poor blood transport comes **stasis of blood in the atrium** and the atrial appendages. There is a risk of forming thrombus and a **risk of thromboembolism.**
- **Rapid, irregular ventricular rate**: with multiple wavelets bombarding the atrioventricular (AV) node. The AV node's slowed, *decremental* conduction properties (more rapid stimulation slows conduction) prevent atrial fibrillation from becoming ventricular fibrillation. Nonetheless, the normal response to AF is a rapid, irregular rate, usually leading to rapid irregular palpitations.
- **Decreased cardiac output** follows from the rapid rate, the irregularity, and possibly the loss of atrial contribution to ventricular filling. Depressed cardiac output leads to a variety of symptoms, including lightheadedness, fatigue, lack of energy, dyspnea. Dyspnea may also be caused by pulmonary congestion associated with decreased output.

THERAPY MODALITIES

- **Anticoagulation.** Since thromboembolism is a major potential consequence of AF, each patient requires consideration of systemic anticoagulation with warfarin. The stasis of atrial fibrillation predisposes to thrombus formation, but it is the return of organized atrial activity that is most likely to cause dislodgement of any thrombus existing in the atrium (particularly the atrial appendages).
  - The risk of stroke in nonrheumatic atrial fibrillation is closely related to comorbidities. The CHADS2 scoring system is used to estimate the stroke risk (see **Table 31-1** and **Table 31-2**).[98]

TABLE 31-1. Calculating the CHADS2 Score

Risk Factor	CHADS2 "Points"
Congestive Heart Failure	1
Hypertension	1
Age 75 or Older	1
Diabetes Mellitus	1
History of Stroke or TIA	2
CHADS2 Score	Sum

- CHADS2 score of 0 usually prompts aspirin therapy only.
- CHADS2 score of 1 may be treated with aspirin or warfarin (or dabigatran).
- CHADS2 score of 2 or more is an indication for warfarin with an INR target of 2.0 to 3.0 (or dabigatran).
- The CHA2DS2-VASc Score is an additional system that accounts for some additional risk factors for stroke (such as age between 65 and 74, vascular disease, and sex).[99] As with the CHADS2 score, the CHA2DS2-VASc score is correlated with recommendation for anticoagulation (see **Table 31-3**).
  - 0: aspirin therapy or no anticoagulant and no antiplatelet agent
  - 1: treated with either aspirin or warfarin (or dabigatran)
  - 2 or more: treated with warfarin (or dabigatran)
- Contraindications (primarily risk of bleeding, including risk of falls with head trauma) to warfarin therapy may override the indications.
- In patients with persistent atrial fibrillation in whom cardioversion is planned, anticoagulation—at least for the short term—should be considered to minimize the risk of thromboembolism.
  - It is the new atrial activation pattern of sinus rhythm (not the jolt of a cardioversion shock) that increases the risk of embolism of a thrombus.

TABLE 31-2. CHADS 2 Score and Risk of Stroke in Non-valvular Atrial Fibrillation

CHADS2 Score	Risk of Stroke (per year)	Recommended Anticoagulation
0	1.9%	Aspirin therapy
1	2.8%	Aspirin or warfarin (or dabigatran)
2	4.0%	Warfarin (or dabigatran)
3	5.9%	Warfarin (or dabigatran)
4	8.5%	Warfarin (or dabigatran)
5	12.5%	Warfarin (or dabigatran)
6	18.2%	Warfarin (or dabigatran.

TABLE 31-3. Calculating the CHA2DS2-VASc Score

Risk Factor	CHA2DS2-VASc "Points"
Congestive Heart Failure or Systolic LV Dysfunction	1
Hypertension	1
Age 75 or Greater	2
Diabetes Mellitus	1
Prior Stroke, TIA, or Thromboembolism	2
Vascular Disease	1
Ages 65-74 years	2
Sex	2 (for female)
CHA2DS2-VASc Score	Sum

- This means that pharmacologic cardioversion has a risk of thromboembolism, just as electrical cardioversion does.
  - Even when pre-cardioversion transesophageal echo reveals no left atrial thrombus, full atrial activity may not return for 3–4 weeks, making it possible for thrombus to form even after the cardioversion. Anticoagulation is therefore indicated after cardioversion, even if transesophageal echo reveals no thrombus.
- There is no evidence that returning a patient to sinus rhythm removes the risk of thromboembolism or stroke. Therefore, the indications for anticoagulation apply regardless of other treatment. Many will discontinue anticoagulation if there is no evidence of recurrent atrial fibrillation for an extended period of time. However, it is still possible for the next presentation of recurrent atrial fibrillation to be in the form of a stroke.
- **Dabigatran**, a direct thrombin inhibitor, has been approved by the Food and Drug Administration (FDA) for use in atrial fibrillation.[100] INR monitoring is not required.
- Rate control and rhythm control. Long-term strategies for treatment of AF include both **rate control** only and attempted **rhythm control**. Large trials have shown no mortality benefit to the rhythm control strategy.[101,102] Rhythm control is more likely to require recurring hospital visits and cardioversions and changes in medications. Rhythm control is more appropriate in patients who are symptomatic despite rate control.
  - Rate control:
    - Pharmacologic rate control:
      - Beta-blockers
      - Some calcium channel blockers
        - Diltiazem (a benzothiazepine)
        - Verapamil (a phenylalkylamine)
        - NOT dihydropyridines (e.g., nifedipine, amlodipine), which have very little rate-slowing activity

- ○ Nonpharmacologic rate control:
  - Catheter ablation of the AV node creates complete heart block.
    - Requires pacemaker implantation and the patient usually becomes "pacemaker-dependent"
      - ▫ Attempts at "AV node modification" to slow the ventricular rate without requiring a pacemaker have been disappointing.
- • Rhythm control:
  - ○ Pharmacologic rhythm control. The potent antiarrhythmic agents have significant side effects and toxicities, particularly proarrhythmia. Many clinicians admit the patient to initiate these drugs; others follow ambulatory ECG monitoring during initiation of the drug (watching for: arrhythmias, QT prolongation, QRS widening, bradycardia).
    - Class Ic antiarrhythmic agents
      - ▫ Drugs
        - ▫ Flecainide
        - ▫ Propafenone
          - ▲ Has some rate-slowing effects
      - ▫ Contraindicated in the presence of structural heart disease, particularly MI or other scar
      - ▫ Use-dependence: Conduction slowing (due to Na^+ channel blockade) is more prominent at faster rates.
        - ▫ Toxic widening of the QRS with rapid rates
        - ▫ Use a rate-controlling (AV nodal blocking) drug with these agents, particularly flecainide:
          - ▲ Beta-blockers
          - ▲ Diltiazem or verapamil
        - ▫ When initiating IC agents, watch QRS with exercise. Discontinue use if QRS widens with increased rate.
      - ▫ Forms of proarrhythmia
        - ▫ May convert AF to slow flutter that may be conduct 1:1 with rapid ventricular rate (and toxic wide QRS): "flecainide flutter."
        - ▫ In presence of scar, shortening of the wavelength may facilitate reentry and VT.
    - Class III antiarrhythmic agents:
      - ▫ Drugs
        - ▫ Sotalol
          - ▲ Significant beta-blockade
        - ▫ Dofetilide
        - ▫ Amiodarone
          - ▲ Extraordinarily large volume of distribution, long half-life
          - ▲ Nonspecific in effect (Class I, II, III, and IV) effects
          - ▲ Multiple noncardiac toxicities, including pulmonary, thyroid, and hepatic

- Most are cumulative dose dependent (though there are more rare shorter term toxicities, especially pulmonary).
  - ▲ No renal toxicity; no contraindication in renal disease
  - ▢ Dronedarone
    - ▲ Developed to be similar to amiodarone, without the Iodine moieties and the associated toxicities.
- Forms of proarrhythmia
  - ▢ QT prolongation (due to K+ channel blockade)
    - ▲ Especially sotalol, dofetilide
  - ▢ Bradycardia for amiodarone, sotalol, dronedarone
- Class Ia agents (quinidine, procainamide, disopyramide) are now rarely used because of an unfavorable risk/benefit profile.
- ○ Nonpharmacologic rhythm control
  - Surgical MAZE procedure.
    - Multiple ablation or atriotomy lines of block
    - Frequently performed in conjunction with valve replacement or other surgery
    - Less invasive versions are continuously being developed to improve utility of this surgery
    - Experienced surgeon is required.
  - Catheter ablation
    - Based primarily on isolating pulmonary vein ostia, since much paroxysmal atrial fibrillation is triggered by spontaneous activity in the pulmonary veins.
    - 60–80% long-term relief from atrial fibrillation. Higher success in paroxysmal AF, lower in persistent or long-term persistent AF.
    - Unlike other ablative therapies, early recurrence of AF may not predict longer term failure of the procedure.
    - Targets other than the pulmonary vein antra include complex fractionated atrial electrograms (CFAEs [said: "cafes"]) and atrial myocardium in the coronary sinus.
    - Low risk of significant complications:
      - ▢ Thromboembolism
      - ▢ Perforation/pericardial tamponade
      - ▢ Atrio-esophageal fistula
        - ▲ Often delayed in development (about 2 weeks)
        - ▲ Rare but frequently lethal due to air embolism, bacteremia, massive esophageal bleeding
        - ▲ Any esophageal symptoms after catheter ablation should be evaluated carefully.
          - CT first, NOT esophagogastroduodenoscopy (EGD) (which insufflates the esophagus)
        - ▲ Fever and leukocytosis are among the most sensitive findings.

- "Hybrid" catheter and surgical ablation allows for the strengths of each modality to be exploited. Surgical access may improve ablation efficacy. Endocardial mapping can assess effect of ablation and establishment of lines of conduction block.

URGENT/IMMEDIATE TREATMENT OF AF

- As always, assess the patient, not just the ECG or the rhythm.
- Always consider the patient's anticoagulation status. The risk of thromboembolism is high if the duration of the fibrillation is more than 72 hours (or unknown) without therapeutic anticoagulation with warfarin or heparin. The risk or thromboembolism is not related to means of cardioversion. The "jolt" from a direct current shock is not the cause of thromboembolism; return of organized atrial contraction is. Do not think that use of a pharmacologic agent (including ibutilide, dofetilide, amiodarone), or a low energy shock, or even pace-termination of atrial flutter will avoid the risk of stroke or other thromboembolism. So, starting an antiarrhythmic drug without excluding the presence of left atrial thrombus poses a similar risk to a DC shock. (Occasionally the need for the antiarrhythmic drug may outweigh the risk, especially since [with exception of ibutilide] cardioversion from AF by an antiarrhythmic drug is uncommon. An example would be a patient in persistent atrial fibrillation who requires amiodarone for recurrent life-threatening ventricular arrhythmias.)
  - If the duration is *known* and is less than 72 hours. The duration of the patient's symptoms may poorly reflect the duration of the arrhythmia. Your judgment concerning accuracy of symptoms may be required. The patient should understand the increased risk of thromboembolism/stroke if he/she is incorrect concerning the duration of the arrhythmia.
  - For longer/unknown duration of AF, therapeutic anticoagulation (without lapses) for a minimum of 3 weeks is conventionally required.
  - Transesophageal echo (TEE) can establish the absence of left atrial thrombus. If no thrombus is seen *and* if the patient is therapeutically anticoagulated, cardioversion can be safely performed (of course, it is never risk-free).
  - For patients at risk for thromboembolism, the risk extends beyond the time of the actual cardioversion. Anticoagulation is indicated for at least 3 weeks (in the absence of a more powerful contraindication). This is based on the time required for near-full recovery of atrial contraction.
- If the hemodynamic situation is severe, urgent cardioversion is indicated. This is fairly rare. Often, relative hypotension is related to rapid ventricular response.
- **Rate control therapy** is the most common treatment modality for rapid atrial fibrillation: Though rate-slowing agents (except digoxin) tend to

lower blood pressure, lowering the ventricular rate may have a more prominent *positive* effect on blood pressure. Careful administration with short-acting medicines and careful monitoring of the ECG and blood pressure is required. *Beware sinus bradycardia (or long sinus pause) occurring at the time of spontaneous cardioversion to sinus rhythm.* This is a variant of sick sinus syndrome exposed by the rate-slowing drugs. Less common, but an important consideration, is bradycardia due to AV node dysfunction after the return to sinus rhythm. In fast-acting, rate-slowing agents:

- IV metoprolol: usually given in 5 mg increments
- IV diltiazem: 20 mg (0.25 mg/kg) bolus over 2 minutes (may be repeated), and a continuous infusion, starting at 10 mg/hour, which can be increased or decreased in 5 mg/hour increments
- IV esmolol: 0.5 mg/kg over 1 minute, then 50–200 mcg/kg/min
- IV verapamil: 5–10 mg (0.075–0.15 mg/kg) over 2 minutes and repeated as needed
- IV digoxin should be avoided due to poor efficacy and narrow therapeutic window with high risk of toxicity. Can be loaded with 0.5 mg IV then 0.25 mg every 6 hours twice, followed by once daily dosing.

ATRIAL FLUTTER

Flutter is more organized than fibrillation, and the term typically implies a single reentrant wave of activation in the atrium, though it does not exclude a focal source. *Flutter* usually implies a more rapid rate than *atrial tachycardia*. There is no strict division between the 2 in terms of rate, but an atrial rate > 180 bpm (cycle length: 333 ms) would likely be considered slow flutter. Slower atrial rhythms might be designated atrial tachycardia.

By far the most common atrial flutter is mediated by a reentrant wave that circulates on the atrial side of the tricuspid valve. Since size of the tricuspid annulus is similar among people, the rate of this *typical atrial flutter* is commonly about 300 bpm (cycle length: 200 ms). Most commonly, the activation wave proceeds up the septum, across the roof, down the right atrial free wall, then across the *IVC-tricuspid isthmus* (the narrow strip of atrial floor between the IVC-RA junction and the tricuspid valve annulus)—*counterclockwise* (if you are looking at the tricuspid annulus from the apex of the heart). Flutter may also utilize the same circuit in the opposite, *clockwise*, direction. Other flutters are called *atypical* and may be related to a surgical scar or other abnormality in the atria.

Atrial flutter is described in detail in the section concerning atrial tachyarrhythmias. Clinically, it is treated identically to atrial fibrillation with the following additional considerations:

- Atrial mechanical activation may be more organized, but indications for anticoagulation are essentially the same as for atrial fibrillation. This includes the need to ensure the absence of left atrial thrombus prior to cardioversion and the indication for anticoagulation after return to sinus rhythm.

- Since the atrial rate is regular, the ventricular rate is often rapid and regular. For typical flutter, for example, 2:1 AV block is common. Since the atrial rate is about 300 bpm, the ventricular rate will be 150 bpm. Rate control often requires creation of 3:1 block to yield a ventricular rate of 100 bpm (or 4:1 AV block to yield a rate of 75 bpm). Titration of rate-controlling drugs may be more difficult than for atrial fibrillation.
- Particularly for typical, isthmus-dependent flutter, catheter ablation is an earlier option. Ablation for typical flutter has a well established track record for efficacy. A line of conduction block across the IVC-tricuspid isthmus eliminates the circuit, and reentry is prevented.

32 ■ CATHETER ABLATION OF ARRHYTHMIAS

INTRODUCTION

Catheter ablation for tachycardias is usually performed as a therapeutic extension of a diagnostic electrophysiology study (EP study), which may include extensive computer-based "electroanatomic" mapping in concert with conventional mapping techniques, such as entrainment mapping, activation mapping, and pacing mapping. The goal of these mapping procedures is to locate a site that is critical to the arrhythmia:

- The origin (focus) of a focal arrhythmia (such as an ectopic atrial tachycardia focus, or a right ventricular outflow tract ventricular tachycardia [VT] focus)
- A critical isthmus of myocardium that completes a circuit for reentrant arrhythmias (such as atrial flutter, scar-related ventricular tachycardia, the "slow pathway" of Atrioventricular Nodal Reentrant Tachycardia [AVNRT], or the accessory pathway of Wolff-Parkinson-White syndrome)
- Ablation of the AV node is a time-tested therapy for controlling the ventricular rate in atrial fibrillation.
  - Pacemaker is also required.
  - AV node ablation does not control the fibrillation itself.
- More extensive ablation techniques have arisen for situations in which a single effective site cannot be established:
  - Atrial fibrillation ablation currently relies on extensive ablation in the left atrium
  - The substrate modification approach for scar-related VT
    - Ablation in regions potentially mediating VT, in the absence of inducing and mapping a specific VT

The goal of ablation then is to render the critical myocardium inactive. Ablation denatures the proteins, killing the cells and causing a (usually) very well circumscribed scar, which for practical purposes, is electrically inactive.

THE CATHETERS

- An ablation catheter must be precisely manipulable to reach whatever area of the heart is necessary.
  - All are deflectable to produce a curve near the distal tip, allowing steering.
  - Various curve radii are available.
  - Most can be introduced via an 8 French introducer sheath.

- Since it is desirable to map the ideal site and then ablate, the ablation catheter is also the roving mapping catheter, typically with 4 recording electrodes.
  - The distal electrode delivers the ablation energy. Its dimensions therefore, may sacrifice some mapping function for ablation function. Larger electrodes are frequently desired for ablation.

ENERGY SOURCES

Radiofrequency energy is the most widely used energy for ablation.

- Alternating current is delivered at the tip electrode with an indifferent electrode (a high surface area patch) on the patient's skin.
- Resistive heating occurs as the energy penetrates the tissue.
- Heating to greater than about 50°C results in lesion formation.
- The energy generator is programmed to a maximum energy delivered and a maximum catheter tip temperature.
  - High temperatures under the surface of the myocardium may reach boiling, with a rapid expansion of water vapor and an explosion ("steam pop") which may result in significant damage and perforation.
- The typical lesion is a few millimeters wide and deep.
  - Deeper and larger lesions can be produced with larger tip electrodes.
  - Irrigated catheters keep the tip temperature cool, avoiding reaching the temperature maximum and higher temperature to be reached within the myocardium for deeper lesions.
  - Larger, deeper lesions increase the risk of undesired damage to neighboring structures (the conduction system, coronary arteries) and/or perforation.
- Inadvertent damage to the conduction system (e.g., heart block, requiring pacemaker) is an important risk.

CRYOTHERMAL ENERGY

- Liquid nitrogen circulated through the catheter tip brings it to −80°C.
  - The tip adheres to the myocardium.
- Primary advantage is the early reversibility if an adverse effect is seen.
  - When ablating near the conduction system, if AV block or PR prolongation is seen, some time is required before the damage becomes permanent.
    - If ablation is discontinued promptly, the effect will usually reverse as the tissue rewarms.

Other energy sources, such as microwave, laser, and high energy ultrasound are essentially in developmental stages.

■ REFERENCES

(1) Gibbons RJ, Balady GJ, Bricker JT, et al. ACC/AHA 2002 guideline update for exercise testing: a report of the American College of Cardiology/American Heart Association Task Force on Practice Guidelines (Committee on Exercise Testing). *J Am Coll Cardiol.* 2002;40(8):1531–1540.

(2) American College of Cardiology Foundation Appropriate Use Criteria Task Force; American Society of Echocardiography; American Heart Association; American Society of Nuclear Cardiology; Heart Failure Society of America; Heart Rhythm Society; Society for Cardiovascular Angiography and Interventions; Society of Critical Care Medicine; Society of Cardiovascular Computed Tomography; Society for Cardiovascular Magnetic Resonance; American College of Chest Physicians, Douglas PS, Garcia MJ, Haines DE, et al. ACCF/ASE/AHA/ASNC/HFSA/HRS/SCAI/SCCM/SCCT/SCMR 2011 Appropriate use criteria for echocardiography. *J Am Soc Echocardiogr.* 2011;24(3): 229–267.

(3) Hendel RC, Berman DS, Di Carli MF, et al. ACCF/ASNC/ACR/AHA/ASE/SCCT/SCMR/SNM 2009 appropriate use criteria for cardiac radionuclide imaging: a report of the American College of Cardiology Foundation Appropriate Use Criteria Task Force, the American Society of Nuclear Cardiology, the American College of Radiology, the American Heart Association, the American Society of Echocardiography, the Society of Cardiovascular Computed Tomography, the Society for Cardiovascular Magnetic Resonance, and the Society of Nuclear Medicine. *Circulation.* 2009;119(22):e561–587.

(4) Taylor AJ, Cerqueira M, Hodgson JM, et al. A report of the American College of Cardiology Foundation Appropriate Use Criteria Task Force, the Society of Cardiovascular Computed Tomography, the American College of Radiology, the American Heart Association, the American Society of Echocardiography, the American Society of Nuclear Cardiology, the North American Society for Cardiovascular Imaging, the Society for Cardiovascular Angiography and Interventions, and the Society for Cardiovascular Magnetic Resonance. *Circulation.* 2010;122(21):e525–555.

(5) Hendel RC, Patel MR, Kramer CM, et al. ACCF/ACR/SCCT/SCMR/ASNC/NASCI/SCAI/SIR 2006 appropriateness criteria for cardiac computed tomography and cardiac magnetic resonance imaging: a report of the American College of Cardiology Foundation Quality Strategic Directions Committee Appropriateness Criteria Working Group, American College of Radiology, Society of Cardiovascular Computed Tomography, Society for Cardiovascular Magnetic Resonance, American Society of Nuclear Cardiology, North American Society for Cardiac Imaging, Society for Cardiovascular Angiography

and Interventions, and Society of Interventional Radiology. *J Am Coll Cardiol.* 2006;48(7):1475–1497.

(6) Fleisher LA, Beckman JA, Brown KA, et al. ACC/AHA 2007 guidelines on perioperative cardiovascular evaluation and care for noncardiac surgery: a report of the American College of Cardiology/American Heart Association Task Force on Practice Guidelines (Writing Committee to Revise the 2002 Guidelines on Perioperative Cardiovascular Evaluation for Noncardiac Surgery) developed in collaboration with the American Society of Echocardiography, American Society of Nuclear Cardiology, Heart Rhythm Society, Society of Cardiovascular Anesthesiologists, Society for Cardiovascular Angiography and Interventions, Society for Vascular Medicine and Biology, and Society for Vascular Surgery. *J Am Coll Cardiol.* 2007;50(17):e159–241.

(7) Auerbach A, Goldman L. Assessing and Reducing the Cardiac Risk of Noncardiac Surgery. *Circulation.* 2006;113:1361.

(8) The Seventh Report of the Joint National Committee on Prevention, Detection, Evaluation, and Treatment of High Blood Pressure (JNC 7). *Hypertension.* 2003;42:1206.

(9) Julius S, Alderman MH, Beevers G, et al. Cardiovascular risk reduction in hypertensive black patients with left ventricular hypertrophy: the LIFE study. *J Am Coll Cardiol.* 2004;43:1047–1055.

(10) Mehta SR, Tanguay JF, Eikelboom JW, et al. Double-dose versus standard dose clopidogrel and high-dose versus low-dose aspirin in individuals undergoing percutaneous coronary intervention for acute coronary syndromes (CURRENT-OASIS 7): A randomised factorial trial. *Lancet.* 2010;376:1233–1243.

(11) Kastrati A, Mehilli J, Neumann FJ, et al. Abciximab in patients with acute coronary syndromes undergoing percutaneous coronary intervention after clopidogrel pretreatment: The ISAR-REACT 2 randomized trial. *JAMA.* 2006;295:1531–1538.

(12) Stone GW, McLaurin BT, Cox DA, et al. Bivalirudin for patients with acute coronary syndromes. *N Engl J Med.* 2006;355:2203–2216.

(13) Stone GW, Witzenbichler B, Guagliumi G, Peruga JZ, Brodie BR, Dudek D, Kornowski R, Hartmann F, Gersh BJ, Pocock SJ, Dangas G, Wong SC, Kirtane AJ, Parise H, Mehran R, the HORIZONS-AMI Trial Investigators. Bivalirudin during primary pci in acute myocardial infarction. *N Engl J Med.* 2008;358:2218–2230.

(14) Keeley EC, Boura JA, Grines CL. Primary angioplasty versus intravenous thrombolytic therapy for acute myocardial infarction: A quantitative review of 23 randomised trials. *Lancet.* 2003;361:13–20.

(15) Stone GW. Angioplasty strategies in st-segment elevation myocardial infarction. *Circulation.* 2008;118:552–566.

(16) Maisel AS, Krishnaswamy P, Nowak RM. Rapid measurement of B-type natriuretic peptide in the emergency diagnosis of heart failure. *N Eng J Med.* 2002;347:161–167.

(17) Hunt SA, Abraham WT, Chin MH, et al. ACC/AHA 2005 guideline update for the diagnosis and management of chronic heart failure

in the adult: a report of the American College of Cardiology/American Heart Association Task Force on Practice Guidelines (Writing Committee to Update the 2001 guidelines for the evaluation and management of heart failure): collaboration with the American College of Chest Physicians and the International Society for Heart and Lung Transplantation: endorsed by the Heart Rhythm Society. *Circulation.* 2005;112(12):e154–235.

(18) Poole-Wilson PA, Swedberg K, Cleland JG, et al. Comparison of carvedilol and metoprolol on clinical outcomes in patients with chronic heart failure in the Carvedilol Or Metoprolol European Trial (COMET): randomized controlled trial. *Lancet.* 2003;362:7–13.

(19) Packer M, Coats A, Fowler MB, et al. Effect of carvedilol on survival in severe chronic heart failure. *N Engl J Med.* 2001;344:1651–1658.

(20) The Cardiac Insufficiency Bisoprolol Study II (CIBIS-II): a randomized trial. *Lancet.* 1999;353:9–13.

(21) Hjalmarson A, Goldstein S, Fagerberg B, et al. Effects of controlled-release metoprolol on total mortality, hospitalizations, and well-being in patients with heart failure: The Metoprolol CR/XL Randomized Intervention Trial in congestive heart failure (MERIT-HF). *JAMA.* 2000;283:1295.

(22) The SOLVD Investigators. Effect of enalapril on survival in patients with reduced left ventricular ejection fractions and congestive heart failure. *N Engl J Med.* 1991;325:293–302.

(23) Packer M, Poole-Wilson PA, Armstrong PW, et al. Comparative effects of low and high doses of the angiotensin-converting enzyme inhibitor, lisinopril, on morbidity and mortality in chronic heart failure. *Circulation.* 1999;100:2312–2318.

(24) Pitt B, Poole-Wilson PA, Segal R, et al. Effect of losartan compared with captopril on mortality in patients with symptomatic heart failure: randomized trial. The Losartan Heart Failure Survival Study ELITE II. *Lancet.* 2000;355:2312–2318.

(25) Cohn JN, Tognani G, et al. A randomized trial of the angiotensin-receptor blocker valsartan in chronic heart failure. *N Engl J Med.* 2001;345:1667–1675.

(26) Yusuf S, Pfeffer MA, Swedberg K, et al. Effects of candesartan in patients with chronic heart failure and preserved left-ventricular ejection fraction: The CHARM Preserved Trial. *Lancet.* 2003;362:772–776.

(27) Cohn JN, Archibald DG, Zieshe S, et al. Effect of vasodilator therapy on mortality in chronic congestive heart failure. Results of a Veterans Administration Cooperative Study. *N Engl J Med.* 1986;314:1547–1552.

(28) Taylor AL, Ziesche S, Yancy S, et al. Combination of isosorbide dinitrate and hydralazine in blacks with heart failure. *N Engl J Med.* 2004;351:2049–2057.

(29) VMAC Investigators. Intravenous nesiritide vs nitroglycerin for treatment of decompensated congestive heart failure: a randomized controlled trial. *JAMA.* 2002;287:1531–1540.

(30) The Digitalis Investigation Group. The effect of digoxin on mortality and morbidity in patients with heart failure. *N Engl J Med.* 1997;336:525–533.

(31) Rathore SS, Curtis JP, Wang Y, et al. Association of serum digoxin concentration and outcomes in patients with heart failure. *JAMA.* 2003;289:871–878.

(32) Pitt B, Zannad F, Remme WJ, et al. The effect of spironolactone on morbidity and mortality in patients with severe heart failure. *N Engl J Med.* 1999;341:709–717.

(33) Pitt B, Remme WJ, Zannad F, et al. Eplereone, a selective aldosterone blocker, in patients with left ventricular dysfunction after myocardial infarction. *N Engl J Med.* 2003;348:1309–1321.

(34) Cuffe MS, Califf RM, Adams KF, et al. Short-term intravenous milrinone for acute exacerbations of chronic heart failure: a randomized controlled trial. *JAMA.* 2002;287:1541–1547.

(35) Bardy GH, Lee KL, Mark DB, et al. Amiodarone or an implantable cardioverter-defibrillator for congestive heart failure. *N Engl J Med.* 2005; 352: 225–237.

(36) Cleland JG, Daubert JC, Erdmann E, et al. The effect of cardiac resynchronization on morbidity and mortality in heart failure. *N Engl J Med.* 2005;352:1539–1549.

(37) Rose EA, Geljins AC, Moskowitz AJ, et al. Long-term mechanical left ventricular assistance for end-stage heart failure. *N Engl J Med.* 2001;345:1435–1443.

(38) Felker GM, Thompson RE, Hare JM, et al. Underlying causes and long-term survival in patients with initially unexplained cardiomyopathy. *N Engl J of Med.* 2000;342:1077–1078.

(39) Li JS, Sexton DJ, Mick N, et al. Proposed modifications to the Duke criteria for the diagnosis of infective endocarditis. *Clin Infect Dis.* 2000;30:633–638.

(40) Wilson W, Taubert KA, Gewitz M, et al. Prevention of Infective Endocarditis: Guidelines from the American Heart Association: A Guideline from the American Heart Association Rheumatic Fever, Endocarditis, and Kawasaki Disease Committee, Council on Cardiovascular Disease in the Young, and the Council on Clinical Cardiology, Council on Cardiovascular Surgery and Anesthesia, and the Quality of Care and Outcomes Research Interdisciplinary Working Group. *Circulation.* 2007; 116:1736–1754.

(41) Krahn AD, Klein GJ, Yee R, et al. Randomized assessment of syncope trial: conventional diagnostic testing versus a prolonged monitoring strategy. *Circulation.* 2001;104:46–51.

(42) Middlekauff HR, Stevenson WG, Stevenson LG, et al. Syncope in advanced heart failure: high risk of sudden death regardless of origin of syncope. *J Am Coll Cardiol.* 1993;21:110–116.

(43) Knight BP, Goral R, Pelosi F, et al. Outcome of patients with nonischemic dilated cardiomyopathy and unexplained syncope treated with an implantable defibrillator. *J Am Coll Cardiol.* 1999;33:1964–1970.

(44) Sanchez JM, Katsiyiannis WT, Gage BF, et al. Implantable Cardioverter-defibrillator therapy improves long-term survival in patients with unexplained syncope, cardiomyopathy, and a negative electrophysiologic study. *Heart Rhythm.* 2005;2:367–373.

(45) Smith TW, Cain ME. Sudden cardiac death: Epidemiologic and financial worldwide perspective. *J Interv Card Electrophys.* 2006;17:199–203.

(46) The ASTRAL Investigators. Revascularization versus medical therapy for renal-artery stenosis. *N Engl J Med.* 2009; 361(20):1953–1962.

(47) Peripheral Arterial Disease (Lower Extremity, Renal, Mesenteric, and Abdominal Aortic): Guidelines for the Management of Patients With. *J Am Coll Cardiol.* 2006;47:1239–1312.

(48) von Kodolitsch Y, Schwartz AG, Nienaber CA. Clinical prediction of acute aortic dissection. *Arch Intern Med.* 2000;160(19):2977.

(49) Mehta RH, Suzuki T, Hagan PG, Bossone E, Gilon D, Llovet A, Maroto LC, Cooper JV, Smith DE, Armstrong WF, Nienaber CA, Eagle KA, IRAD Investigators. Predicting death in patients with acute type a aortic dissection. *Circulation.* 2002;105:200–206.

(50) Thoracic Aortic Disease: Guidelines for the Diagnosis and Management of Patients With. *J Am Coll Cardiol.* 2010;55:e27–130.

(51) Reed WW, Hallett JW, Jr., Damiano MA, Ballard DJ. Learning from the last ultrasound. A population-based study of patients with abdominal aortic aneurysm. *Arch Int Med.* 1997;157:2064–2068.

(52) Greenhalgh RM, Brown LC, Powell JT, Thompson SG, Epstein D. Endovascular repair of aortic aneurysm in patients physically ineligible for open repair. *NEJM.* 2010;362(20):1872–1880.

(53) Greenhalgh RM, Brown LC, Powell JT, Thompson SG, Epstein D, Sculpher MJ. Endovascular versus open repair of abdominal aortic aneurysm. *NEJM.* 2010;362(20):1863–1871.

(54) Hankey GJ, Warlow CP, Sellar RJ. Cerebral angiographic risk in mild cerebrovascular disease. *Stroke; a journal of cerebral circulation.* 1990;21:209–222.

(55) Mayberg MR, Wilson SE, Yatsu F, et al. Carotid endarterectomy and prevention of cerebral ischemia in symptomatic carotid stenosis. *JAMA.* 1991;266:3289–3294.

(56) Brott TG, Hobson RW, 2nd, Howard G, Roubin GS, Clark WM, Brooks W, Mackey A, Hill MD, Leimgruber PP, Sheffet AJ, Howard VJ, Moore WS, Voeks JH, Hopkins LN, Cutlip DE, Cohen DJ, Popma JJ, Ferguson RD, Cohen SN, Blackshear JL, Silver FL, Mohr JP, Lal BK, Meschia JF. Stenting versus endarterectomy for treatment of carotid-artery stenosis. *N Engl J Med.* 2010;363:11–23.

(57) Nocturnal Oxygen Therapy Trial Group. Continuous or nocturnal oxygen therapy in hypoxemic chronic obstructive lung disease: a clinical trial. *Ann Intern Med.* 1980;93(3):391–398.

(58) Long term domiciliary oxygen therapy in chronic hypoxic cor pulmonale complicating chronic bronchitis and emphysema. *Lancet.* 1981;317(8222):681–686.

(59) Corsico AG, D'Armini AM, Cerveri I, et al. Long-term Outcome after Pulmonary Endarterectomy. *Am J Respir Crit Care Med*. 2008;178(4):419–424.

(60) Coronary Revascularization: Appropriate Use Criteria for. *J Am Coll Cardiol*. 2009;53:530–553.

(61) Serruys PW, Morice M-C, Kappetein AP, Colombo A, Holmes DR, Mack MJ, Stahle E, Feldman TE, van den Brand M, Bass EJ, Van Dyck N, Leadley K, Dawkins KD, Mohr FW, the SI. Percutaneous coronary intervention versus coronary-artery bypass grafting for severe coronary artery disease. *N Engl J Med*. 2009;360:961–972.

(62) Epstein AE, DiMarco JP, Ellenbogen KA, et al. ACC/AHA/HRS 2008 guidelines for device-based therapy of cardiac rhythm abnormalities: a report of the American College of Cardiology/American Heart Association Task Force on Practice Guidelines (Writing Committee to Revise the ACC/AHA/NASPE 2002 Guideline Update for Implantation of Cardiac Pacemakers and Antiarrhythmia Devices). *J Am Coll Cardiol*. 2008;51:e1–62.

(63) Baldasseroni S, Opasich C, Gorini M, et al. Left bundle-branch block is associated with increased 1-year sudden and total mortality rate in 5517 outpatients with congestive heart failure: A report from the Italian Network on Congestive Heart Failure. *Am Heart J*. 2002;143:398–405.

(64) Breithardt OA. Sinha AM, Schwammenthal E, et al. Acute effects of cardiac resynchronization therapy on function mitral regurgitation in advanced heart failure. *J Am Coll Cardiol*. 2003;41:765–770.

(65) St. John Sutton MG, Plappert T, Abraham WT, et al. Effect of cardiac resynchronization therapy on left ventricular size and function in the chronic heart failure. *Circulation*. 2003;107:1985–1990.

(66) Cazeau S, Leclercq C, Lavergne T, et al. Effects of multisite biventricular pacing in patients with heart failure and intraventricular conduction delay. *New Engl J Med*. 2001;344:873–880.

(67) Auricchio A, Stellbrink C, Sack S, et al. Long-term clinical effect of hemodynamically optimized cardiac resynchronization therapy in patients with heart failure and ventricular conduction delay. *J Am Coll Cardiol*. 2002;39:2026–2033.

(68) Abraham WR, Fisher WG, Smith AL, et al. Cardiac resynchronization in chronic heart failure. *New Engl J Med*. 2002;346:1845–1853.

(69) Young, JB, Abraham WT, Smith AL, et al. Combined cardiac resynchronization and implantable cardioversion defibrillation in advanced chronic heart failure: The Miracle ICD Trial. *JAMA*. 2003; 289: 2685–2694.

(70) Bristow MR, Saxon LA, Boehmer J, et al. Cardiac resynchronization therapy with or without an implantable defibrillator in advanced chronic heart failure. *New Engl J Med*. 2004;2140–2150.

(71) Cleland, JGF, Daubert J-C, Erdmann E, et al. The effect of cardiac resynchronization on morbidity and mortality in heart failure. *New Engl J Med*. 2005;352:1539–1549.

(72) Bradley DJ, Bradley EA, Baughman KL, et al. Cardiac Resynchronization and Death from Progressive Heart Failure: A Meta-analysis of Randomized Controlled Trials. *JAMA.* 2003; 289:730-740.

(73) Moss AJ, Hall WJ, Cannom DS, et al. Cardiac-resynchronization for the prevention of heart-failure events. *New Engl J Med.* 2009; 361:1329–1338.

(74) Tang ASL, Wells GA, Talajic M, et al. Cardiac resynchronization therapy for mild-to-moderate heart failure. *New Engl J Med.* 2010;363:2385–2395.

(75) Burri H, Sunthorn H, Shah D, et al. Optimization of device programming for cardiac resynchronization therapy. *PACE.* 2006;29:1416–1425.

(76) Ellenbogen KA, Gold MR, Meyer TE, et al. Primary results from the SmartDelay determined AV optimization: a comparison to other AV delay methods used in cardiac resynchronization therapy (SMART-AV) trial: a randomized trial comparing empirical, echocardiographically-guided, and algorithmic atrioventricular delay programming in cardiac resynchronization therapy. *Circulation.* 2010;122:2660–2668.

(77) Epstein AE, DiMarco JP, Ellenbogen KA, et al. ACC/AHA/HRS 2008 guidelines for device-based therapy of cardiac rhythm abnormalities: a report of the American College of Cardiology/American Heart Association Task Force on Practice Guidelines (writing committee to revise the ACC/AHA/NASPE 2002 Guideline Update for Implantation of Cardiac Pacemakers and Antiarrhythmia Devices). *J Am Coll Cardiol.* 2008;51:e1–e62.

(78) United States Food and Drug Administration. FDA News Release: FDA Approves Devices for Heart Failure Patients. http://www.fda.gov/NewsEvents/Newsroom/PressAnnouncements/ucm226123.htm. Accessed August 21, 2011.

(79) Chung ES, Leon AR, Tavazzi L, et al. Results of the predictors of response to CR (PROSPECT) trial. *Circulation.* 2008;117:2608–2616.

(80) Beshai JF, Grimm RA, Nagueh, SF, et al. *New Engl J Med.* 2007; 357:2461–2471.

(81) The Antiarrhythmics Versus Implantable Defibrillators Investigators. A comparison of antiarrhythmic-drug therapy with implantable defibrillators in patient resuscitated from near-fatal ventricular arrhythmias. *N Engl J Med.* 1997;337:1576–1583.

(82) Connolly SJ, Gent M, Roberts RS, et al. Canadian implantable defibrillator study (CIDS): a randomized trial of the implantable cardioverter defibrillator against amiodarone. *Circulation.* 2000;101:1297–1302.

(83) Kuck K-H, Cappato R, Siebels J, et al. Randomized comparison of antiarrhythmic drug therapy with implantable defibrillators in patient resuscitated from cardiac arrest. *Circulation.* 2000;201:748–754.

(84) Connolly SJ, Hallstrom AP, Cappato R, et al. Meta-analysis of the implantable cardioverter defibrillator secondary prevention trials. *Eur Heart J.* 2000;21:2071–2078.

(85) Moss AJ, Hall WJ, Cannom DS, et al. Improved survival with an implanted defibrillator in patients with coronary disease at high risk for ventricular arrhythmia. *N Engl J Med.* 1996;335:1933–1940.

(86) Buxton AE, Lee KL, Fisher JD, et al. A randomized study of the prevention of sudden death in patients with coronary artery disease. *N Engl J Med.* 1999;341:1882–1890.

(87) Moss AJ, Zareba W, Hall WJ, et al. Prophylactic implantation of a defibrillator in pateints with myocardia infarction and reduced ejection fraction. *N Engl J Med.* 2002;346:877–883.

(88) Bansch D, Antz M, Baczor S, et al. Primary prevention of sudden cardiac death in idiopathic dilated cardiomyopathy: the cardiomyopathy trial (CAT). *Circulation.* 2002; 105:1453–1458.

(89) Strickberger SA, Hummel JD, Bartlett TG, et al. Amiodarone versus implantable cardioverter defibrillator: randomized trial in patients with nonischemic cardiomyopathy and asymptomatic nonsustained ventricular tachycardia—AMIOVERT. *J Am Coll Cardiol.* 2003; 41:1707–1712.

(90) Bristow MR, Saxon LA, Boehmer J, et al. Cardiac resynchronization therapy with or without an implantable defibrillator in advanced chronic heart failure. *N Engl J Med.* 2004;350:2140–2150.

(91) Kadish A, Dyer A, Daubert JP, et al. Prophylactic defibrillator implantation in patients with nonischemic dilated cardiomyopathy. *N Engl J Med.* 2004;350:2151–2158.

(92) Bardy GH, Lee KL, Mark DB, et al. Amiodarone or implantable cardioverter defibrillator for congestive heart failure. *N Engl J Med.* 2005; 352:225–237.

(93) Bigger JT. Prophylactic use of implanted defibrillators in patients at high risk for ventricular arrhythmias after coronary-artery bypass graft surgery. *N Engl J Med.* 1997;337:1569–1575.

(94) Hohnloser SH, Kuck K-H, Dorian P, et al. Prophylactic use of an implantable cardioverter-defibrillator after acute myocardial infarction. *N Engl J Med.* 2004; 351:2481–2488.

(95) Nanthkumar K, Epstein AE, Kay GN, et al. Prophylactic implantable carderverter-defibrillator therapy in patients with left ventricular systolic dysfunction. *J Am Coll Cardiol.* 2004;44:2166–2172.

(96) Epstein AE, DiMarco JP, Ellenbogen KA, et al. ACC/AHA/HRS 2008 guidelines for device-based therapy of cardiac rhythm abnormalities: a report of the American College of Cardiology/American Heart Association Task Force on Practice Guidelines (Writing Committee to Revise the ACC/AHA/NASPE 2002 Guideline Update for Implantation of Cardiac Pacemakers and Antiarrhythmia Devices). *J Am Coll Cardiol.* 2008;51:e1–e62.

(97) Centers for Medicare and Medicaid Services National Coverage Decision 20.4 Implantable Automatic Defibrillators. http://www.cms.gov/medicare-coverage-database/details/ncd-details.aspx?NCDId=110&ver=3. Accessed August 22, 2011.

(98) Gage BF, Waterman AD, Shannon W, et al. Validation of clinic classification schemes for predicting stroke: results from the National Registry of Atrial Fibrillation. *JAMA.* 2001;285:2864–2870.

(99) Lip GYH, Nieuwlaat R, Pisters R, et al. Refining clinical risk stratification for predicting stroke and thromboembolism in atrial fibrillation using a novel risk factor-based approach: the Euro Heart Survey on Atrial Fibrillation. *Chest.* 2010;137:273–272.

(100) Connolly SJ, Ezekowitz MD, Yusuf S, et al. Dabigatran versus warfarin in patients with atrial fibrillaiton. *New Engl J Med.* 2009;361:1139–1151.

(101) The Atrial Fibrillation Follow-up Investigation of Rhythm Management (AFFIRM) Investigators. A comparison of rate control and rhythm control in patients with atrial fibrillation. *New Engl J Med.* 2002;347:1825–1833.

(102) Van Gelder IC, Hagens VE, Bosker HA, et al. A comparison of rate control and rhythm control in patients with recurrent persistent atrial fibrillation. *New Engl J Med.* 2002;347:1834–1840.

(103) U.S. Preventive Services Task Force. *Screening for Peripheral Arterial Disease: Recommendation Statement.* AHRQ Publication No. 05-0583-A-EF, August 2005. Agency for Healthcare Research and Quality, Rockville, MD. http://www.uspreventiveservicestaskforce.org/uspstf05/pad/padrs.htm

■ FURTHER READING

(1) 2007 Chronic Angina Focused Update of the ACC/AHA 2002 Guidelines for the Management of Patients With Chronic Stable Angina. *J Am Coll Cardiol.* 2007; 50:2264–2274.

(2) 2010 ACCF/AHA Guideline for Assessment of Cardiovascular Risk in Asymptomatic Adults: Executive Summary. *J Am Coll Cardiol.* 2010; 56:2182–2199.

(3) ASA/ACCF/AHA/AANN/AANS/ACR/ASNR/CNS/SAIP/SCAI/SIR/SNIS/SVM/SVS Guideline on the Management of Patients With Extracranial Carotid and Vertebral Artery Disease. *J Am Coll Cardiol.* 2011; 57:16–94.

(4) Baumgartner H, Hung J, Bermejo J, et al. Echocardiographic Assessment of Valve Stenosis: EAE/ASE Recommendations for Clinical Practice. *J Am Soc Echo.* 2009; 22(1): 1–23.

(5) Bonow RO, Carabello BA, Chatterjee K, et al. ACC/AHA 2006 guidelines for the management of patients with valvular heart disease. *J Am Coll Cardiol.* 2006; 48(3): e1–e148.

(6) Brickner EM, Hillis LD, Lange RA. Congenital Heart Disease in Adults: First of Two Part. *N Engl J Med.* 2000; 256–263.

(7) Brickner EM, Hillis LD, Lange RA. Congenital Heart Disease in Adults: Second of Two Parts. *N Engl J Med.* 2000; 342: 334–342.

(8) Delacretaz E. Clinical Practice: Supraventricular Tachycardia. *N Engl J Med.* 2006; 354:1039–1051.

(9) Ellenbogen KA, Wilkoff BL, Kay GN, Lau CP. *Clinical Cardiac Pacing, Defibrillation, and Resynchronization Therapy, 4th Edition.* Philadelphia: Saunders. 2011.

(10) Ellenbogen KA, Wood M. *Cardiac Pacing and ICDs, 5th Edition.* Oxford: Blackwell Publishing. 2008.

(11) Epstein AE, DiMarco JP, Ellenbogen KA, Estes NAM III, Freedman RA, Gettes LS, Gillinov AM, Gregoratos G, Hammill SC, Hayes DL, Hlatky MA, Newby LK, Page RL, Schoenfeld MH, Silka MJ, Stevenson LW, Sweeney MO. ACC/AHA/HRS 2008 guidelines for device-based therapy of cardiac rhythm abnormalities: a report of the American College of Cardiology/American Heart Association Task Force on Practice Guidelines (Writing Committee to Revise the ACC/AHA/NASPE 2002 Guideline Update for Implantation of Cardiac Pacemakers and Antiarrhythmia Devices). *Journal of the American College of Cardiology* 2008;51:e1–e62.

(12) Fogoros, RN. *Electrophysiologic Testing, 4th ed.* Oxford: Blackwell Publishing. 2006. pp. 304.

(13) Fuster V, Walsh RA, Harrington RA (eds.). *Hurst's The Heart, 13th ed.* New York: McGraw-Hill. 2011. pp. 2500.

(14) Gaca AM, Jaggers JJ, Dudley LT, Bisset GS III. Repair of Congenital Heart Disease: A Primer—Part 1. *Radiology.* 2008; 247: pp. 617–631.

(15) Gaca AM, Jaggers JJ, Dudley LT, Bisset GS III. Repair of Congenital Heart Disease: A Primer—Part 2. *Radiology.* 2008; 248:44–60.

(16) Huikuri HV, Castellanos A, Myerburg RJ. Sudden Death Due to Cardiac Arrhythmias. *N Engl J Med.* 2001; 345: 1473–1482.

(17) Jarcho JA. Biventricular Pacing. *N Engl J Med.* 2006; 355:288–294.

(18) Josephson ME. Atrioventricular Conduction, in *Clinical Cardiac Electrophysiology: Techniques and Interpretations, 4th ed.* Philadelphia: Lippincott, Williams, & Wilkins 2008. pp. 93–113.

(19) Josephson ME. Clinical Cardiac Electrophysiology, 4th ed. Philadelphia: Lippincott Williams & Wilkins. 2008. pp. 922.

(20) Josephson ME. Sinus Node Function, in *Clinical Cardiac Electrophysiology: Techniques and Interpretations, 4th ed.* Philadelphia: Lippincott, Williams, & Wilkins 2008. pp. 69–92.

(21) Khairy P, Poirer N, Mercier LA. Univentricular Heart. *Circuation.* 2007; 115: 800–812.

(22) McLaughlin VV, Archer SL, Badesch DB, Barst RJ, Farber HW, Lindner JR, Mathier MA, McGoon MD, Park MH, Rosenson RS, Rubin LJ, Tapson VF, Varga J. Accf/aha 2009 expert consensus document on pulmonary hypertension. *Circulation.* 2009;119:2250–2294.

(23) Murdoch DR, Corey GR, Hoen B, et al. Clinical Presentation, Etiology, and Outcome of Infective Endocarditis in the 21st Century: The International Collaboration on Endocarditis-Prostective Cohort Study. *Archives of Internal Medicine.* 2009; 169: 463–473.

(24) O'Keefe, JH, Hammill SC, Freed MS, Pogwizd SM. *The ECG Criteria Book, 2nd ed.* Sudbury, MA: Jones and Bartlett Publishers.

(25) Otto, CM, Bonow RO. Valvular Heart Disease. In: Libby P, Bonow RO, Mann DL, et al, eds. *Braunwald's Heart Disease: A Textbook of Cardiovascular Medicine, 8th ed.* Philadelphia: Elsevier Saunders; 2008:1625–1712.

(26) Priori SG, Zipes, DP (eds). Sudden Cardiac Death: A handbook for clinical practice.Oxford: Blackwell Publishing. 2006. p. 292.

(27) Reynolds MR, Thosani AJ, Pinto DS, Josephson ME. Chapter 49: Sudden Cardiac Death. In Hurst's *The Heart, 13th ed.* Fuster V, Walsh RA, Harrington RA. (eds). New York: McGraw Hill. 2011.

(28) Rhodes JF, Hijazi ZM, Sommer RJ. Pathophysiology of Congenital Heart Disease in the Adult: Part 2: Simple Obstructive Lesions. *Circulation.* 2008; 117:1228–1237.

(29) Saxon LA, Ellenbogen KA. Resynchronization Therapy for the Treatment of Heart Failure. *Circulation.* 2003; 108:1044–1048.

(30) Smith, TW. *Tarascon Electrocardiologica.* Sudbury, MA: Jones and Bartlett Publishers. In press.

(31) Sommer RJ, Hijazi ZM, Rhodes JF. Pathophysiology of Congenital Heart Disease in the Adult: Part 1: Shunt Lesions. *Circulation.* 2008; 117: 1090–1099.

(32) Sommer RJ, Hijazi ZM, Rhodes JF. Pathophysiology of Congenital Heart Disease in the Adult: Part III: Complex Congenital Heart Disease. *Circulation.* 2008; 117:1340–1350.

(33) Surawicz B, Knilans TK. Ambulatory Electrocardiography, in Surawicz B, Knilans TK:: *Chou's Electrocardiography in Clinical Practice, 6th ed.* Philadelphia: Saunders, 2008. pp. 631–645.

(34) Surawicz B, Knilans TK. *Chou's Electrocardiography in Clinical Practice, 6th ed.* Philadelphia: Saunders Elsevier. 2008. pp. 752.

(35) The Seventh Report of the Joint National Committee on Prevention, Detection, Evaluation, and Treatment of High Blood Pressure (JNC 7). *Hypertension.* 2003;42:1206.

(36) TP III Update 2004: Implications of Recent Clinical Trials for the ATP III Guidelines. *JAMA.* 2001;285:2486–2497.

(37) Wagner, G. *Marriott's Practical Electrocardiography.* Philadelphia: Lippincott, Williams and Wilkins. 2008. pp. 488.

(38) Wagner, G. Atrioventricular Block in *Marriott's Practical Electrocardiography, 11th ed.* Wagner G. (ed.) Philadlphia: Lippincott, Williams & Wilkins. pp.401–422.

(39) Wilber DJ, Packer DL, Stevenson (eds.) *Catheter Ablation of Cardiac Arrhythmias: Basic Concepts and Clinical Applications, 3rd ed.* Oxford: Blackwell Futura. 2008. pp. 392.

(40) Zimetbaum PJ, Josephson ME. (eds). *Practical Clinical Electrophysiology.* Philadelphia: Lippincott Williams & Wilkins. 2009. pp. 304.

(41) Zoghbi WA, Enriquez-Sarano M, Foster E, et al. Recommendations for Evaluation of the Severity of Native Valvular Regurgitation with Two-dimensional and Doppler Echocardiography. *J Am Soc Echo.* 2003; 16(7): 777–802.

SECTION IV

SUPPLEMENT: BEDSIDE PROCEDURES

33 ■ THE SELDINGER TECHNIQUE FOR VASCULAR ACCESS

Sven-Ivar Seldinger introduced his method of venous access in 1953. Access is obtained to the lumen of the vein or artery with a hollow needle and secured with a soft-tipped guidewire. A flexible catheter can then be passed into the vessel over the guidewire, using it for support.

- The technique described here is essential to much of invasive cardiology and critical care. It is used for subclavian, internal jugular, and femoral vein access. All cardiologists and internists should feel comfortable wielding a needle and guidewire for this procedure. Use sterile technique and sterile gloves.
- Explore the surface landmarks in detail before scrubbing and draping.
- Infiltrate the skin with lidocaine, keeping in mind that most pain sensors are at the skin surface.
- Vascular ultrasound guidance is utilized by some to localize the vessel and other important structures (e.g., carotid or femoral artery) during cannulation.
- Carefully advance the needle into the vessel, with constant withdrawing force on the syringe plunger (**Figure 33-1A**).
  - Practice doing this with one hand so that the other hand can be used to explore landmarks and retract the skin to ease the needle puncture.

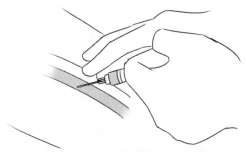

FIGURE 33-1A. Cannulating left formal vein.

The fingers are palpating the artery and the introducer needle is advanced at a 45° angle to the skin until a flash of purple blood is obtained.
- When the needle tip is in the vein, blood will flash into the syringe.
  - It is preferable to puncture the vein only once, but if the venous pressure is low, the distensible vein may collapse, and the needle will pass through both walls of the vein. If the deepest comfortable forward progress has been made with no blood return, continue the negative pressure on the syringe and slowly withdraw the needle until blood flashes into the syringe.
- STOP movement when blood flashes into the syringe.
- HOLD the needle still while continuing to withdraw with the syringe to ensure continued blood return.
- DO NOT move the needle while removing the syringe from the needle.
- Advance the guidewire into the vessel (**Figure 33-1B**).
  - If it does not move smoothly, you must remove it, reattach the syringe and re-obtain access.

Once the vein is cannulated, the syringe is disconnected from the introducer needle to confirm the return of purple, nonpulsatile blood and then a flexible wire is advanced through the needle with the J tip directed toward the heart.
- Remove the needle, keeping the guidewire in place.
- *DO NOT let the guidewire advance fully into the vessel and embolize.*

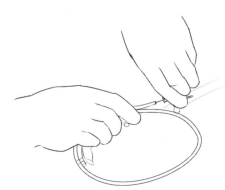

FIGURE 33-1B. Threading the wire through the introducer needle.

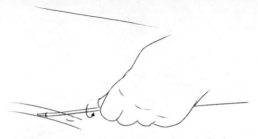

FIGURE 33-1C. Dilating the skin and subcutaneous tissue over the wire.

- Place your access catheter (or introducer sheath) over the wire (**Figure 33-1C**).
  - If necessary, use a dilator to prepare for introduction of the catheter.
    - If your catheter has an internal dilator to be removed after insertion, you're using a *Modified Seldinger* technique.

A dilator is advanced over the wire with a twisting motion to dilate a tract through the skin, soft tissue, and vein. The dilator is then withdrawn over the wire, leaving the wire in place.

- Receive and hold the wire from the back end of the catheter *before* advancing the catheter into the body (**Figure 33-1D**).
- Remove the wire (and dilator).
- Evacuate air from the catheter, flush the catheter, and secure it appropriately.
- In many cases, an immediate x-ray is desirable to document placement and check for complications (e.g., pneumothorax, if subclavian or internal jugular vein approach).

A triple-lumen catheter is inserted over wire and advanced to a predesignated depth of insertion. The wire is then withdrawn through the distal port of the catheter. Each catheter port will then be flushed with sterile saline.

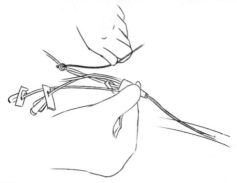

FIGURE 33-1D. A central venous catheter is introduced over wire.

TIPS

- Arterial puncture is frequently done without a syringe, and the blood flash will be pulsatile.
  - Take care not to splash yourself, particularly your eyes.
- Align the numbers (or something) marked on the syringe with the bevel on the needle so you can keep track of where the bevel is when it is buried in the patient.
- Some prefer to have lidocaine (or saline) in the syringe.
  - Others find that a fluid makes the blood flash appear redder than it is, raising the possibility of arterial cannulation when the vein is targeted. Therefore, a syringe with saline that is emptied by flushing it through the needle is preferred.
- Some advocate the use of a smaller "finder" needle (e.g., 21 gauge) to find the vein. That needle is then left in place while the operator attempts to track the larger access needle over the smaller needle.
  - Others find this very awkward and cumbersome, trying to keep the finder needle and syringe in place while advancing a large needle.
    - The presence of the finder needle also obscures the surface landmarks.
    - The finder needle is also very unlikely to stay still while operator is manipulating the access needle; damage may be done to the vessel or other structures.

- If the vessel is entered during local anesthetization, the location of the vessel is now known and access should be relatively easy, even without the "finder" technique. (Avoid injecting lidocaine into a vein.)
- Avoid lateral movement of the needle when it is deep in the tissue.
  - The bevel is sharp, and moving it laterally turns it into a scalpel being moved blindly.
  - All motion (except when the needle is at the surface) should be advancing or withdrawing.
- Avoid air embolism. Anytime a vein is accessed, there is a risk of air entry through an open canal (particularly for subclavian and internal jugular access, if the patient takes a deep breath).
  - Close the access as soon as possible.
  - For the higher pressure arteries, air embolism is much less likely because there should be pulsatile blood flow.
- Avoid withdrawing the wire when using the needle; it is possible to shear off and embolize a portion of the wire. If the wire must be withdrawn, do so very carefully or remove the entire needle wire assembly and start again.
- Removing a central venous line is not a trivial procedure. Avoid air embolism.
  - For subclavian and internal jugular lines, prevent air from entering the vein
    - The patient should be supine.
    - Prevent a sudden inspiration as the line is removed.
      - Having the patient hum while sliding line out is a tried and true method.
    - Cover the site immediately.

34 ■ CENTRAL VENOUS CATHETERIZATION[1-11]

INDICATIONS FOR CENTRAL VENOUS CATHETERS

- Central venous pressure (CVP) monitoring
- Central parenteral nutrition infusion
- No peripheral access
- Temporary hemodialysis access
- Plasmapheresis
- Infusion of vasopressor medications
- Infusion of potentially caustic solutions: various chemotherapy meds or hypertonic saline
- Introducer access for a pulmonary artery catheter or transvenous pacemaker
- Emergency venous access during a cardiac arrest

CONTRAINDICATIONS OF CENTRAL VENOUS CATHETER PLACEMENT

- Patient refuses or is too combative
- Venous thrombosis of target vein
- Superior vena cava syndrome (for subclavian or internal jugular vein catheterization)
- Inferior vena cava filter (relative contraindication for femoral vein catheterization)
- Soft tissue infection, burns or abrasions involving the entry site for central line
- Trauma to the site
- Uncorrected bleeding diathesis AND noncompressible vessel (subclavian vessels)
  - PTT > 1.5 × upper limit of normal
  - INR > 1.5 in patient on warfarin
  - Platelets < 50K
  - Uremia
  - Caution with chronic antiplatelet therapy

EQUIPMENT

- Sterile gown and gloves
- Mask with face shield
- Surgeon's cap
- Sterile prep: chlorhexidine or povidone-iodine swabs
- Sterile drape

- 5-ml syringe × 2
- 25-gauge and 22-gauge needles
- Sterile syringes filled with sterile saline
- 1% lidocaine for local anesthesia
- J-tipped flexible guidewire
- No. 11 scalpel
- Dilator
- Central venous catheter
- Silk or nylon suture
- Sterile occlusive dressing

GENERAL TECHNIQUE FOR CENTRAL LINE PLACEMENT IN ALL LOCATIONS

- Informed consent.
- Perform a "time out" to confirm the correct patient, side, and procedure.
- Wash hands and then don a surgeon's cap and mask, and a sterile gown and gloves.
- Wide sterile prep of the procedure area with either chlorhexidine or povidone-iodine.
  - Chlorhexidine is preferred to povidone-iodine.
- Wide sterile drape of the procedure area.
- Flush all catheter ports with sterile saline.
- 15–20° Trendelenberg position for internal jugular or subclavian vein catheterizations.
- Modified Seldinger technique utilized for placement of central venous catheter:
  - Anesthetize skin and underlying soft tissue.
  - Advance introducer needle connected to syringe under constant negative pressure until a flash of blood is seen (Figure 33-1A).
  - Disconnect syringe from needle and assure non-pulsatile, purple venous blood return.
  - Introduce guidewire through the needle with J tip directed toward the heart to a depth of 20 cm (Figure 33-1B).
  - Withdraw needle, leaving wire in place.
  - Use scalpel to nick the skin over the wire (**Figure 34-1**).
  - Place dilator over the wire and advance dilator through the skin and into the vein with a rotating motion (Figure 33-1C).
  - Withdraw the dilator, leaving the wire in place.
  - Introduce the central venous catheter over the wire (Figure 33-1D).
  - Withdraw the wire into the catheter and grasp the wire tip beyond the most distal catheter port.
  - Advance the catheter over wire to the appropriate depth of insertion:
    - Right subclavian vein: 13–16 cm
    - Left subclavian vein: 14–17 cm
    - Right internal jugular vein: 12–14 cm
    - Left internal jugular vein: 13–16 cm

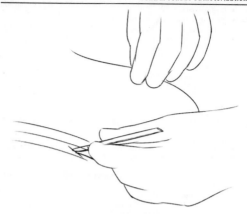

FIGURE 34-1. Nicking skin with scalpel over the wire.

A scalpel is used to nick the skin over the wire after the needle is withdrawn from the wire. Always maintain control of guidewire.
- Withdraw the wire and cap the distal port.
- Flush all catheter ports again with sterile saline.
- Secure catheter in place with suture (**Figure 34-2**).
- Apply a clear, sterile dressing over catheter insertion site.

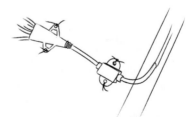

FIGURE 34-2. Securing the central venous catheter in place.

A central venous catheter is secured in place in four locations with suture. A sterile, transparent occlusive dressing is then placed over the catheter at the insertion site.

- Check a chest x-ray after placement of a subclavian or internal jugular vein catheter to confirm appropriate catheter tip location and to check for a pneumothorax.
- Ultrasound guidance of internal jugular or femoral vein catheterization by experienced operators reduces the incidence of mechanical complications (relative risk 0.32), insertion attempts, and procedure time.

INTERNAL JUGULAR VEIN CATHETERS

- Central Approach
  - Landmarks (**Figure 34-3**)
    - Sternal and clavicular heads of sternocleidomastoid muscle form a triangle with the clavicle as the base of the triangle
    - Ipsilateral nipple (or midclavicular line in women)
  - Positioning
    - Turn head 30° to contralateral side
  - Entry site and needle direction
    - Insert just below the apex of the triangle, 1 cm lateral to the carotid pulse.
    - Aim needle toward the ipsilateral nipple 30–45° to the skin.
    - Vein should be entered within 3 cm.

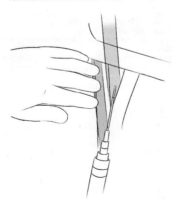

FIGURE 34-3. Central approach to internal jugular vein catheterization.

The fingers are overlying the carotid pulse. The anterior cervical triangle is bordered by the sternal and clavicular heads of the sternocleidomastoid muscle and inferiorly by the clavicle. The insertion site is 1 cm inferior to the apex of the triangle and just lateral to the carotid pulse. The needle is inserted at a 30–40° angle to the skin and aiming toward the ipsilateral nipple.

- Posterior Approach
  - Landmarks
    - Posterolateral border of the clavicular head of the sternocleidomastoid muscle
    - Sternal notch
  - Positioning
    - Turn head 30° to contralateral side.
  - Entry site and needle direction
    - Entry site is just above where the external jugular vein crosses the posterolateral edge of the sternocleidomastoid muscle (about 5 cm above the clavicle).
    - Aim towards the sternal notch 15° anterior to horizontal.
    - Vein should be entered within 5 cm.

SUBCLAVIAN VEIN CATHETERS

- Infraclavicular Approach
  - Landmarks (**Figure 34-4**)
    - Curve of the clavicle (or intersection of clavicle and first rib)
    - Sternal notch
  - Positioning
    - Turn head 30° to contralateral side.
  - Entry site and needle direction
    - Entry site is 1 cm lateral and 0.5 cm inferior to the curve of clavicle.
    - Aim 1 finger-width above the sternal notch with needle as parallel to the bed as possible; may use thumb of non-syringe hand to help push needle under clavicle.
    - Vein should be entered within 5 cm.

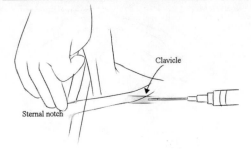

FIGURE 34-4. Infraclavicular approach to subclavian vein catheterization.

- Supraclavicular Approach
  - Landmarks
    - Lateral boarder of the sternocleidomastoid muscle
    - Sternal notch and ipsilateral sternoclavicular joint
  - Positioning
    - Turn head 30° to contralateral side.
  - Entry site and needle direction
    - Entry site is 1 cm lateral and 1 cm cephalad from the point at which the clavicular head of the sternocleidomastoid muscle inserts onto the clavicle.
    - Aim needle toward sternal notch at an angle 10–15° anterior to the horizontal plane.
    - Vein should be entered within 2–3 cm.

Insertion site for infraclavicular subclavian line placement is 1 cm lateral and 0.5 cm inferior to the curve of the clavicle. The introducer needle is kept as parallel to the ground as possible and is directed toward the tip of the finger that is located in the sternal notch.

FEMORAL VEIN CATHETERS

- Landmarks (**Figure 34-5**)
  - Medial to femoral artery pulsation about 2 cm below inguinal ligament
  - Vein located 2/3 distance from anterior superior iliac spine to the pubic tubercle
- Positioning
  - Supine position with leg slightly abducted and toes pointing toward ceiling

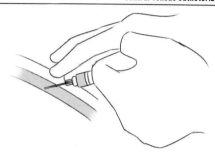

FIGURE 34-5. Femoral vein catheterization.

- Entry site and needle direction
  - Entry site is 1 cm medial to femoral artery pulsation.
  - Aim parallel to femoral pulse (toward umbilicus if no pulse); 30–45° angle to skin.
  - Vein should be entered within 5 cm.
  - If no pulse is palpable (e.g., cardiac arrest), the vein is approximately 2/3 the distance from the anterior superior iliac crest to the ipsilateral pubic tubercle; the pulse palpable with CPR is felt at the femoral vein, so aim for the palpated pulse.

The fingers are palpating the left femoral pulse and the introducer needle is advanced 1 cm medial to the femoral pulse at a 45° angle aiming toward the umbilicus.

COMPLICATIONS

TABLE 34-1. Complications of Central Venous Catheter Placement

Complication	Subclavian vein	Internal jugular vein	Femoral vein
Catheter-related blood stream infection (per 1000 line days)	4	8.6	15.3
Pneumothorax	1.5–3.1%	0.1–0.2%	N/A
Hemothorax	0.4–0.6%	< 0.1%	N/A
Catheter malposition	1.8–9.3% (7%)	1.8–14% (5%)	N/A
Line-related vein thrombosis (per 1000 catheter days)	0–13 (8)	1.2–3	8–34 (21)

TABLE 34-1. Complications of Central Venous Catheter Placement (continued)

Complication	Subclavian vein	Internal jugular vein	Femoral vein
Arterial puncture	0.5–3.1%	3.0–6.3%	6–9%
Hematoma	1.2–2.1%	0.1–2.2%	3.8–4.4%
Arrhythmia	Atrial dysrhythmias in 28–41%; ventricular ectopy in up to 25%		N/A
Cardiac perforation	Very rare		N/A
Air embolus	Negligible if performed in Trendelenberg position		
Lost guidewire	Negligible if operator maintains control of guidewire		

Data from *NEJM*. 2007; 356: e21, *NEJM*. 2003; 348: 1123–1133, and *Ann Thoracic Med*. 2007; 2: 61–3.

CODING

36556	Introduction of non-tunnelled central venous catheter (> 5 years old)
36555	Introduction of non-tunnelled central venous catheter (< 5 years old)
36800	Dialysis catheter placement
36597	Reposition central venous catheter
76937	Ultrasound guidance for central lines

REFERENCES

(1) *NEJM*. 2007; 356: e21.
(2) *Arch Int Med*. 2004; 164: 842–850.
(3) *Arch Surg*. 2004; 139: 131–136.
(4) *NEJM*. 2003; 348: 1123–1133.
(5) *Crit Care Med*. 2005; 33: 13.
(6) *BMJ*. 2003; 327: 361.
(7) *JAMA*. 2001; 286: 700.
(8) *Acad Emer Med*. 2002; 9: 800.
(9) *Anesth*. 2002; 97: 528.
(10) *Crit Care Med*. 2007; 35S: S178–S185.
(11) *Ann Thoracic Med*. 2007; 2: 61–63.

35 ■ ARTERIAL LINE PLACEMENT[1-4]

INDICATIONS

- Management of shock states
- Continuous blood pressure monitoring
- Continuous cardiac output monitoring
- Frequent arterial blood gas sampling
- Consider if need for very frequent blood draws
  - Severe diabetic ketoacidosis
  - Severe hyponatremia
  - Severe hypernatremia

CONTRAINDICATIONS

- Insufficient collateral circulation from the ulnar artery
  - Assess collateral circulation with a modified Allen test
  - Modified Allen test
    - Compress ulnar and radial arteries with fist clenched
    - Raise clenched fist above patient's head for one minute
    - Lower arm, relax fist, release ulnar artery but continue radial artery compression
    - Normal perfusion should return within six seconds
- Severe Raynaud's syndrome
- Thromboangiitis obliterans (Buerger disease)
- Overlying cellulitis or full-thickness burns to area of insertion
- Major injury to the extremity
- Need for thrombolytic therapy
- Lymphatic obstruction in the extremity proximal to the cannulation site
- Presence of an arteriovenous shunt in the extremity (relative contraindication)
- Bleeding diathesis (relative contraindication)
  - Coagulopathy (INR > 2 or PTT > 2× upper limit of normal)
  - Platelets < 50,000

EQUIPMENT

- 20-gauge radial artery catheter-over-wire kit or 20-gauge angiocatheter
- Pressure transducer tubing
- Pressure transducer
- 4-0 silk or nylon suture
- Armboard

- Tape
- 1% lidocaine for skin anesthesia
- Flexible guidewire (for femoral/brachial arterial lines)
- No. 11 scalpel (for femoral/brachial arterial lines)
- Sterile occlusive dressing

TECHNIQUE FOR RADIAL ARTERIAL LINE

- Informed consent.
- Perform a "time out" procedure to confirm correct patient, site, and procedure.
- Use an armboard with mild wrist extension for radial arterial line placement.
- Wash hands and then don sterile attire.
- Radial artery is palpated ~2 cm proximal the wrist crease (**Figure 35-1**).
- Use lidocaine without epinephrine around artery (minimizes arterial vasospasm).
- Take your time locating the maximal impulse.
  - Your first shot is your best shot.
- Advance needle at a 30–45° angle until arterial flash seen; then lower catheter angle to 10–15° (**Figure 35-2**).
  - Advance wire through needle (radial arterial line kit) (see **Figure 35-3** and **Figure 35-4**) or catheter over needle (angiocatheter).
- Advance catheter over wire if using a radial arterial line kit (**Figure 35-5**).

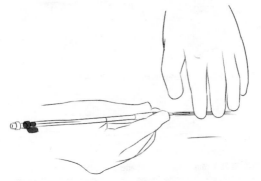

FIGURE 35-1. Radial arterial line catheter insertion.

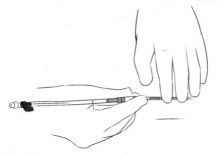

FIGURE 35-2. Arterial flash is seen.

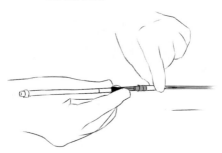

FIGURE 35-3. Wire threaded through arterial catheter needle.

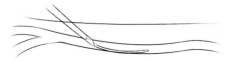

FIGURE 35-4. Wire threaded through arterial catheter and needle.

Adapted from Custalow CB. *Color Atlas of Emergency Department Procedures.* Philadelphia, PA: Saunders; 2004: 131, Figure 4.

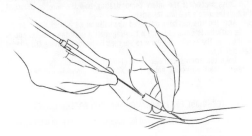

FIGURE 35-5. Advancing a radial catheter over wire.

Adapted from Custalow CB. *Color Atlas of Emergency Department Procedures*. Philadelphia, PA: Saunders; 2004: 132, Figure 5.

- Remove wire and needle, leaving catheter in place.
- Attach pressure transducer tubing to catheter hub and assure that a good arterial waveform is seen on the monitor (**Figure 35-6**).
- Secure catheter in place with suture.
- Place a clear, sterile occlusive dressing over insertion site.

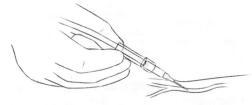

FIGURE 35-6. Connecting arterial catheter to pressure transducer tubing.

The radial artery pulse is palpated with two fingers to determine the optimal catheter insertion site and artery direction. An arterial line catheter is inserted just distal to the felt radial pulse at a 30° angle.

The radial artery catheter is inserted until an arterial flash is seen within the catheter lumen. At this point, stop advancing the catheter and advance the wire through the needle.

Once an arterial flash is seen, the catheter is held steady as the wire is advanced fully through the needle into the artery.

Cross section of the artery demonstrating how the wire is advanced through the needle and into the artery.

After the wire has been advanced, the catheter kit is held steady as the white catheter is advanced with a twisting motion until the catheter hub is at the skin. The needle and the wire are then withdrawn, leaving the arterial catheter in place.

Once the arterial catheter is in place, pressure transducer tubing is screwed onto the catheter hub and an arterial waveform should be seen on the monitor screen.

TECHNIQUE FOR FEMORAL OR BRACHIAL ARTERIAL LINES

- Consider using an ultrasound for brachial artery or femoral arterial line placement.
  - Real-time ultrasound guidance requires a sterile sheath and sterile ultrasound gel.
- Brachial artery typically cannulated about 5 cm above the elbow.
- Femoral artery typically cannulated 2–3 cm below the inguinal crease.
- Modified Seldinger technique utilized to place brachial or femoral arterial lines:
  - Introducer needle is used to cannulate the artery at a 30–45° angle.
  - Syringe is detached from the needle and pulsatile blood is confirmed.
  - Thread guidewire through the needle.
  - Withdraw the needle, leaving the wire in place.
  - Use a scalpel to nick the skin over the wire.
  - Advance the catheter over the wire until the hub is at the skin; then withdraw the wire.
- Attach pressure transducer tubing to catheter hub and assure that a good arterial waveform is seen on the monitor.
- Secure catheters in place with suture.
- Place a clear, sterile occlusive dressing over insertion site.

COMPLICATIONS

- Major Complications
  - Arterial thrombosis (< 1%)
  - Catheter embolization (very rare)
  - Pseudoaneurysm (especially in femoral location, very rare)
  - Arteriovenous fistula (especially in femoral location, very rare)
- Minor Complications
  - Catheter-related bloodstream infection (0.5%)
  - Bleeding (2%)
  - Hematoma
  - Median nerve impairment (especially with prolonged wrist hyperextension)

CODING

36620   Percutaneous arterial line placement
76937   Vascular ultrasound

REFERENCES

(1) *NEJM*. 2006; 354: e13–e14.
(2) Roberts JR, Hedges JR, eds. *Clinical Procedures in Emergency Medicine*. 5th ed. Philadelphia, PA: Saunders; 2009: 349–363.
(3) Chen H, Sonnenday CJ, eds. *Manual of Common Bedside Surgical Procedures*. 2nd ed. Philadelphia, PA: Lippincott Williams & Wilkins; 2000: 69–80.
(4) *Anesthesiology*, 2004; 100: 287–291.

36 ■ RIGHT HEART CATHETERIZATION

The major role of right heart catheterization is the accurate measurement and characterization of intracardiac hemodynamics including filling pressures, cardiac output, resistances, and oxygen saturations.

Pressure transduction is achieved by attaching a small-volume-displacement strain gauge–type pressure transducer to a fluid-filled catheter that is then advanced through the cardiac chambers. Inspection of the morphology of the waveforms can give insight into various cardiac disorders such as shock, pericardial disease, and valvular heart disease.

Left atrial and left ventricular filling pressure can be measured directly or are most commonly estimated by advancing a balloon-tipped, end-hole catheter to wedge in a branch of the pulmonary artery allowing transduction of left atrial pressure. This so-called pulmonary capillary wedge pressure (PCWP) may overestimate left ventricular end diastolic volume (preload) when there is mitral stenosis or regurgitation, PEEP or Auto-PEEP, acute respiratory failure, COPD with pulmonary hypertension, or pulmonary venoconstriction. PCWP underestimates left ventricular preload with decreased LV compliance (MI, LVH, diastolic dysfunction, pericardial disease), severe AI, and high intrapericardial or intrathoracic pressure. Note: LVEDP is proportional to the gradient between intracardiac and intrapericardial pressure while PCWP is proportional to the difference between intracardiac and atmospheric pressure. Normal intracardiac pressures are listed in **Table 36-1**.

In addition to intracardiac pressure and associated waveforms, right heart catheterization can be utilized to derive cardiac output and vascular resistance using 2 major methods.

- **Thermodilution.** A thermal indicator method of measuring output that uses 2 thermistors to measure temperature change and derive flow rate. Does not require withdrawal of blood or arterial puncture.

TABLE 36-1. Normal Hemodynamic Parameters

Pressures	Average (mm Hg)
Right Atrium/ Central Venous Pressure	5-12 cm H_2O
Right Ventricle	20-30/6-12 mm Hg
Pulmonary Artery	20-30/8-12 mm Hg
Pulmonary Capillary Wedge	8-12 mm Hg
Left Ventricle	90-140/5-12 mm Hg
Aorta	90-140/7060-90 mm Hg
Cardiac Output	4-8 L/min
Cardiac Index	2.8-4.2 L/min/m²
Systemic Vascular Resistance	800-1200 (dynes-sec/cm⁵)
Pulmonary Vascular Resistance	100-300 (dynes-sec/cm⁵)

- **Fick oxygen method.** This method is based on the Fick principle that uses the concept that the total uptake of a substance (in this case oxygen) by an organ is the product of the blood flow (cardiac output) and the arteriovenous concentration of the substance.

HEMODYNAMIC EQUATIONS

Blood pressure:

$$\text{MAP} = \frac{\text{Systolic BP} + (2 \times \text{Diastolic BP})}{3} = \text{DBP} + \frac{\text{SBP} - \text{DBP}}{3}$$

Fick cardiac output:

$$\text{CO} = \frac{O_2 \text{ Consumption}}{(\text{Arterial} - \text{Venous}) \ O_2 \text{ Content}}$$

$$= \frac{VO_2(\text{mL}/\text{min})}{(\text{Arterial } O_2 \text{ Sat} - \text{Venous } O_2 \text{ Sat}) \times 1.36 \times \text{Hb}(\text{gm}/\text{dL}) \times 10}$$

$$O_2 \text{ Consumption} = VO_2(\text{mL}/\text{min})$$

$$\text{Assumed} \approx 125 \text{ mL}/\text{min} \times \text{BSA}(\text{m}^2)$$

The AVO$_2$ difference is calculated based on the difference between arterial and mixed venous O$_2$ content.

$$O_2 \text{ Content} = \text{saturation} \times 1.36 \times \text{hemoglobin (g/100 mL)}$$

$$\text{AVO}_2 \text{ Difference} = (\text{Arterial saturation} - \text{Mixed Venous Saturation}) \times 1.36 \times \text{Hemoglobin} \times 10$$

Example: If arterial saturation is 98%, mixed venous saturation is 68%, hemoglobin is 12.0 g/100 mL, and O$_2$ Consumption is 250 mL O$_2$/min) then:

$$\text{CO} = \frac{250}{(0.98 - 0.68) \times 1.36 \times 12.0 \times 10} = \frac{250}{49} = 5.1 \text{ L}/\text{min}$$

Cardiac index: $\text{CI} = \dfrac{\text{CO}}{\text{BSA}}$ (Normal 2.5–4.2 L/min/m^2)

Stroke volume: $\text{SV} = \dfrac{\text{CO}}{\text{HR}}$

- **Ohm's Law.** Vascular resistances are based upon Ohm's law which relates volume flow to pressure change and resistance ($R = \Delta P/Q$). An application of this law allows calculation of systemic and pulmonary vascular resistance

Pulmonary vascular resistance
(PVR, dyne/sec/cm^5) = $\dfrac{80 \times (\text{Mean PA Pressure} - \text{Mean PCWP})}{\text{Cardiac Output (L/min)}}$

Systemic vascular resistance
(SVR, dyne/sec/cm^5) = $\dfrac{80 \times [\text{MAP (mmHg)} - \text{RA Pressure(mm Hg)}]}{\text{Cardiac Output (L/min)}}$

The data from right heart catheterization aids in diagnosis and evaluation of various cardiac disorders:

- Differentiation of shock states (see Appendix B: Cardiac Emergencies, Shock)
- Differentiation of cardiogenic vs. noncardiogenic pulmonary edema (ARDS)
- Diagnosis of right ventricular infarction during acute myocardial infarction
  - If the ratio of RA pressure to pulmonary capillary wedge pressure is > 0.8, then right ventricular involvement is suggested.
- Left to right intracardiac shunt detection and quantification
  - Oximetric measurements. Oxygen content in the blood is measured sequentially in the inferior and superior vena cava, right atrium, right ventricle, and pulmonary artery. Left-to-right shunting can be detected by noting an increase in saturation ("step-up") in one of the cardiac chambers and the amount of shunt (Qp/Qs) can be quantified.
- Calculation of valve orifice area in aortic or mitral stenosis
  - Gorlin formula uses flow and pressure gradient data to calculate valvular orifice area.
  - Hakki A, et al,[1] proposed a simplified valve area formula based on their observation that the product of heart rate, systolic ejection period or diastolic ejection period, and the Gorlin formula constant was nearly the same for all patients.
    - *Equation:* Cardiac output/square root of the peak-to-peak gradient
- Measurement of vasodilator responsiveness in patients with pulmonary hypertension
  - The response of PVR, cardiac output, and filling pressures to administration of 100% FiO$_2$ and then addition of inhaled nitric oxide or another selective pulmonary vasodilator are assessed.
- Evaluation of constrictive pericarditis, restrictive cardiomyopathy cardiac tamponade (see Chapter 22: Pericardial Disorders)

Right heart catheterization can also be useful in guiding therapy:

- Management of severely decompensated heart failure or cardiogenic shock where the right heart catheter can be utilized to "tailor" medical therapy to optimize intracardiac hemodynamics
- Patients with severe pulmonary hypertension where pulmonary vasodilating medications are being titrated
- Assessing the efficacy of therapeutic interventions in patients with multiple causes of shock (e.g., cardiogenic shock with sepsis and hemorrhage) where noninvasive methods of estimating filling pressures, output, and resistances are insufficient or inconsistent.

CONTRAINDICATIONS

Absolute:
- Right ventricular assist device
- Prosthetic right heart valve
- Right ventricular mural thrombus or mass
- Latex allergy (may use latex-free catheter)
- Infection or full-thickness burn at insertion site

Relative:
- Severe coagulopathy
- Thrombocytopenia
- LBBB (see Complications)
- Right-sided endocarditis with vegetation by echocardiogram
- Uncontrolled ventricular or atrial dysrhythmia
- Prior pneumonectomy

PROCEDURE FOR RIGHT HEART CATHETERIZATION

- Right internal jugular and left subclavian vein access allow the natural curve of the catheter to guide it into the pulmonary artery easily, but the left subclavian is not compressible if bleeding or arterial puncture occur.
- Femoral vein, left internal jugular, right subclavian, and brachial veins are also options for access.
- The Seldinger technique (see Appendix A: Bedside Procedures, Seldinger Technique for Vascular Access) with or without ultrasound guidance is used to gain central venous access.
- Catheters are available in 5 French and 7 French sizes with additional ports for medication administration, pacing, and/or continuous oximetric monitoring. The appropriate catheter should be selected.
- After the pulmonary artery catheter lumens are flushed with sterile saline, and the distal port is attached to a pressure transducer, confirmation that the baseline pressure is zeroed at the level of the right atrium.
- The catheter is shaken to ensure a deflection can be noted on the pressure display.

- The balloon is inflated with to ensure no leak and proper deflation.
- If the catheter will be left in place, a sterile sleeve is applied over the catheter.
- The catheter is inserted into the access sheath.
  - After it is inserted 10–15 cm, the balloon is inflated.
  - Pressure monitoring and/or fluoroscopy are used to monitor the location of the catheter.
  - Waveforms at RA, RV, PA, and the wedge position are recorded.
    - The RA is approximately 30 cm from the right internal jugular or subclavian vein and 35–40 cm from the femoral vein.
    - The wedge position is typically at 45–60 cm.
  - At the wedge position in the pulmonary artery, deflate the balloon, then ensure that a PA tracing is present. Re-inflate balloon to verify that catheter becomes wedged again.
  - *Do not advance with the balloon deflated to prevent vascular/cardiac injury.*
  - *Do not pull back with the balloon inflated.*
  - *Never leave the catheter in wedge position longer than necessary.*
  - *Do not overinflate the balloon.*
- Secure the catheter.
  - Suture the access sheath in place
  - Extend and lock the sterile sleeve to the access sheath.
  - Obtain chest X-ray. Ideal position is 3–5 cm from midline
- Interpretation of pressure tracings
  - Normal pulmonary capillary wedge and RA tracing contains three waves per cardiac cycle.
    - The A-wave corresponds to atrial contraction and is followed by an x descent.
    - The C-wave is usually difficult to appreciate and results from bulging of the tricuspid or mitral valve during ventricular contraction.
    - The V-wave corresponds to atrial filling during ventricular contraction and is followed by the y descent.
    - Large V-waves are a sign of mitral or tricuspid regurgitation or ventricular septal perforation.
      - A "giant" V-wave is if the peak V-wave is twice the mean pulmonary capillary wedge pressure.
    - The x descent is preserved and y descent is diminished in the setting of elevated and equalized diastolic filling pressures during cardiac tamponade.
    - The x and y descents may be exaggerated in constriction, restriction, and right ventricular infarction.
    - Increased A-wave with blunted x descent is seen in mitral stenosis.
    - A "dip and plateau" or "square root" sign may be seen in the right ventricular pressure tracing in constriction or right ventricular infarction.

- ○ Measure wedge pressures at end-expiration or end-inspiration in intubated patients.
- ○ In an intubated patient, subtract ½ of PEEP from PCWP.
- Interpretation of hemodynamic profiles (see Appendix B: Cardiovascular Emergencies, Shock)
- Complications of right heart catheterization include:
  - Access site bleeding/thrombosis/infection
  - Carotid artery puncture
  - Pneumothorax (especially with subclavian access in ventilated patients)
  - Air embolism
  - Pulmonary artery rupture (0.2%)
  - Right bundle branch block which may lead to complete heart block if there is a preexisting LBBB (0.1–5% risk)
  - Pacemaker lead dislodgement
  - Pulmonary infarction
  - Tricuspid/pulmonic valve damage and/or endocarditis

REFERENCES

(1) Hakki A, et al. A simplified valve formula for the calculation of stenotic cardiac valve areas. *Circulation*. 1981;63:1050–5.

37 ■ URGENT TEMPORARY PACING

Temporary pacing may be required when the need for pacing is more immediate than the ability to implant a permanent pacemaker. Examples of indications for urgent pacing are:

- Complete heart block with unreliable escape rhythm
- Profound sinus bradycardia with symptoms despite physiologic stimuli
- Episodic asystole due to sinus pauses or high degree AV block

Transcutaneous pacing uses 2 electrode patches on the skin, typically to the anterior and posterior chest. The transcutaneous pacing device is usually also a defibrillator, typical defibrillation electrode pads are used.

- Transcutaneous pacing captures a fairly large mass of skeletal chest muscle in addition to the heart. Therefore, transcutaneous pacing is painful. To minimize the pain:
  - Sedate the awake patient.
  - Discontinue pacing as soon as possible.
  - Keep the transcutaneous pacing rate low.
  - Keep the pacing energy low, just above the capture threshold.

Transvenous pacing requires a catheter electrode, usually with a pair of electrodes at the tip.

- The catheter is placed via an introducer sheath. Usual sites are:
  - The internal jugular vein (right is preferred over left)
  - The subclavian vein (left is preferred over right)
  - The femoral vein (right is preferred over left)
  - If feasible, use of a femoral vein is preferred, leaving the upper body veins undisturbed for probable permanent pacemaker implantation.
- Most catheters used for temporary pacing are balloon-tipped to assist with steering the catheter into the right ventricle
  - Advancing a pacing catheter to the heart without fluoroscopy is possible but should be reserved for acute emergencies only.
    - The risk of perforation is high.
    - Catheter placement can be guided by electrograms and by pacing. The goal is to capture the right ventricle.
  - Using fluoroscopy, the operator can guide the catheter tip into the right ventricular apex.
    - The balloon can assist in getting the catheter into the right atrium and across the tricuspid valve. The balloon may then tend to follow blood into the RV outflow tract.
    - It may be necessary to deflate the balloon.
  - The balloon should remain down after placement in order to maximize stability of the catheter.
  - After placing the catheter, secure it to the skin with sutures and a dressing.

- The pacing catheter is connected to the temporary pacing pulse generator. Urgent temporary pacing is almost always ventricular pacing only. (In post-surgical patients, temporary epicardial pacing wires may be present in both the atrium and ventricle, and dual chamber pacing is possible.)
  - Check the pacing and sensing threshold of any new transvenous pacemaker.
  - The pacing output (usually in mA [milliamps]) should be set well above the threshold. There is no need to save battery in temporary device.
  - Set the pacing rate no higher than needed.
    - If the indication for pacing is intermittent pauses/brady, the rate should be set relatively low so that need for pacing can be tracked.
- If, for example, the rate is set at 80 bpm, the underlying rate cannot be monitored.
  - Do not check the underlying rhythm by simply turning the generator off (or unplugging the cables).
- A prolonged pause is very likely—not a good assessment of the underlying rhythm.
- Instead, gradually lower the rate, waiting for the intrinsic beats to occur.

38 ■ CARDIOVERSION

Direct current (DC) cardioversion (DCCV) is easy and quick to perform. However, its facility should not cause the physician to underestimate the potential risks.

Cardioversion can be performed electively for atrial fibrillation and atrial flutter and other hemodynamically well tolerated rhythms. It may also be required urgently for life-threatening or hemodynamically compromising rhythms.

RISKS

- Skin burning. May be treated with topical moisturizer or analgesic.
- Thromboembolism or CVA. This applies to atrial fibrillation/flutter, in which poor atrial transport is transformed to good atrial transport by cardioversion. Atrial tachycardia and other SVTs which do not reduce atrial contraction and VT/VF do not predispose to formation of left atrial thrombus.
  - Appropriate anticoagulation for atrial fibrillation minimizes (but does not remove) the risk.
  - Atrial fibrillation alone (without cardioversion) also carries a risk of embolism/CVA.
- Arrhythmia. A cardioversion can result in a malignant arrhythmia instead of sinus, particularly if the timing of the shock is incorrect. The new rhythm must be treated, with an immediate additional shock if appropriate.
- Pain. A cardioversion shock is painful if performed without anesthesia.
- Pulmonary edema after cardioversion is a rare complication, usually in the setting of underlying heart disease.

ELECTIVE CARDIOVERSION

- Informed consent. Specific risks are noted above.
- Anesthesia. Deep sedation to general anesthesia is desirable. An anesthesiologist can typically achieve short-term general anesthesia without intubation ventilation using agents such as propofol.
- Set-up
  - Defibrillator. Most modern defibrillators deliver a biphasic waveform, which has been shown to improve efficacy.
    - Some attempt to use low energy, but lower energy is more likely to fail, requiring repeated shocks of higher energy.
    - Synchronization—very important
      - *For any rhythm in which a QRS can be identified and tracked by the defibrillator, the shock should be synchronized.*

- An unsynchronized shock may occur during the "vulnerable period" during repolarization and induce VF.
  - For VF or polymorphic VT, an unsynchronized shock should be delivered.
- Electrodes. High-surface-area adhesive electrodes have largely supplanted hand-held paddles.
  - Adhesive electrodes should be placed in an anterior-posterior (AP) configuration.
    - For AF, the anterior patch should be placed just to the right of the sternum, and the posterior patch should be placed between the spine and the left scapula.
  - Hand-held paddles are usually placed to the right of the sternum and at the apex of the heart.
  - Pressure on the electrodes reduces impedance and increases the rate of success. A fist pressing on the anterior adhesive electrode is effective. Use a glove if you must, but the top of the electrode is already well insulated.
- Steps:
  - Prepare the electrodes, and telemetry. Be familiar with the device.
  - Set the cardioversion energy to 200 J (or other selected energy).
  - Turn synchronization ON.
  - Ensure that the device is synchronizing to the QRS properly.
  - Ensure appropriate sedation/anesthesia.
  - Charge the defibrillator.
  - Have everyone "clear" contact with the patient.
  - While watching the telemetry to ensure appropriate synchronization: Press and hold the "shock" button until the shock is delivered (there may be a delay while the device awaits a sync-able QRS).
  - Continue to watch telemetry to ensure cardioversion to sinus.
    - Be prepared to recharge immediately in the event of malignant arrhythmia.
    - Be prepared to administer atropine or to initiate transcutaneous pacing for sustained pauses of profound bradycardia

URGENT CARDIOVERSION

- For hemodynamically unstable rhythms, cardioversion follows essentially the same steps.
  - If time does not allow for sedation/anesthesia, the patient is likely to be unconscious and the shocks are delivered as part of ACLS protocol.
  - Semi-urgent cardioversion in an awake patient should allow time for sedation/anesthesia.
  - If the rhythm is VF or polymorphic VT to which the device is unlikely to be able to sync, synchronization should be turned off.

39 ■ PERICARDIOCENTESIS[1-6]

ETIOLOGIES OF PERICARDITIS ASSOCIATED WITH LARGE PERICARDIAL EFFUSIONS

- Common causes of cardiac tamponade in the United States: idiopathic or viral pericarditis; malignancy; rheumatic diseases; and uremia
- Other causes: infectious (tuberculous [cause of up to 14% of cardiac tamponade in developing countries], bacterial, fungal, rickettsial or fungal); Dressler's syndrome; post-irradiation; chest trauma; postpericardiotomy; hypothyroidism; and meds (hydralazine, isoniazid, methyldopa, phenytoin, and procainamide).

INDICATIONS

- Diagnostic
  - To determine the etiology of an unexplained pericardial effusion
- Therapeutic
  - Relief of cardiac tamponade (a pulsus paradoxus > 12 mm Hg or a ratio of paradoxical pulse/pulse pressure that exceeds 50% are both abnormal)

CONTRAINDICATIONS

- Small asymptomatic pericardial effusion (less than 200 ml)
- Loculated pericardial effusion
- Absence of an anterior pericardial effusion
- Acute traumatic hemopericardium
- Coagulopathy
  - INR > 1.4 or PTT > 1.5 times the upper limit of normal
- Thrombocytopenia (platelet count < 50,000)

COMPLICATIONS

- Cardiac puncture
- Laceration of a coronary artery
- Liver laceration
- Cardiac arrhythmias
- Hemothorax
- Pneumothorax
- Infection
- Air embolus

EQUIPMENT

- Prepackaged pericardiocentesis kit containing: introducer needle, J wire, dilator, catheter guide, 8 Fr drainage catheter, drainage bag, three-way stopcock, 60-ml aspirating syringe, and sterile collection tubes
- Echocardiogram (for echocardiogram-guided pericardiocentesis)
- Sterile prep: chlorhexidine or povidone-iodine swabs
- Sterile drape or towels
- Sterile gown and gloves
- Surgeon's cap and mask
- 1% lidocaine with or without epinephrine, with 10-ml syringe and needles
- Sterile ECG monitoring cord with alligator clip
- Cardiac monitor
- Sterile bandage
- No. 11 scalpel
- 2-0 nylon suture

TECHNIQUE

- Informed consent.
- Perform a "time out" to confirm the correct patient and procedure.
- Place patient supine with the head of bed elevated to 45°.
- Sterile prep and drape of the lower chest and subxiphoid area.
- Anesthetize the insertion site 0.5 cm left of the xiphoid tip with 1% lidocaine.
- Attach one end of the sterile ECG cord to the pericardiocentesis needle using an alligator clip and the other end to the V1 or V5 precordial lead using another alligator clip.
- Assure proper functioning of the cardiac monitor.
- Advance the introducer needle connected to a syringe at a 30–45° angle to the skin with constant negative pressure. Aim toward the left shoulder (**Figure 39-1**).
  - Echocardiogram used for real-time ultrasound-guided pericardiocentesis.
  - Typical depth of insertion from the skin to the pericardium is 6–8 cm.
  - Negative deflection of the QRS complex, or ST segment depression, occurs when the needle touches the pericardial sac.
  - Stop advancing the needle when pericardial fluid is obtained.
  - Pericardial fluid does not clot in cases of hemopericardium.
  - ST segment elevation signifies needle contact with the epicardium/myocardium, and the needle should be withdrawn several millimeters.
  - Once pericardial fluid is aspirated, disconnect the syringe from the needle and thread a J wire through the needle (see **Figure 39-2** and **Figure 39-3**).

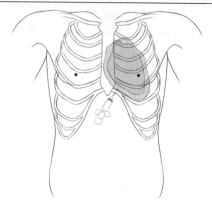

FIGURE 39-1. Subxiphoid approach to pericardiocentesis.

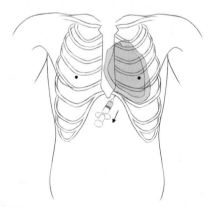

FIGURE 39-2. Aspiration of pericardial fluid.

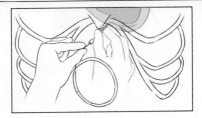

FIGURE 39-3. Threading wire through the needle.

Pericardiocentesis needle is inserted 1 cm below and to the left of the xiphoid notch directed toward the left shoulder.

Pericardial fluid is aspirated. In equivocal cases, pericardial fluid can be differentiated from blood because it does not clot.

Once pericardial fluid is aspirated, the syringe is disconnected and a flexible wire is advanced through the needle. The needle is then withdrawn leaving the wire in place.

- Remove the needle and leave the wire in place
- Make a 3-mm skin incision along the wire using a scalpel
- Introduce dilator over the wire and then remove the dilator, leaving the wire in place (**Figure 39-4**).
- Introduce the drainage catheter over wire until it is within the pericardial space, then remove the wire and secure the catheter in place with suture (see **Figure 39-5** and **Figure 39-6**).
- Manually aspirate fluid or attach the catheter to a sterile drainage bag
- Obtain a postprocedure electrocardiogram, echocardiogram, and chest x-ray

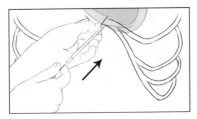

FIGURE 39-4. Advancing dilator over wire.

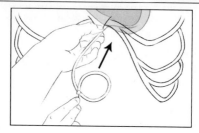

FIGURE 39-5. Pericardiocentesis catheter is introduced over wire.

A dilator is advanced over the wire to dilate a soft tissue tract into the pericardium.

A pericardiocentesis catheter is advanced over wire to an appropriate depth of insertion.

After the pericardiocentesis catheter is introduced, the wire is withdrawn and the pericardiocentesis catheter is secured in place.

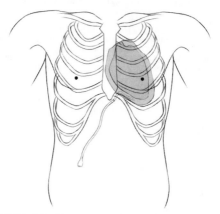

FIGURE 39-6. Pericardiocentesis catheter in place.

LABORATORY ANALYSIS OF PERICARDIAL FLUID

- Blood work: Complete blood count, renal panel, troponin I; ANA, rheumatoid factor, TSH and PPD skin test.
- Pericardial Fluid Analysis
  - Routine studies: cell count and differential, protein, glucose, lactate dehydrogenase, pH, cultures and gram stain
  - Optional studies: cultures for fungi and acid-fast bacilli, AFB RNA by PCR, adenosine deaminase level and cytology

CODING

33010   Pericardiocentesis, initial
33011   Pericardiocentesis, subsequent
76930   Ultrasound guidance for pericardiocentesis

REFERENCES

(1) *Mayo Clin Proc.* 2002; 77: 429.
(2) *Curr Treatment Options Cardiovasc Med.* 1999; 1: 79.
(3) *Clin Cardiology.* 2008; 31: 531–537.
(4) *Canadian J Cardiol.* 1999; 15: 1251.
(5) *Intensive Care Med.* 2000; 26: 573.
(6) *NEJM.* 2004; 351: 2195.

40 ■ INTRA-AORTIC BALLOON PUMP SUPPORT

INDICATIONS

- **Myocardial ischemia**: refractory unstable angina or postinfarction angina; refractory polymorphic VT; support for PCI
- **Cardiogenic shock**: pump failure; acute mitral regurgitation or acute ventricular septal rupture (as a bridge to definitive treatment)
- **Pre- and Postoperative:** myocardial depression and weaning from bypass

CONTRAINDICATIONS

- Aortic valve insufficiency > mild-moderate
- Severe obstructive aortic or iliofemoral artery disease
- Aortic dissection, aortic aneurysm
- No definitive treatment for underlying pathology

OPERATING THE INTRA-AORTIC BALLOON PUMP (IABP)

- **Balloon deflation**: nadir of end-diastolic pressure should occur just before arterial upstroke (aortic valve opening) begins
  - Late deflation: ventricle contracts against inflated balloon
  - Premature deflation: suboptimal afterload reduction
- **Balloon inflation**: should occur just after dicrotic notch
  - Early inflation: ventricle contracts against inflated balloon
  - Late inflation: excessive diastolic hypotension and suboptimal augmentation of coronary flow
- Anticoagulation is optional as long as pump is not in "standby"
- During CPR the IABP should be turned off or set in "standby" mode

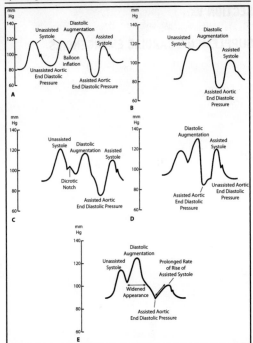

FIGURE 40-1. Timing examples: Arterial pressure waveforms with 1:2 counter pulsation.

A: Normal timing
B: Early inflation
C: Late inflation
D: Early deflation
E: Late deflation

Reprinted from Am J Cardiol, Vol. 97, Issue 9, Trost JC and Hillis D, Intra-aortic balloon counterpulsation, pages 1391–1398, Copyright 2006, with permission from Elsevier.

SECTION V

SUPPLEMENT: CARDIAC EMERGENCIES

41 ■ HYPERTENSIVE EMERGENCIES[1]

- Defined by end-organ damage, *e.g.*, encephalopathy, renal dysfunction, CHF, cardiac ischemia, decreased placental perfusion
- DBP usually > 120 mm Hg but BP can be as low as 160/100 in previously normotensive patient (*e.g.*, pregnant woman, drug reaction in young adult)
- "Hypertensive urgency:" elevated BP without end-organ damage; usually appropriate to treat as outpatient with oral medications

ETIOLOGY

- Chronic HTN
- Renal or renovascular disease
- Drug ingestion (cocaine, amphetamines)
- Non-adherence or withdrawal (esp. clonidine, β-blocker)
- Pheochro-mocytoma
- Scleroderma or other collagen-vascular disease
- S/p carotid artery or neurosurgery
- Head or spinal cord injury
- Guillain-Barré syndrome

TABLE 41-1

Clinical Scenario	Goal of Treatment	1St Line Rx	Comments
Hypertensive encephalopathy	20–25% reduction in MAP over 2–3 hr (but keep DBP > 100 mm Hg)	SNP, FD, CVP, labetalol, nicardipine	Treatment may worsen neuro function. Avoid clonidine, βB (CNS effects).
Ischemic stroke	If BP > 220/120 lower 15–25% in first day	Labetalol, nicardipine	SNP, FD, and NTG may increase ICP. Goal BP 185/110 if thrombolytics.
Intracerebral hemorrhage	Gradually reach 160/80, MAP < 110, CPP > 60 with ICP monitor, or prestroke level	Labetalol, SNP, nicardipine	Monitor for worsening neuro function after lowering BP

TABLE 41-1 (continued)

Clinical Scenario	Goal of Treatment	1St Line Rx	Comments
Subarachnoid hemorrhage	Same as intracerebral hemorrhage	Nimodipine 60 mg PO/PNGT q 4 hr (to prevent spasm) ± labetalol	Avoid SNP, FD, and NTG (increase ICP)
Pulmonary edema	DBP ≤ 100 mm Hg or resolution of symptoms	SNP *plus* NTG *plus* diuretic	Avoid (-) inotropes in LV dysfunction. Search for myocardial ischemia. In CAD or PAD, seek RAS.
Myocardial infarction or unstable angina	DBP ≤ 100 mm Hg or resolution of symptoms	NTG, βB. Add SNP if DBP remains elevated	
Aortic dissection	SBP 100–120 or MAP 80 mm Hg (watch urine output)	SNP or CVP or FD *plus* βB or labetalol	Decrease dP/dT. Avoid vasodilator monotherapy.
Sympathomimetic crisis (cocaine, amphetamines, pheochromocytoma, MAOI reaction, βB or clonidine withdrawal)	DBP ~100–105 (but ≤ 25% reduction in presenting BP) over 2–6 hr	Phentolamine (1st) then βB *or* labetalol. Benzodiazepine for cocaine-like drugs. Alternative: NTG ± Ca blocker.	Avoid βB or labetalol alone (unopposed α stimulation). Restart βB or clonidine if withdrawing.
Pregnancy (eclampsia)	DBP 90–105 or MAP ≤ 126 mm Hg	Hydralazine, labetalol, nifedipine	*PO:* methyldopa. Avoid SNP, ACE-I.
Postoperative	Preop BP	SNP, labetalol, diuretic	Treat pain, volume overload, & ↓O₂
Acute renal insufficiency	DBP ~100–105 (but ≤ 25% reduction in presenting BP)	FD, Ca channel blockers, CVP	Avoid diuretics. Maintain renal blood flow.

SNP=sodium nitroprusside   FD=fenoldopam   βB=β-blocker   CVP=clevidipine   NTG=nitroglycerin   ICP=intracranial pressure

Data from Magee LA, et al. Hydralazine for treatment of severe hypertension in pregnancy: meta-analysis. *BMJ.* 2003;327:955–960.

REFERENCES

(1) Marik PE, Varon J. Hypertensive crises: challenges and management. *Chest.* 2007;131:1949–1962.

42 ■ SHOCK

Shock results from poor tissue perfusion and oxygenation, with microcirculatory inadequacy to sustain tissue oxygen needs, leading to cellular dysoxia. In critically ill patients, tissue hypoxia is due to inadequate or disordered regional distribution of blood flow both between and within organs. Therefore, therapy in shock should be aimed, at least in part, at restoring with urgency an adequate organ perfusion pressure. Lack of end-organ perfusion is often but not always manifested in hypotension, oliguria, change in mental status, cool extremities and metabolic acidosis. Shock can be classified as cardiogenic, distributive, and hypovolemic.

TABLE 42-1. Differentiating Forms of Shock

Cause	PCWP	CO	SVR	Mixed Venous (SVO$_2$)	Comments
Cardiogenic					Typically with elevated CVP compared to distributive shock
Myocardial dysfunction	⇑	⇓	⇑	⇓	Most common cause of CS, typically in setting of ischemia/infarction. Hemodynamic Goals: PCWP 15-18 , MAP > 65mmHg, CI >2.2, SVR 1000-1200
Acute MR	⇑	⇓ (forward)	⇑	⇓	Most common with inferior-posterior MI. Up to 50% of pts may not have sig murmur. Large PCW V waves. Aggressive afterload reduction and consider IABP. Spectrum can vary from ischemic MR to acute papillary muscle rupture
Acute VSD	⇑	⇓	⇑	⇓	CO$_{RV}$>CO$_{LV}$. O$_2$ "step-up" at RV. Large PCW V waves. Typically 3-5 days post MI. Most commonly in pts with wrap-around LAD with LAD occlusion with inf ST elevations and also pure inf STEMI. New harsh holosystolic murmur at LLSB w/ thrill. Consider nitroprusside for pronounced afterload reduction

TABLE 42-1. Differentiating Forms of Shock

Cause	PCWP	CO	SVR	Mixed Venous (SVO₂)	Comments
LV Free Wall Rupture	⇑	⇓	⇑	⇓	Most common 5-14 days post STEMI, though can be earlier. Tamponade physiology
RV Infarction	⇔/⇓	⇓	⇑	⇓	Typically with Inferior MI. RA pressure >> PCWP. Goal PCW >18mmHg
Tamponade	⇑	⇓	⇑	⇓	RAP=RVEDP=PAD=PCWP, ⇑ Pulsus Paradoxus.
Distributive					
Sepsis (early)	⇔/⇓	Usually ⇑	⇓	⇑	CO may ⇓ due to sepsis-mediated LV dysfunction, esp in later phases (mixed cardiogenic-septic physiol)
Anaphylaxis, liver disease, spinal shock, adrenal insuff.	⇔/⇓	⇑	⇓	⇑	Epinephrine for anyphylaxis after treating underlying cause; pure α agonist in spinal shock
Hypovolemic					
Hemorrhage, dehydration	⇓	⇓	⇑	⇓	Invasive monitoring needed only if co-existing LV dysfunction

For interpretation of PA catheters- see PA catheter section
For details on management of STEMI, indications for urgent revascularization and severe heart failure-see relevant sections.

TABLE 42-2. Relative Action of Adrenergic, Non-adrenergic Drugs and Non-pharmacologic Therapies for Shock

Drug/Therapy	Receptor	HR	Inotropy	SVR	Comments
Dopamine- Low Dose	DA	0	0	⇔⇓	Renal and splanchnic vasodilation
Dopamine- High Dose	$\beta_1 \Rightarrow \alpha_1$	⇑	⇑⇑	⇑⇑	1st line tx for CS (pro-arrythmic, may increase tachycardia in pts more than other 1st line drugs)
Dobutamine	$\beta_1, \beta_2 > \alpha_1$	⇔⇑	⇑⇑	⇓⇓	Inotrope and vasodilator, may lower BP. Pro-arrythmic

TABLE 42-2. Relative Action of Adrenergic, Non-adrenergic Drugs and Non-pharmacologic Therapies for Shock

Drug/Therapy	Receptor	HR	Inotropy	SVR	Comments
Norepinephrine	$\alpha_1, \alpha_2, \beta_1$	⇔⇑	⇑⇑	⇑⇑⇑	2nd drug of choice in CS. Some evidence supporting its use over dopamine in CS.
Phenylephrine	α_1	0	0	⇑⇑⇑⇑	For refractory hypotension, especially vasculogenic (low SVR)
Epinephrine	$\alpha_1, \alpha_2, \beta_1, \beta_2$	⇑⇑⇑	⇑⇑⇑⇑	⇑⇑⇑	For anyphylaxis or refractory cardiac failure (e.g. post CABG). Proarrhythmic
Isoproterenol	β_1, β_2	⇑⇑⇑⇑	⇑⇑	⇔⇓	Primarily increases HR. May cause reflex hypotension
Milrinone	PDE inhibitor	⇔⇑	⇑⇑	⇓⇓	Similar response as dobutamine, less frequently used, less prone to dysrhythmias
Vasopression	ADH analog				2nd line agent to be used in refractory SS. May induce coronary ischemia.
Intra-Aortic Balloon Pump	Counter-pulsation Device	No Effect	⇑⇑⇑	⇓⇓	Consider in pump failure, Acute MR or Acute VSD
Left Ventricular Assist Devices			⇑⇑⇑⇑ (mechanically)		Primarily for forms of cardiogenic shock. Some devices with capability of oxygenating venous blood

The dose should be titrated up to achieve effective blood pressure or end-organ perfusion as evidenced by such criteria as urine output or mentation.

TABLE 42-3. Drug Choices in Shock

Hemodynamics	Initial Treatment	Comments
PCWP (or CVP) ⇓	Aggressive volume expansion	Consider pressors initially, but reevaluate once PCWP >18 or CVP >12
CO⇓, SVR⇑	Dobutamine	Milrinone alternatively dopamine plus nitroprusside
CO⇓, SVR⇔ or⇓	Dopamine	Alternatively Norephinephrine
SVR⇓, CO⇑	Dopamine or Norephinephrine	Can add epinephrine or phenylephrine for refractory hypotension

43 ■ DIAGNOSING THE WIDE COMPLEX TACHYCARDIA

Symptomatic wide complex tachycardia in the clinical setting should initially be assumed to be ventricular tachycardia (VT), and may require urgent treatment if there is hemodynamic instability. The ECG challenge is to differentiate VT from supraventricular rhythms with wide QRS complexes. Longer term treatment may rely on a confident diagnosis.

The differential diagnosis of wide complex tachycardia follows from the differential diagnosis of wide QRS complex (see Chapter 3: Electrocardiography):

- VT
- Supraventricular tachycardia (SVT) with aberrancy (bundle branch blocks, fascicular blocks, combinations of blocks)
- Pre-excitation
  - Atrial tachyarrhythmias in the WPW syndrome
  - Antidromic AV reentrant tachycardia [see Chapter 18: Tachyarrhythmias, Supraventricular Tachycardias (SVTs)]

We present an algorithm for differentiating VT from the others. It is a practical guide developed from the work and observations of Josephson ME, et al,[1] and Wellens HJJ[2].

When faced with a wide complex tachycardia: *Treat the patient, not the ECG!*

- Hemodynamic instability may require volume resuscitation, sedation and cardioversion, or urgent cardioversion. ACLS protocols may be required.

Know that *the rate, the blood pressure, and the tolerance of the patient for the rhythm are not very useful in determining whether or not the rhythm is VT.*

- Administration of drugs such as verapamil or adenosine, based on the assumption of SVT can have dangerous results.
- On the other hand, knowledge that patient has underlying coronary disease or dilated cardiomyopathy, certainly make VT more likely.

The default diagnosis is: VT. The ECG is then examined more closely for details to support or refute the diagnosis of VT.

Search for signs of V-A dissociation. Finding V-A dissociation (i.e., with faster ventricular activity than atrial activity) essentially clinches the diagnosis of VT. Evidence of V-A dissociation includes:

- Sighting P-waves that are clearly dissociated from the QRSs (and slower).
  - Note that seeing 1:1 V-A *association* neither confirms nor excludes VT.
- *Capture beats (Dressler beats)*: a narrow QRS that is conducted from a supraventricular origin implies that the supraventricular source is dissociated from the tachycardia, which must be ventricular.

- *Fusion beats*, that is, fusion between a dissociated supraventricular source and the ventricular source of the wide complex, are evidence of the same phenomenon as capture beats.

Examine the QRS morphology. V-A dissociation is highly specific for VT, but it often cannot be found, since the wide QRS may obscure P-waves. QRS morphology features are not as specific, but can provide strong clues to the source of the tachycardia. The criteria are indicative of whether the QRS complex follows typical patterns of aberrancy (more likely in SVT) or deviates significantly from typical patterns (more likely in VT).

- First, look at lead V$_1$: Is it primarily positive or negative?
  - If positive, say "This wide complex tachycardia has a *right bundle branch block pattern*." (Do not say, "*right bundle branch block*," which specifically indicates a supraventricular source with aberrancy.)
  - If negative, say "This wide complex tachycardia has a *left bundle branch block pattern*." (Do not say, "*left bundle branch block*," which specifically indicates a supraventricular source with aberrancy).
- If there is a *right* bundle branch block *pattern*, any of the following are evidence of VT:
  - In lead V$_1$:
    - R-wave of higher amplitude than R' (the first "rabbit ear" is bigger than the second)
    - Monophasic R-wave (a big wide R-wave without rabbit ears)
    - qR (an initial Q-wave, essentially in place of the first rabbit ear)
  - In lead V$_6$:
    - R-wave amplitude less than S-wave amplitude (sometimes said: R < S or R:S ratio < 1)
- If there is a *left* bundle branch block *pattern*, any of the following are evidence of VT:
  - In lead V$_1$ or V$_2$:
    - R-wave > 30 ms long (that is almost 1 small box)
    - Time from initial negative deflection to nadir of the S-wave (the "downslope of the S") > 60 ms
    - *Notching* of the S-wave downslope
  - In lead V$_6$:
    - Any Q-wave (qR or QS).

Other Morphology observations may be useful but are still less specific:
- *Concordance* of the QRS (i.e., all negative deflections or all positive deflections) across the precordial leads is suggestive of VT.
- Extreme (sometimes called *northwest*) axis of the QRS is more consistent with VT.
- Extremely wide QRSs are more likely ventricular in origin.

Caveats concerning the use for the morphology criteria:
- Pre-excitation (including antidromic AV reentrant tachycardia) produces a QRS that is the same as a ventricular origin at the site of the insertion of the accessory pathway. The morphology is likely to suggest VT.
  - Knowledge of the patient's baseline ECG is handy.

- Pre-excited atrial fibrillation is typically *irregular with irregularly variable QRS widths.*
- Antiarrhythmic drugs can cause dramatically atypical aberrancy that might suggest VT.
  - Particularly Class IA antiarrhythmic drugs (flecainide and propafenone)
    - Particularly with toxicity and rapid rates. The Class IA drugs have *use-dependency*, meaning they have stronger effects (including toxic effects) at rapid rates.
- Metabolic disturbances can create highly atypical aberrancy that might suggest ventricular origin.
  - The classic example is **hyperkalemia**, which also suppresses P-waves.
    - **However**, the rate in hyperkalemia is usually not tachycardic.

When still in doubt after application of the guides above, say, "This is probably VT," and treat the patient appropriately.

- If after exhaustive analysis, the diagnosis is still not clear, consider electrophysiology study. If the rhythm can be induced, analysis with intracardiac electrograms and various mapping techniques can aid in diagnosis.

REFERENCES

(1) Josephson ME, et al. Electrocardiographic criteria for ventricular tachycardia in wide complex left bundle branch block morphology tachycardias. *Am J Cardiol.* 1988;61:1279-83.
(2) Wellens HJJ. Ventricular tachycardia: diagnosis of broad QRS complete tachycardia. *Heart.* 2001;86:579-85.

INDEX

Page numbers followed by "f" indicates figures and by "t" indicates tables.

333

CODE ALGORITHMS

BASIC LIFE SUPPORT FOR MEDICAL PROFESSIONALS[1]

For unresponsive patients not breathing or not breathing normally.

Cardiac arrest in children and infants, usually asphyxiation requiring ventilations + compressions. Consider foreign-body airway obstruction.

TABLE 1

	Adults	Children	Infants
Upon recognition	Get help; Get AED; Start CPR: Compression, Airway, Breathing sequence		
Compression Rate	100/min	100/min	100/min
Compression Depth	≥ 5cm; allow complete recoil	≥ $\frac{1}{3}$ anteroposterior depth (~5 cm); allow complete recoil	≥ $\frac{1}{3}$ anteroposterior depth (~4 cm); allow complete recoil
Interruptions	Minimize, < 10 sec; Rotate compressors q 2 min		
Airway	Head tilt and chin lift; Possible trauma → jaw thrust		
Untrained rescuers	Compressions-only, no ventilations		
Compressions: Ventilation (No airway device)	30:2	30:2 single rescuer 15:2 two rescuers	30:2 single rescuer 15:2 two rescuers
Compressions: Ventilation (Airway device)	8–10 breaths/min lasting ~1 sec, asynchronous with chest compressions, visible chest rise		
Defibrillation	AED/Defibrillator as soon as possible, minimize interruptions in compressions. Resume CPR immediately after each shock.		

Pulse checks allocated < 10 sec unless definite pulse identified.

Place in (lateral recumbent) recovery position after clearly normal breathing and effective circulation restored.

Drowning victims (unresponsive) should receive rescue breathing.

ADVANCED CARDIAC LIFE SUPPORT

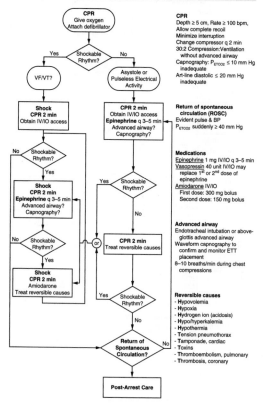

FIGURE 1. Adult cardiac arrest.

Adapted from Neumar RW, et al. Adult advanced cardiovascular life support. *Circulation*. 2010;122:S729–S767.

ADDITIONAL COMMENTS ON ADULT CARDIAC ARREST

Ventilation, CO_2 detectors, and oximetry

Use **suction** devices

Colorimetric CO_2 detectors may be misleading if contaminated with acidic gastric contents or drugs (*e.g.*, epinephrine via ETT)

CO_2 may be low in lung hypoperfusion (cardiac arrest) or severe airflow obstruction

Ominous **prognosticators**:
- P ETCO$_2$ < 10 mm Hg (persistently) via ETT
- Central vein O$_2$ saturation < 30%
- Diastolic BP < 20 mm Hg during CP

Avoid hyperventilation

Drug delivery

IV Access: central line unnecessary if large-bore peripheral access is obtained

IV access **should not delay** CPR and defibrillation

Remember intraosseous and **endotracheal** delivery option

Think ahead: Prepare drugs before rhythm and pulse checks

Flush drugs with 10–20 mL IV fluid bolus

Drugs **can** be **administered via ETT**: epinephrine, atropine, lidocaine, vasopressin, naloxone; use 2–2.5 × usual dose diluted in 5–10 mL NS or D5W

Do not pause compressions for ventilation with advanced airway

Ventricular tachycardia or ventricular fibrillation

Amiodarone is a first line drug that increases ROSC

Lidocaine does not increase ROSC

Magnesium IV is indicated only for Torsades related to prolonged QT (1–2 g in 10 mL)

Echo may have value in identifying treatable causes of cardiac arrest especially after ROSC

Consider differential diagnosis: H's and T's on algorithm

Accelerated idioventricular rhythm: May not require treatment if associated with perfusion

Epinephrine: High doses are generally ineffective, except possibly in β-blocker or Ca-blocker overdose

Vasopressin: Intended to be administered only once

Asystole or pulseless electrical activity

Emergency echocardiography: May be useful when cardiac tamponade or myocardial mechanical complications (wall or papillary rupture, VSD) are suspected

Pacing: No utility in arrest except selected events such as iatrogenic asystole

Consider differential diagnosis of reversible etiologies (H's and T's on algorithm)

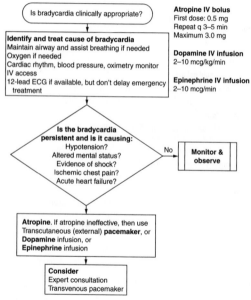

FIGURE 2. Bradycardia.

Adapted from Neumar RW, et al. Adult advanced cardiovascular life support. *Circulation.* 2010;122:S729–S767.

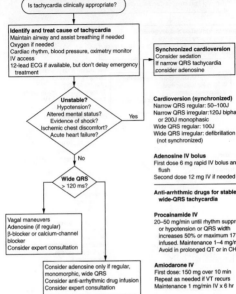

FIGURE 3. Tachycardia.

Adapted from Neumar RW, et al. Adult advanced cardiovascular life support. *Circulation.* 2010;122:S729–S767.

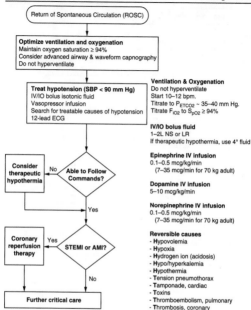

FIGURE 4. Immediate care after cardiac arrest.

Adapted from Peberdy MA, et al. Post-cardiac arrest care: 2010 AHA Guidelines. *Circulation.* 2010; 122:S768–786.

REFERENCES

(1) Adapted from Travers AH, *et al.* CPR overview: 2010 AHA Guidelines. *Circulation.* 2010;122:S676–S684 and Berg MD, *et al.* Pediatric basic life support: 2010 AHA Guidelines. *Circulation.* 2010;122:S862–S875.